SINGLE-PHOTON EMISSION COMPUTED TOMOGRAPHY

SINGLE-PHOTON EMISSION COMPUTED TOMOGRAPHY

BARBARA Y. CROFT, PH.D.

Assistant Professor
Division of Medical Imaging
Department of Radiology
University of Virginia School of Medicine
Charlottesville, Virginia

YEAR BOOK MEDICAL PUBLISHERS, INC.
Chicago • London

Copyright © 1986 by Year Book Medical Publishers, Inc. All rights reserved. No part of this publication may be reproduced, stored in a retrieval system, or transmitted, in any form or by any means, electronic, mechanical, photocopying, recording, or otherwise, without prior written permission from the publisher. Printed in the United States of America.

0 9 8 7 6 5 4 3 2 1

Library of Congress Cataloging-in-Publication Data
Croft, Barbara Y., 1940–
 Single-photon emission computed tomography.

 Includes bibliographies and index.
 1. Tomography, Emission. I. Title.
 [DNLM: 1. Tomography, Emission Computed. WN 160 C941s]
 RC78.7.T62C76   1986   616.07'575
 85-26320
 ISBN 0-8151-2007-9

Sponsoring Editor: James D. Ryan, Jr.
Manager, Copyediting Services: Frances M. Perveiler
Production Project Manager: Max Perez
Proofroom Supervisor: Shirley E. Taylor

Preface

Single-photon emission computed tomography (SPECT) has been practiced in a few medical centers since the mid-1960s, but has only recently come into widespread use with the commercial development of rotating gantries for the Anger camera. In the meantime, x-ray-transmission computed tomography, based on the same principles, has become an everyday diagnostic modality. Because of the late blooming of SPECT, there is no one book that offers a full discussion of the subject from theory through data collection and quality assurance to clinical practice. This book provides such information, concentrating on 180-degree and 360-degree tomography, with no attempt to include any form of limited-angle tomography. I do not intend to overemphasize the place of SPECT, although my enthusiasm for the technique is great for reasons I hope will become clear. The book is meant for professionals in nuclear medicine—physicians, physicists, and anyone desiring to know more about SPECT.

The book begins with the history of tomography. Chapter 2 addresses theory from two perspectives: first, a nonmathematical qualitative discussion for those interested in understanding computed tomography without complex math, and second, a deeper, more thorough treatment using mathematics where appropriate. Chapter 3 describes the various kinds of instrumentation used for SPECT, bringing in the threads of rectilinear-scanner and Anger-camera based instruments. Chapter 4 is a discussion of the computers needed and used in SPECT, although it is not an exhaustive treatment; that would be another book. Chapter 5 describes data acquisition and processing and the reasons for choosing particular methods. Chapter 6 is a critique of SPECT and a discussion of likely future directions, including guidelines for those about to purchase an instrument. Quality assurance is the focus of chapter 7. The extreme importance of this topic to SPECT makes this chapter important reading for any practitioner. Chapter 8 discusses the clinical applications of SPECT that are in use or described in the literature; to avoid being overwhelmed, the reader should keep in mind that not all of these are practiced at any one medical center.

A clinician interested in the actual practice of SPECT is advised to read the first part of Chapter 2 on theory, and Chapters 5, 7, and 8. Those purchasing SPECT for the first time are advised to study Chapter 6 for some ideas to consider in deciding which equipment best meets their needs. Chapters 5, 7, and 8 are recommended to technologists developing protocols for patient examinations and quality assurance.

Where possible, the references have been drawn from journals and books that should be readily available; more obscure sources are included only if they are the only written discussions available and for the sake of completeness. Full papers are preferred over abstracts. Many of the citations carry older dates, because nuclear medicine is evolutionary, with the dreams and theories of one era becoming the realities of another.

I wish to thank my first editors, Patricia O'Connell, Michael Sims, and Sarah Jeffries, for their help and improvements; my second editors, notably James D. Ryan, Jr., and Frances M. Perveiler, for their understanding and encouragement; my colleagues for their discussions, suggestions, and contributed images, especially David Teates and Stephen Graham; my illustrator, Craig Harding, and his colleagues in the University of Virginia Hospitals' Division of Biomedical Communications; and most especially my husband, Joseph E. Croft, for his collaboration in the effort and his understanding of a temperamental author's needs. My trusty IBM PC and WordStar have made the mechanics much simpler and even fun.

BARBARA Y. CROFT, PH.D.

Contents

PREFACE	v
1 / HISTORY AND COORDINATE SYSTEM	1
HISTORY	1
COORDINATE SYSTEM	4
2 / THEORY OF TOMOGRAPHY	9
GENERAL DESCRIPTION OF THE MATHEMATICS OF SPECT	11
TOMOGRAPHIC PROCESS	11
DIGITAL DATA AND THEIR EFFECTS	20
POISSON STATISTICS AND THE ACCURACY OF SPECT	23
ACCURACY OR QUANTIFICATION AND SPECT	28
SUMMARY	32
THEORETICAL TREATMENT	32
BACK-PROJECTION METHODS	34
SIMPLE BACK PROJECTION	34
FILTERED BACK PROJECTION OR CONVOLUTION	35
ATTENUATION-CORRECTED FILTERED BACK PROJECTION	38
FILTRATION OF BACK-PROJECTED IMAGES	43
FOURIER METHODS	43
ALTERNATIVES TO REAL SPACE OPERATIONS ALREADY DISCUSSED	43
METHODS FOR SOLVING THE GENERAL PROBLEM	44
OTHER ANALYTIC SOLUTIONS	45

Contents

ITERATIVE SOLUTIONS	45
ITERATIVE REAL SPACE METHODS	47
ALGEBRAIC RECONSTRUCTION TECHNIQUES	47
SIMULTANEOUS ITERATIVE RECONSTRUCTION TECHNIQUE	48
LEAST-SQUARE ITERATIVE TECHNIQUE	48
MAXIMUM LIKELIHOOD TECHNIQUE	48
COMPARISON OF RESULTS	49

3 / INSTRUMENTATION ... 54

ANGER CAMERA SPECT SYSTEMS	54
ANGER CAMERA HEAD AND ELECTRONICS	55
GANTRY AND TABLE—MECHANICAL OPERATIONS	68
ISSUES—SENSITIVITY AND SPEED	80
COMPTON SCATTERING DEVICES	82
OTHER 360–DEGREE TOMOGRAPHIC DEVICES	83
MARK IV	83
ABERDEEN SECTIONAL SCANNER	88
CLEON 710	89
HARVARD BODY SCANNER	90
TOMOMATIC 64	90
SPRINT	91
HEADTOME II	92
HYBRID POSITRON-SPECT INSTRUMENTS	93
LIMITED-ANGLE TOMOGRAPHY	94

4 / COMPUTER NEEDS FOR SPECT ... 101

TYPICAL COMPUTER SYSTEM	102
CENTRAL PROCESSING UNIT	102
POWER AND AIR CONDITIONING	104
MACHINE LANGUAGE AND OPERATING SYSTEM	105
MAGNETIC STORAGE	108
INTERFACE TO CAMERA	110
DISPLAY HARDWARE AND SOFTWARE	111
LONG-TERM STORAGE—FILM AND MAGNETIC MEDIA	112
NUCLEAR MEDICINE AND SPECT SOFTWARE	112
OPERATIONS	118

5 / Data Acquisition and Processing 123
Acquisition Variables 123
Uniformity, Linearity, and Other Corrections. 123
Center of Rotation and Absolute Pixel Size 124
Collimator. 125
Energy Setting and Windows 128
Matrix Size, Angular Increment, and Implications 132
180 vs. 360 Degrees of Data Collection 133
Time per Angle or Total Examination Time. 133
Gating. 134
Patient-Following Orbit 135
Patient Positioning 136
Processing 142
Uniformity and Linearity Corrections 142
Patient-Contour Following 143
Creation and Use of the Cine Presentation 143
Creation and Use of the Sinogram Presentation. 144
Manual Realignment. 145
Summing 145
Filtering 146
Attenuation and Scatter Corrections 149
Back Projection and Interpolation 152
Various Other Views. 155
Smoothing and Contrast Enhancement 156
Display. 157
Quantification 160
Image Storage, Networking, PACS, and SPECT 164

6 / Whys and Wherefores of SPECT 168
Reasons for Using SPECT 168
Problems With SPECT 169
General Clinical Application of Special
SPECT Properties. 171
Research of the Future. 172
Connection With TCT, NMR, and Ultrasound. 173
Choosing and Purchasing a SPECT System. 173

x   Contents

7 / QUALITY ASSURANCE: ACCEPTANCE TESTING AND QUALITY CONTROL 177
- HUMAN FACTORS 178
- THE SYSTEM 179
- CAMERA QUALITY CONTROL 181
  - ENERGY PEAKING AND WINDOW SETTING 184
  - SENSITIVITY AND UNIFORMITY 186
  - LINEARITY 193
  - RESOLUTION 195
- COMPUTER AND INTERFACE QUALITY CONTROL 196
  - CENTER OF ROTATION—X-AXIS OFFSET AND STRAIGHTNESS 197
  - X AND Y AXIS DISTANCE CALIBRATION 200
  - TIMING OF CAMERA AND COMPUTER 200
  - ADCs AS DATA-TRANSFER DEVICES 201
  - COMPUTER-TO-CAMERA INTERFACE FOR GANTRY CONTROL 202
  - GATING 203
- SPECT SOFTWARE QUALITY CONTROL AND SOFTWARE FOR QUALITY CONTROL 204
- SPECT QUALITY CONTROL 206
  - MECHANICAL MOTION 207
  - SENSITIVITY, UNIFORMITY, LINEARITY, RESOLUTION, ATTENUATION CORRECTION, VOLUME CALIBRATION, AND ENERGY EFFECTS 209
  - FORMATTER AND OTHER HARD COPY DEVICES 214
- SPECIFIC KINDS OF PROBLEMS: THEIR DIAGNOSIS AND CURE 215
  - ARTIFACTS TO LOOK FOR ON PATIENT EXAMINATIONS 215
- INSTALLATION AND ACCEPTANCE TESTING 218
  - MECHANICAL SET-UP 218
  - USUAL ANGER CAMERA TESTS 220
  - CAMERA-COMPUTER INTERFACE TESTS 220
  - ANGULAR DEPENDENCE OF IMAGES 220
  - SOFTWARE INSTALLATION AND TESTING 223
  - ACQUISITION VARIABLES 227
- ROUTINE QUALITY CONTROL 228
  - DAILY 228
  - WEEKLY 229

- MONTHLY 230
- QUARTERLY 232
- SEMIANNUALLY. 232
- ANNUALLY. 232

8 / Clinical Uses of SPECT 235
- GENERAL TECHNICAL DETAILS 235
  - PATIENT AND INSTRUMENT PREPARATION 236
  - CONDUCTING A TYPICAL STUDY 238
  - QUALITY ASSURANCE FOR CLINICAL SPECT 239
  - TROUBLESHOOTING 239
- HEAD 240
  - BLOOD-BRAIN BARRIER 242
  - CEREBRAL BLOOD FLOW 245
  - RECEPTOR BINDING 250
  - CEREBROSPINAL FLUID SPACE 251
  - PITUITARY GLAND 251
- LUNGS 253
- HEART 257
- LIVER AND SPLEEN 269
- BONE 275
- GALLIUM AND TUMOR IMAGING 278
- KIDNEYS 280
- THYROID 282
- GASTROINTESTINAL TRACT 283
- RADIOTHERAPEUTIC RADIOPHARMACEUTICALS
  AND FUTURE USES 284

INDEX 299

1

History and Coordinate System

Tomography, from the Greek *tomo*, slice or section (as in microtome) and *graph*, delineation, means the creation of slice images. The several landmarks in the development of tomography are worth examining individually for what they tell us about the way the human mind works and the bearing of technologic progress on medicine.

HISTORY

The first landmark was the x-ray, from which evolved the medical specialty of radiology. Some 20 years after the first x-rays, it was realized that if one plane in the human body was kept fixed while the x-ray source and the film were moved through like angles, an unblurred image of the plane would result. It took 20 more years for planar tomography to become one of the practical techniques that radiologists had at their disposal. Planar tomography is flawed, however. First, there is no way to prevent structures outside the plane of interest from also appearing on the image. A second and related problem is the fact that the technique creates images of low contrast because all of the irradiated tissue contributes to the image in some way. Finally, the radiation dose to patients is not insignificant.

X-radiology depends on differences in x-ray attenuation of the tissues viewed with an external source of x-rays, while nuclear medicine exploits differences in the distribution of internally administered radionuclides. There is a real difference in the number of unknown factors in the two specialties. In radiology, the strength of the x-ray beam is a constant; what is unknown is the distribution of the attenuation in the body. In addition, the absolute strength of the x-ray beam puts the technique in a statistical category that allows the rapid production of images of high resolution even with detectors of poor sensitivity. In nuclear medicine, the strength of the source and its position, as well as the distribution of attenuation, are all unknown. Considerations of radiation dose do not permit making patients radioactive enough to use detectors with exquisite resolution, so nuclear medical images are always count poor.

The nuclear medicine equivalent to planar transmission tomography, the rectilinear scanner, was actually in use before the nuclear medicine equivalent to the flat plate x-ray, the Anger camera. Although it provided a larger image, the Anger camera was technologically more complex than the rectilinear scanner; hence the delay in its early widespread use. The rectilinear scanner achieved planar tomographic images by using a collimator focused on the plane of interest. Not a great deal was made of its tomographic capabilities by most users, although Kuhl (1958) saw that the focused collimator could be used to advantage in large organs like the liver by "wrapping it around" the organ, that is, using it to view the organ from all angles, instead of imaging from front or back only.

Kuhl and Edwards (1963) were the exceptional users who understood that a great deal could be made of the tomographic capability of a focused collimator, if the more complex motions of wood-shaping power tools were added to the instrument together with an oscilloscope to obtain images, to replace the direct film exposure methods. Kuhl and Edwards' examination of the possibilities of the technique was an elegant extension of the methods of planar transmission tomography. They explored stereoscopic scanning, longitudinal section scanning, and transverse section scanning. By the following year (Kuhl and Edwards 1964), they had created a device for patient imaging and had established emission tomography as an important diagnostic tool.

Neither nuclear medicine nor radiology practitioners saw Kuhl's lead as one to follow immediately. Many other techniques had to be developed, not the least of which were the Anger camera and the technetium-99m generator. The tomographic techniques did become routine in Kuhl's laboratory (Kuhl et al. 1966), however, and Kuhl and Edwards continued with the development of the instrument. In 1968 Kuhl and Edwards published a discussion of the use of the digital computer to acquire and store data from their instrument.

The computer allowed adjustment of intensities in the final image; it also used paper tape for the initially acquired data and for intermediate storage of results to be transmitted to the hard-copy imaging device. (Paper tape is inexpensive but unbelievably slow and cumbersome by today's standards.)

By 1968 the computer was being used in emission tomography, but as a data-storage device and a contrast enhancer. Images were created by back projection of the acquired data onto a common area, but the special computational needs of this process were not recognized. By computer processing—either by convolution in real space or by filtering in Fourier space—the distracting lost contrast of overlying structures could be regained mathematically. It is splitting hairs, perhaps, to place the beginning of computed tomography (CT) at the beginning of such processing, but only at this point did the computer become more than a large device for simplifying back projection (which by itself can be done using an analog process) and removing background by mere subtraction.

A lost landmark in this story is Radon and his solution to the projection problem. Ever since Radon (1917) first explained in German the principles of reconstruction from projections in transform space (a mathematical construct not completely familiar to the medical scientist), it would have been possible to combine the ideas that come together in computed tomography. Neither the instruments nor the wherewithal to do such calculations existed in 1917, however; nor was Radon's work published in a forum that was accessible to great numbers of medical scientists. Also, as Herman (1980) pointed out, there were a great many details of the calculation that would have to be worked out, even using Radon's solution.

The mathematical part of the CT story was picked up elsewhere. Radon's solution did not come to the attention of English-speaking physicists. The whole idea of mathematical processing to synthesize the transaxial image from the projection images was rediscovered by Cormack (1963, 1964). Not only did Cormack set down some rigorous mathematics, he also did some x-ray CT experiments, albeit with what he deemed to be better statistics than would be available in clinical work, and compared attenuation coefficient values with the actual circumstances of the phantom.

Budinger (1974) and Budinger and Gullberg (1974) provided a nice review of the theoretical developments that led to the use of variations on the reconstruction theme and discussed the particular application of such ideas to count-poor nuclear medicine.

In 1973 Hounsfield reported the use of his x-ray CT instrument to image heads. The details of the mathematical process and the instrument are sketchy because of the proprietary interests of the developer, EMI. In 1974, Ledley and associates did much the same thing with the x-ray ACTA scanner, showing lovely color pictures that excited everyone. The x-ray CT rush was on and, because of fierce competition, there was no thought of revealing any of the secrets of the processing.

Once x-ray-transmission computed tomography was a commercial reality, the way was paved for more innovations in nuclear medicine. This had already begun, simultaneous with the first installation of an EMI unit in the Atkinson Morley Hospital in England in late 1971 (Freeman 1973), as is documented in the proceedings of a symposium on tomographic imaging in nuclear medicine held in late 1972 (Freedman 1973).

In the years since then, commercial development of the rotating Anger camera and simultaneous advances in computer technology have brought us to the present when three-dimensional single-photon-emission computed tomography (SPECT) is an everyday reality.

Other landmarks include limited-angle tomography and positron-emission tomography (PET). Multicrystal focused collimator SPECT systems are descendants of Kuhl's original instruments (Kuhl and Edwards 1970). The most recent single-photon tomographic research has been with rings of detectors and various types of collimators, for example the single-photon ring tomograph, SPRINT (Williams and Knoll 1979; Rogers et al. 1982).

Given the relative difficulties of developing instruments for SPECT, in the face of perfectly useful x-ray-transmission computed tomography, why this bother about SPECT? The answer lies in the basic utility of nuclear medicine—using radiotracers to locate and study the body's organ structures and systems by their physical and biochemical properties. We should thus be on the alert not only for techniques that enhance the anatomic capabilities of nuclear medicine, such as SPECT, but for the means to enhance the ability to study function in such a milieu. Knowledge of how an organ functions may take us much farther in the diagnosis of disease than would a mere picture, however exquisitely detailed, of how that organ looks.

COORDINATE SYSTEM

Early in the exposition of SPECT, it is necessary to decide on a system of coordinates for the subsequent discussion. Any references to

History and Coordinate System 5

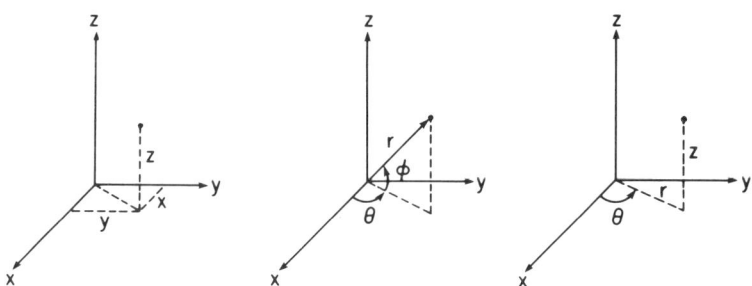

Fig 1–1.—On the left is the three-dimensional Cartesian coordinate system; in the center, the spherical coordinates; and on the right, the cylindrical coordinates.

spatial position can then be made with the assurance that the reader and the author have agreed on the orientation of the images.

The basis for a decision on a system of coordinates should first be explored. Three dimensions are most commonly discussed in terms of Cartesian (x,y,z), spherical (r, θ, π), or cylindrical (r, θ, z) coordinates (Fig 1–1). Most people feel comfortable with Cartesian coordinates. The conventions for forming a Cartesian system are that the axes be at 90 degrees to each other (orthogonal) and that they follow the right-hand rule. By this rule, if you take your right hand and first point the fingers straight in the x direction (Fig 1–2) and then curl them around to point in the y direction, your thumb will point in the positive z direction. Similarly, taking the coordinates *in order*, if the fingers first point in the y direction and then curl around to point in the z direction, the thumb will point in the positive x direction. The left hand will give a different result and is not used. Running the coordinates in any order other than xyzxyzxyz will also give a different result. The convention of using the right-hand rule is, like the one that assigns a negative charge to the electron, just a convention; but once it is used, everything falls into place so long as it is not violated. The right-hand rule prevents problems with incorrect positive (+) and negative (−) signs in calculations that involve directions.

Once it has been decided to use Cartesian coordinates and to follow the right-hand rule, it only remains to decide where to put the origin and which way to point the x axis.

The origin used in this book is the outside of the patient's right heel, with the x axis pointing toward the left heel, the y axis toward the head, and the z axis toward the right toes. See Figure 1–3 for a description of the coordinate system and the coordinates of the image that result. When the transaxial images are created, they are in the

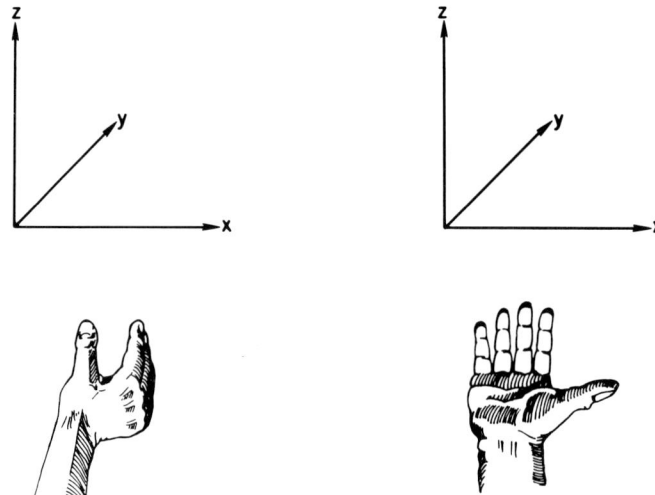

Fig 1–2.—The right-hand rule is designed to give the direction of the third axis in the three-dimensional Cartesian coordinate system, once the planes of the other two axes have been defined.

x-z plane, with the origin in the lower left-hand corner, as though the viewer were standing at the patient's feet looking at the transaxial slice. This choice becomes inconvenient only if spherical or cylindrical coordinate manipulations are desired, because the axis of rotation of such coordinate systems is usually the z axis. In the case of the coordinate system described here and in the case of the body, the axis of rotation is parallel to the y axis. Notice also that since the choice

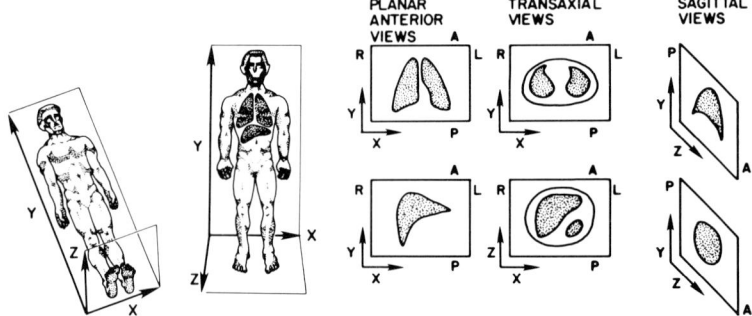

Fig 1–3.—On the left is a supine patient, with the axes indicated. In the middle, the patient is standing, and on the right the axes are marked on the various projections that result from imaging of the patient. The reader is the viewer and can stay right where he is.

of origin is in line with the computer's choice, at the edge rather than in the center of the image, the axis of rotation is not contiguous with any of the axes of the coordinate system.

When exclusively planar images are considered, the x-y plane will be used, no matter at what angle around the patient, unless the meaning does not seem clear without referring to the angle and the z plane. The anterior image of the patient, often used as the sample image in SPECT for delineating the level of the transaxial slices, is in line with the coordinate system, with the x-y origin in the lower left-hand corner.

Clearly, other coordinate system assignments could be used and might work as well or better, depending on their purpose.

BIBLIOGRAPHY

Budinger, T. F. Quantitative nuclear medicine imaging: application of computers to the gamma camera and whole-body scanner. *Recent Adv. Nucl. Med.* 4:41–130, 1974.

Budinger, T. F., and Gullberg, G. T. Three-dimensional reconstruction in nuclear medicine imaging. *IEEE Trans. Nucl. Sci.* 21:2–20, 1974.

Cormack, A. M. Representation of a function by its line integrals, with some radiological applications. *J. Appl. Phys.* 34:2722–2727, 1963.

Cormack, A. M. Representation of a function by its line integrals with some radiological applications. II. *J. Appl. Phys.* 35:2908–2913, 1964.

Freeman, L. M. Computerized transverse axial tomography with x-rays. In *Tomographic Imaging in Nuclear Medicine,* ed. G. S. Freedman. New York: Society of Nuclear Medicine, 1973, pp. 200–204.

Freedman, G. S., ed. *Tomographic Imaging in Nuclear Medicine.* New York: Society of Nuclear Medicine, 1973.

Herman, G. T. *Image Reconstruction from Projections.* New York: Academic Press, 1980.

Hounsfield, G. N. Computerized transverse axial scanning (tomography). I. Description of system. *Br. J. Radiol.* 46:1016–1022, 1973.

Kuhl, D. E. Rotational scanning of the liver. *Radiology* 71:875–876, 1958.

Kuhl, D. E., et al. Transverse section and rectilinear brain scanning with Tc-99m pertechnetate. *Radiology* 86:822–829, 1966.

Kuhl, D. E., and Edwards, R. Q. Image separation radioisotope scanning. *Radiology* 80:653–666, 1963.

Kuhl, D. E., and Edwards, R. Q. Cylindrical and section radioisotope scanning of the liver and brain. *Radiology* 83:926–936, 1964.

Kuhl, D. E., and Edwards, R. Q. Reorganizing data from transverse section scans of the brain using digital processing. *Radiology* 91:975–983, 1968.

Kuhl, D. E., and Edwards, R. Q. The Mark III scanner: a compact device for multiple-view and section scanning of the brain. *Radiology* 96:563–570, 1970.

Ledley, R. S., et al. Computerized axial x-ray tomography of the human body. *Science* 186:207–212, 1974.

Radon, J. Über die bestimmung von funktionen durch ihre integralwerte längs gewisser mannigfaltigkeiten. *Sachsisch. Gesellsch. Wissenschaft. Leipzig Math. Phys.* 69:262–277, 1917.

Rogers, W. L., et al. SPRINT: a stationary detector single photon ring tomograph for brain imaging. *IEEE Trans. Med. Imag.* 1:63–68, 1982.

Rogers, W. L., et al. SPRINT: a single photon ring tomograph. Abstract. *J. Nucl. Med.* 23:P59, 1982.

Williams, J. J., and Knoll, G. F. Initial performance of SPRINT: a single photon system for emission tomography. *IEEE Trans. Nucl. Sci.* 26:2732–2735, 1979.

2

Theory of Tomography

Several fields can benefit from tomographic imaging, including applied mathematics, electron microscopy, radiology (of course), radioastronomy, and vision theory. Numerous attempts have been made by theoreticians in these fields to examine and refine the mathematics involved in tomography. The situation is like that of the troop of blind men examining the elephant: because of their positions around the beast and their previous experience, they feel different things. The result has been lack of unanimity in notation and emphasis. With the added factor of the necessity to test each method under actual conditions of application, advances in theory have been difficult to follow. The only constant factor is that for the great majority of applications, using the digital computer is the only way to create an image from acquired data. The difficulty with computer solutions (or applied mathematical rigor, for that matter) is that neither the algorithms nor the applications are amenable to explanations that use simple examples. One can only begin to treat the ideas to be examined here with simple pictures. As many techniques as possible are illustrated by simple numerical examples and by actual nuclear medicine examples.

An added difficulty in the field of transaxial tomography is that there is money to be made in having the best results. Thus for economic reasons, manufacturers and vendors have a stake in secrecy, so it may not be possible to pinpoint the methods used in each case. The radiology community in general does not have a great interest in tomographic theory, but judges the package as a whole, from imaging table to transaxial image. In articles on x-ray–transmission tomography, for example, it is sufficient to note the manufacturer and model of the instrument used, without an elaborate discussion of algorithms.

Why are we not content with this approach in nuclear medicine? Perhaps the major reason is that our instruments are not so polished, because the market is not so large. Another reason is that the circumstances of imaging, notably the count rate and nuclide, vary so much from one examination to the next that our instruments and computer programs must be prepared to take on more varied circumstances than are seen in x-ray–transmission tomography. For these reasons, practitioners need an understanding of the principles behind the modality to choose the equipment and establish intelligent protocols that will yield the best diagnostic information. The work of Larsson (1980) about the relevant software, its rationale, and its use is an excellent step toward understanding SPECT.

The problem we are confronted with is this: given a number of digital projections of a distribution of radioactivity within a patient (an extended object), acquired at regular angular intervals to cover 180 or 360 degrees, with some nuclear medicine imaging device such as a scanner or Anger camera, can we create an accurate and precise picture of the distribution of the radioactivity in a particular plane of the patient, usually a transaxial plane? As part of this intellectual exercise, we must realize the limitations that this framework imposes, which include, but are not limited to, the following: scatter, resolution, count rate and Poisson statistics, imaging time, geometric limitation of the instrument approaching the patient, size of patient and instrument, energy window, computer storage and time, patient and organ motion, knowledge about individual patient anatomy, computer accuracy, patient physiology, and radioactive decay.

Now that quite a number of specters have been raised (and will be treated in their own time and place), let us return to the main theme, that of the creation of a transaxial slice image from projections of the object. If one slice can be created, then many can be; Anger camera reconstructions are made one x-direction data line at a time. The magnificence of the Anger camera is that the projections (planar images) allow the acquisition of all the x data lines at once, instead of one slice at a time, so the slices automatically go together, with no changes caused by motion occurring between them.

In this chapter, the physics and mathematics of SPECT are discussed. The material is arranged so that one may delve as deeply as desired by reading all the way through, or absorb the general idea without all the details by reading the first part of the chapter and skipping the later sections.

GENERAL DESCRIPTION OF THE MATHEMATICS OF SPECT

Tomographic Process

The transaxial tomographic process is rather like drawing the floor plan of a house by looking in the windows. The viewer is confined to the outside but he can see details inside, and by walking around the house, looking in all the windows, he can perfect his plan. Basically, the back-projection process uses the information gathered from each viewing point, creating a plan from the first view and refining it as the house is circled. Other reconstruction methods wait until all the information is collected and then, figuratively, go back to the office to refine the plans.

For simplicity, we will assume that SPECT planar projection data have been (or are being) collected at regular angular intervals into a series of frames in a digital computer file. We will also assume, for all of our examples, that a parallel-hole collimator is being used, although other collimators can be used.

The processing steps for the data (not necessarily arranged in the same order in every system) are as follows: adjustments for camera and interface properties such as uniformity, linearity, and table positioning; taking geometric mean of data; filtration; attenuation correction; back projection; and more filtering or smoothing. We will discuss each of these steps in some detail.

The adjustments for camera and interface properties may be effected as the computer stores each planar image, or they may be done afterwards with a command from the operator. These are very basic corrections; ordinarily, the actual data in the computer file are changed, and the original data are lost because they are not important. (These corrections are discussed at length in the chapter on data acquisition.)

The detector's response varies as a function of its distance from the collimator face; the response variation is greater in water or tissue than in air. In some SPECT processing, to counteract the degradation of resolution that occurs when imaging tissue, the planar projection data from opposing sides of the patient are added together, giving only half as many projections to be treated as were originally acquired. An average of the data from the opposing sides does not correct for this degradation of resolution with distance as well as the geometric mean does. Figure 2–1 shows the response in water as a function of distance, and the result of taking the geometric mean of opposing data on the response.

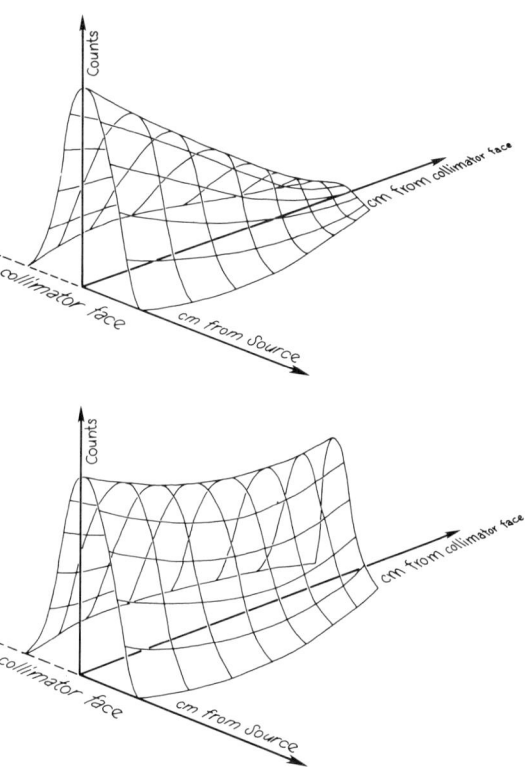

Fig 2–1.—Top, the response of an Anger camera as a function of distance from the collimator face to a line source in water. The sensitivity and resolution of the system are both degraded by the scattering medium. **Bottom,** the result of taking the geometric mean of data taken from opposing sides of line source in water as a function of distance from the collimator face.

Once the basic corrections and adjustments are completed for each pass, the computer's labors begin. Even in an ideal world, a certain amount of image enhancement and filtering should be performed to get the data ready for the creation of the final images. This processing is done by applying specific filters to enhance one spatial frequency range and suppress another. The most basic filtering removes an extra factor of distance that appears in the back-projection process; removal decreases the high background of a simple back-projected image.

The process is called "filtering" because it has much the same effect as putting a mixture of particles of different sizes through a set of filters. The filters divide the mixture into its component parts. The mathematical equivalent of this process picks out component parts for special treatment.

Filtering is done by passing a filter over the data: the filter values are used as multipliers for a patch of data at a time, adding up the

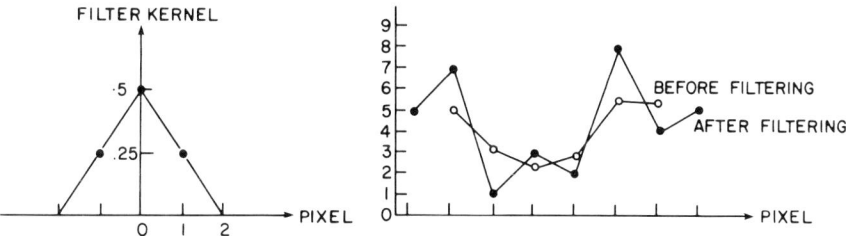

Fig 2–2.—A one-dimensional filter is operating on one-dimensional data. **Left,** the filter is ¼ ½ ¼. **Right,** the data line is
    5   7   1   3   2   8   4   5,
and is designated "Before Filtering." After the filter has been convoluted with the data, the result is
        5.00   3.00   2.25   3.75   5.50   5.25,
which is designated "after filtering." The filter smooths the data, taking out sudden highs and lows, or high-frequency information. The filter is called a low-frequency bandpass filter. No rule has been made for what happens at the edges in this case, so the edges have been ignored.

results of the multiplications, and putting the results back in the place where the filter was centered. This process of patch multiplication is called convolution. Figure 2–2 shows an example of the convolution of a simple smoothing filter with a line of data. The numbers in the filter (1/4, 1/2, 1/4, in this case) are called the "convolution kernel"; their values may be positive or negative. This is a one-dimensional example but the filter may extend in two dimensions.

The equivalent of filtering the information by the convolution process in ordinary x-y space (called "real space") is to transform the data by a Fourier transform function into frequency space and to apply the frequency-dependent filter function before inverse Fourier transformation back into real space. The process of filtering by convolution in real space is completely equivalent to filtering by multiplication by a filter function in frequency space. Making Fourier space plausible to those not familiar with it is not so simple, but perhaps the closest common analogy is that of our thinking about electromagnetic radiation either in terms of its wavelength (real space) or frequency (inverse space).

Filtering for transaxial tomography may be performed in the x direction (the direction of the transaxial slice) or in the y direction (parallel to the axis of rotation), or in an angular sense from one image to the next around the patient. This last resembles the temporal filtering for gated cardiac studies, where successive images are averaged together to smooth the cine presentation. Typically, the planar projection images of a SPECT examination are filtered in the x direction before they are back projected. The transaxial image is filtered in both directions.

The figures accompanying the text show examples of filters used in SPECT; the ramp filter (Fig 2–3) removes extra background from the transaxial images, which the back projection method puts in. Its sharp edge, at the cutoff frequency, which is the reciprocal of twice the pixel (picture unit) cell length, causes bumps in the resulting images (the technical term for the bumps is "ringing," after a sound wave analogy). High values at large frequencies (corresponding to short distances in x-y space) emphasize the high frequencies (which may be only Poisson noise). Therefore, substitutes for the ramp filter are made (Fig 2–3) that incorporate some of the properties of the ramp but roll off smoothly and at lower frequencies. Figure 2–4 shows the convolution kernels for each of these filters, both as continuous curves and at the sampling points used with SPECT data acquired with a 64 × 64 matrix. Note that the process of sampling at a discrete interval means the actual filter function used is not really the equiv-

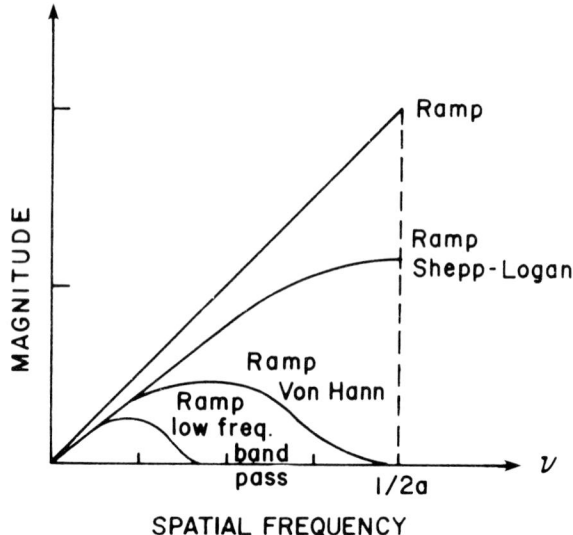

Fig 2–3.—Several filters are illustrated in frequency space. They all combine the ramp necessary for back projection with some other desirable filter property, such as passing low frequencies and screening out high frequencies. The cutoff frequency for the ramp and Shepp-Logan filters is ½a, where a is the distance between pixels in real space (Larsson 1980; Nahmias et al. 1980; Shepp and Logan 1974; Hamming 1977).

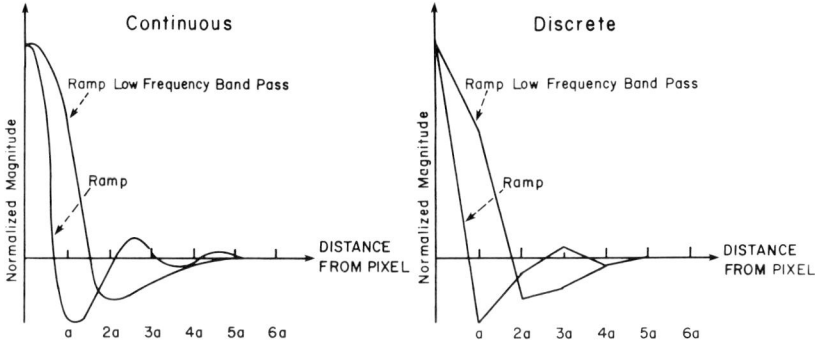

Fig 2–4.—On the left, the kernels of a number of filters are illustrated in continuous real space, with the sampling points displayed. Since the filters are used in a discontinuous or discrete fashion, the sampling points are connected by straight lines, as shown on the right. This in turn means that a transformation back into frequency space would not produce the smooth curves in Figure 2–3; that is, the filters are presented in their idealized frequency space form, but actually used in a discrete form in real space.

alent of the frequency-space version of Figure 2–3. Figure 2–5 illustrates three of these filters used with a clinical image.

The attenuation and scattering of radiation within the patient must be considered next. The deeper in the patient the source of gamma rays is, the more those rays are attenuated on the way to the detector. Thus some correction for attenuation should be made or the center of the patient image will appear less radioactive than the patient actually is. A great deal of controversy and discussion about SPECT centers around attenuation and scattering corrections, because dealing with them properly is a problem. To know how to correct for attenuation, one must know the position and strength of the radioactive source, but to know the position and strength, one must already have done the attenuation correction and created the transaxial image. There are several ways out of this dilemma, ranging from simple approximations to iterative procedures in which the answers to one round of calculations become the input for the next round.

The very simplest thing of all to do is nothing: not bother with attenuation correction and accept the fact that the centers of transaxial images will appear less radioactive than they should. Figure 2–6 shows the difference in a clinical image with and without attenuation correction.

If a correction is desired, the next simplest approximation is to assume that the patient's contour is an ellipse, that any radiation

16 *Chapter 2*

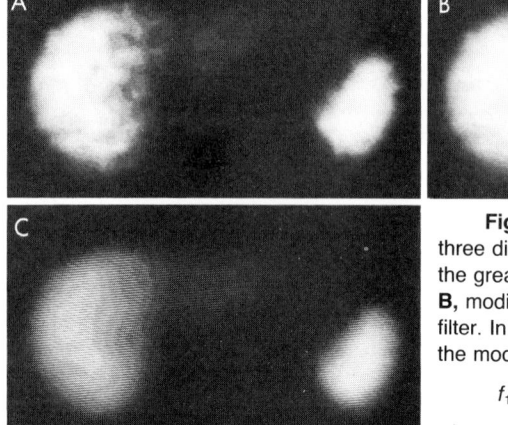

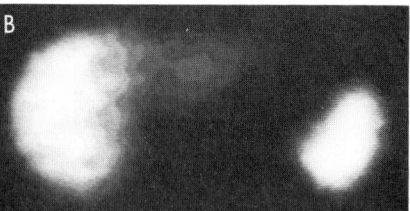

Fig 2–5.—Image of a liver with three different filters. **A**, ramp, showing the greatest amount of detail and noise; **B**, modified Shepp-Logan; **C**, smoothing filter. In real space the formula describing the modified Shepp-Logan filter is

$$f_1(n,a) = -2/(\pi^2 a^2(4n^2-1)),$$

where $n = 0, \pm 1, \pm 2, \ldots$ and a is the length of the side of a pixel. The formula for the smoothing filter is $f(n,a) = 0.4f_1(n,a) + 0.3f_1(n-1,a) + 0.3f_1(n+1,a)$ (Larsson 1980).

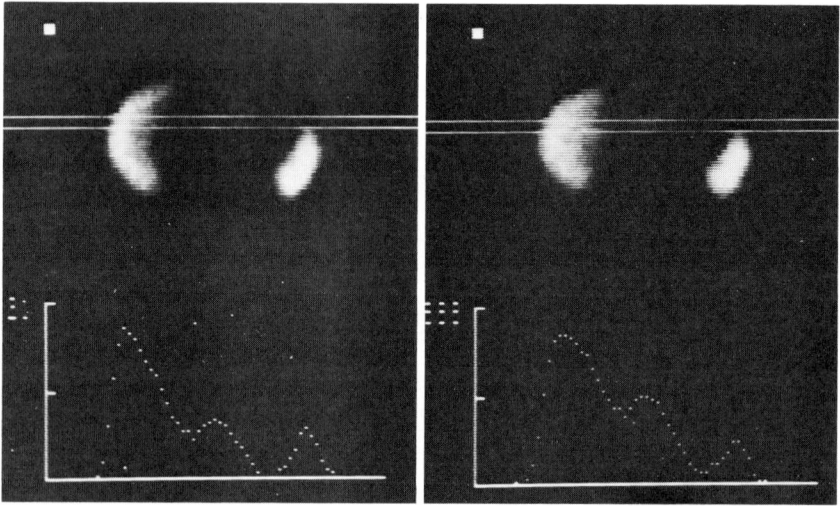

Fig 2–6.—Image of a liver without **Left** and with **Right** attenuation correction. The attenuation coefficient was 0.12 per cm. The graphs show a profile through each image.

seen at a particular angle is really coming from a whole column of radioactive material evenly distributed across the ellipse, and that the attenuation of the tissue is uniform; the corrections are based on these assumptions. In this way each image may be corrected independently of the others once the patient's contour is known. Figure 2–7 illustrates this correction.

Another way to proceed is to go all the way through the processes to the production of the transaxial image (Chang 1978). The transaxial image is then corrected for attenuation at each point by an attenuation-correction matrix. A measured body contour fashions the matrix of attenuation values at each point by considering the projection of that point into each angle through a column of tissue. In the complete process described by Chang, the patient outline and the assumption of a uniform attenuation coefficient are combined to create a correction matrix that is applied to the transaxial image to produce a corrected image. The process may stop at this point. It may continue by reprojecting the corrected transaxial matrix with the correction factors. The created projections are compared with the patient data by subtraction. A set of error projections is the result. The error projections are themselves back projected and the error matrix that is

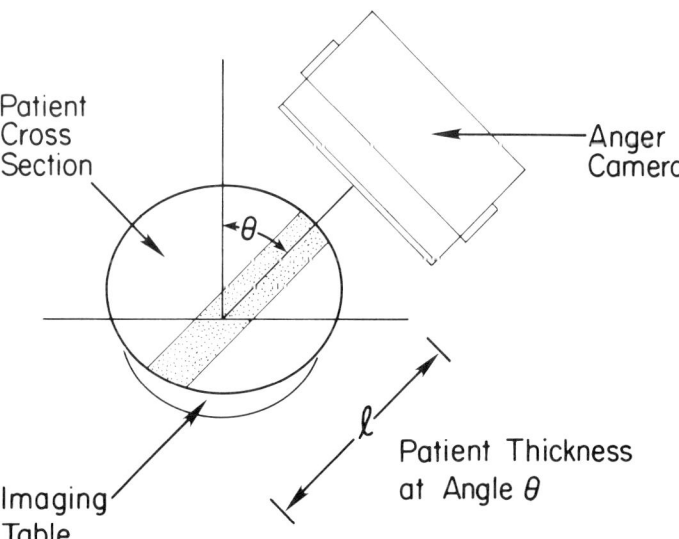

Fig 2–7.—A simple attenuation correction is made by assuming that the transaxial section is uniform and that the radioactivity is distributed evenly in the column of tissue to be back-projected into.

18   *Chapter 2*

created is combined with the corrected transaxial image to create a second corrected transaxial image (Fig 2–8). This process can be repeated over and over (iteration). In practice, it is not repeated, because projection and back projection take time and the results of the first processing seem to be satisfactory. Iteration of the Chang method begins to allow for the fact that the patient's tissues do not have uniform attenuation.

To take into account the real attenuation coefficients for bone, muscle, blood, fat, and other tissues, distributed as they are in a particular patient, one could use either an x-ray–transmission CT image or a gamma-source–transmission CT image as an image of attenuation coefficients. Either possibility extends the time of the examination and increases the radiation dose. It also does not explore the difficulties of achieving uniform x-ray CT images. So far these possibilities have been considered only when the highest degree of

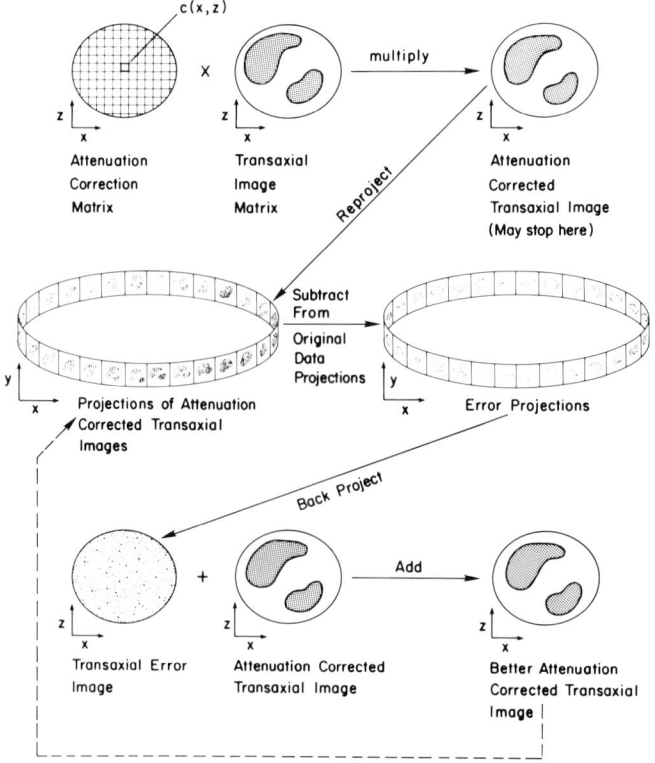

Fig 2–8.—The Chang process for attenuation correction is shown schematically.

quantitative accuracy is required. Another method that shows promise is that of modeling the parts of the human body and then using the transaxial images or a set of quickly acquired single-photon–transmission images to scale the model to the patient, so that an attenuation-correction matrix could be developed for that patient from the model values.

After all the corrections are completed, the transaxial images themselves are created. The back-projection process is simple in conception and operation once the data have been prepared for it. Mathematically, the transaxial slice image is created by putting in the contribution from each angle. It is called "back projection" because the process of acquiring the images is projection, and back projection is the reversal of this process. Indeed, back projection could be performed with the projection data just as they come from the imaging device. The rest of the processing described here is meant to improve the results and make them more quantitative. Figure 2–9 indicates the back-projection process schematically, while Figure 2–10 shows the mathematical process with a very simple matrix. After the initial operation creates a set of transaxial images, iterations of the procedure may be performed to achieve the closest possible relationship between the original projection data and what the transaxial slices would give if they were projected, although each of these steps will take additional time.

Software systems have been developed in which the greatest amount of filtration is done after the images are back projected, using the Chang method for attenuation correction. Certain image-en-

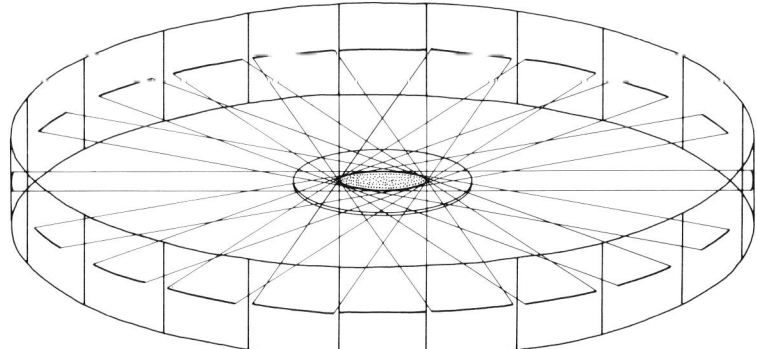

Fig 2–9.—The back-projection process is shown schematically. The projection images are in a ring around the central slice. Information from each of the projection images is back projected into the center, creating a composite image.

20   *Chapter 2*

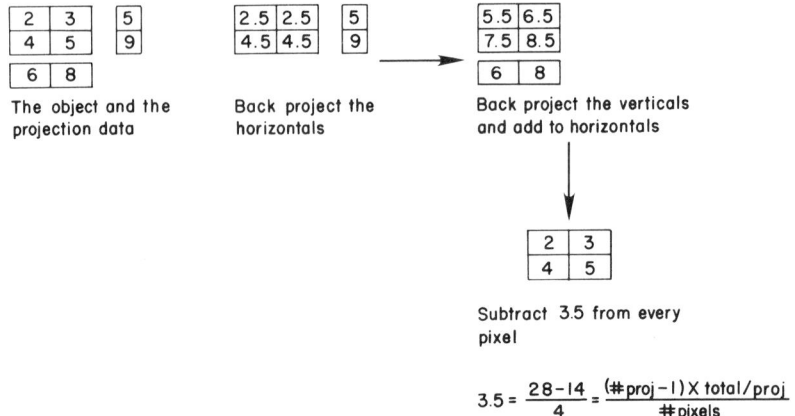

Fig 2-10.—A simple matrix of four numbers is used to illustrate the back-projection process. On the far left, the original distribution is shown; this is unknown during the back projection process and appears as the result. What is known is a set of two projection images. In the back-projection process, the activity in each of the projections is evenly distributed across the central image. The contributions from each of the two directions are added. A constant is subtracted to adjust the contrast and, behold, the original distribution is recovered.

hancement techniques, among them more filtering, are performed on the transaxial images as well. This filtering is usually performed in both the x and z directions to smooth the data or to bring out certain features about which more information is desired.

From the transaxial slices, other projections can be easily formed by recasting the data at any particular angle. If the new slice is at 90 degrees to the transaxial slice (as coronal and sagittal slices are), the formation of the new images is particularly simple. If angulation is involved, interpolation calculations must be made.

The process that has just been described is somewhat idealized, because it does not take into account some of the real-world problems that SPECT solutions encounter. In particular, we should face the effects of using digital data, of Poisson statistics, of attenuation, and of scattering.

Digital Data and Their Effects

For the computer, the analog data from the imaging instrument are forced into a digital matrix representation with a limited number of pixels per image. The projection data are collected at a digital whole number of angles rather than continuously around the patient

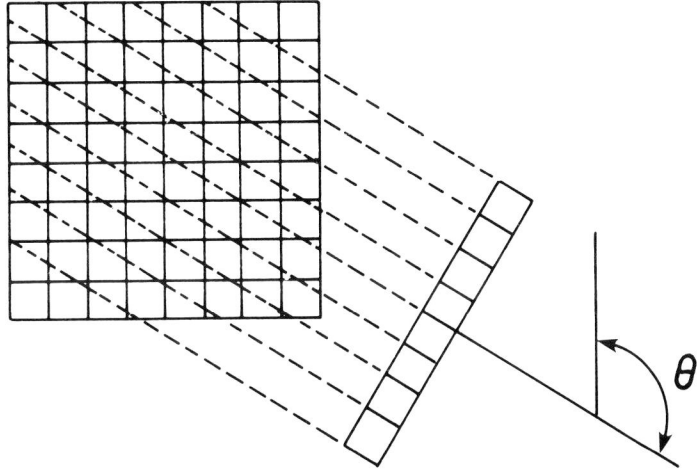

Fig 2–11.—Data from arbitrary angles such as theta will not line up in the back-projected matrix.

(whether the instrument moves continuously or discontinuously). One result of this is that all the mathematics must be done in a discontinuous or discrete manner; filters must be considered to be described more in terms of a bar graph than a smooth line, as had been shown in Figure 2–4. Another result of digital data is the necessity for interpolation whenever the projection is not aligned with the back projection matrix. Figure 2–11 shows that data from angles other than 0 and 90 degrees do not line up with the transaxial matrix pixels. Choices must be made as to how this interpolation will be done. Possibilities (Larsson 1980) range from the choice of the nearest-neighbor pixel value to linear and more complex interpolation methods. Figure 2–12 illustrates nearest-neighbor interpolation.

The thickness of the transaxial slice is under the operator's control. Thicker slices contain more counts (and therefore are less noisy and have greater accuracy), while thin slices have the greatest resolution along the axis of rotation (Fig 2–13). If there is a difference in the amount of activity from one part of a transaxial voxel (volume element) to another, the image incorrectly reflects the actual distri-

22 *Chapter 2*

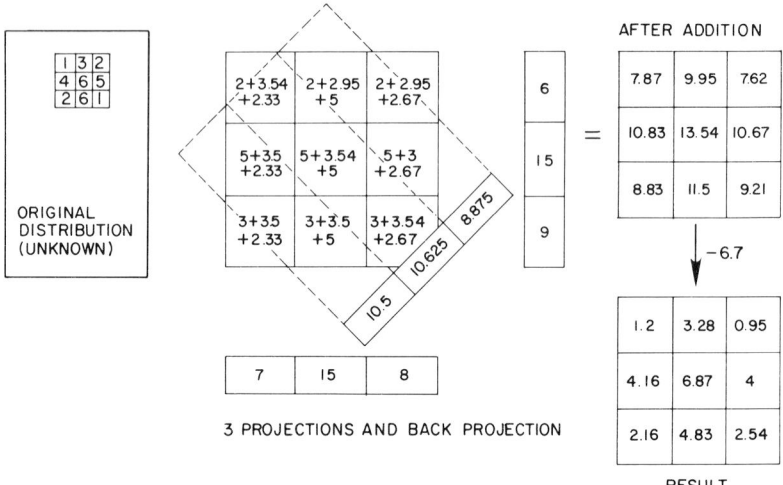

Fig 2–12.—Nearest-neighbor interpolation is illustrated here. Three projections are illustrated. Each is back projected in turn, with the 45–degree projection being back projected according to a nearest-neighbor rule—the nearest full pixel gets the contribution. The original matrix is given on the left, for the reader's information; it is presumed to be unknown during the back-projection process.

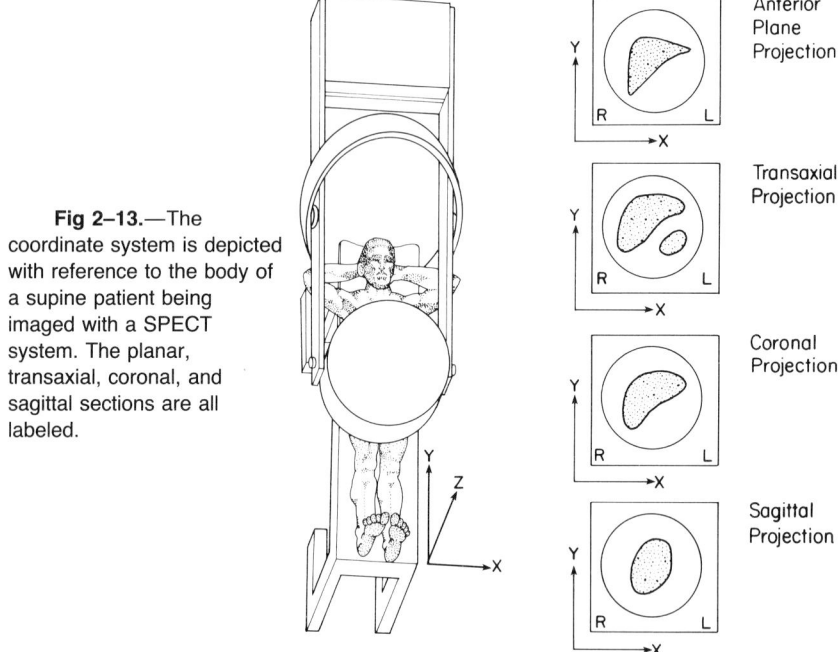

Fig 2–13.—The coordinate system is depicted with reference to the body of a supine patient being imaged with a SPECT system. The planar, transaxial, coronal, and sagittal sections are all labeled.

bution; this is called "partial voluming." If the software creates a slice that is thicker in the y direction than in the x direction, one must think about the process of creating coronal, sagittal, and oblique slices because the thick slices mean less resolution. Coronal and sagittal slices, for example, would have one dimension in which the information has a much greater (and therefore worse) resolution distance than in the other; the problem may be fixed cosmetically by interpolation between transaxial slices, but this does not substitute for having slice voxels that are cubes.

The number of pixels into which the image is divided affects the signal-noise ratio, since the noise is on the order of the square root of the signal; the larger the number of pixels, the smaller the signal-noise ratio and the noisier the data. This problem is best thought of in three dimensions—we should be considering the number of voxels into which the three-dimensional image is divided; this is hard because volume images cannot be printed on paper or film. The implication for filtering is that softer filtering, with less emphasis on high frequencies, must be used for larger numbers of voxels. The result is that sharpness seemingly captured with the greater number of acquisition voxels is lost in processing, because what really matters are numbers of counts and sensitivity, beyond a certain balance point. The number of pixels and angular samples acquired should be tailored to the statistical quality of the data, so that extra noise is not captured only to have to be filtered out.

Poisson Statistics and the Accuracy of SPECT

At the practical level, there are questions of what the theoretical approaches have to say about the resolution, precision, and accuracy of SPECT. Resolution measures how well the position of the activity is determined; better resolution is smaller distance. Precision speaks to the question of how much uncertainty there is in the results; better precision is a smaller number, usually expressed as a fraction or percentage of the result. Accuracy has to do with the comparison of the SPECT results with the actual distribution of activities. Having seen the SPECT images, we have an intuitive sense that the statistical uncertainties do not overwhelm the useful information; therefore, proving that the uncertainty is greater than the data or that resolution is no better than the width of three fingers would be like proving that bumblebees cannot fly. Accuracy, precision, and resolution are all connected through every part of the SPECT system. The discussion presented here should be a framework on which to base considerations of these properties in subsequent chapters.

Chapter 2

Resolution should be approached from two points of view. First, consider the resolution of a system of opposed images combined together through the geometric mean. Figure 2–1 showed that the full width at half maximum (FWHM) for a system incorporating a 30–cm-diameter source was between 1.0 and 1.5 cm, depending on the position of the source in the scattering medium. Next, consider a rotating system: a number of rays N pass through the center of a circle of diameter W. The circumference of the circle is $\pi \times W$. The N rays divide the circumference into arcs of length $\pi \times W/N$. In the simplest way, the length of the arc is equated to the resolution of the system and the diameter of the circle to the width of the patient. In nuclear medicine systems there is usually 360-degree data collection using 2N angles. Thus, the resolution: $R = \pi \times W/2N$. For a numerical estimate, if the patient width is 30 cm and the number of angles in 360 degrees is 64, the resolution is 1.5 cm. Thus 64 angular intervals yield the same order of magnitude for resolution on the outside of the patient cylinder as the FWHM in a scattering medium; inside the patient the angular motion means a smaller distance increment. To be sure that the angular increment will not be responsible for degradation of resolution, one might wish to increase the number of angular increments to 90 or 128 for 30–cm-diameter resolutions of 1.0 or 0.75 cm, respectively, but one must be sure to consider the effect on precision when the counts are divided among 1.5 to 2.0 times as many planar projection images. Note also that we have been discussing the resolution of the outside of the patient. By this very same method, we could show much better resolution inside, and indeed, 64 angles seem quite adequate for most patient examinations. The resolution of the system is never any better than the resolution of the coarsest part; no amount of pushing the pixel size to smaller and smaller limits or using larger numbers of angular increments can help a system whose collimator limits the resolution. The resolution of the system is the square root of the sum of the squares of the resolutions of the individual parts; in SPECT, the individual parts run the gamut from the camera to the final smoothing and the image-presentation device. It can already be seen that the camera and its collimators (combined with the patient as a good-sized source), patient motion, and perhaps the reconstruction algorithm will provide the major sources of degradation of resolution.

The question of precision or adequate statistics seems to be even more troublesome in SPECT than it is in planar imaging. First, consider the imaging of a flood source in a planar fashion. If there are 1 million (1 M) total counts collected, in a planar imaging there would be 330 counts per pixel (a circle in a 64 × 64 matrix) and an expected standard deviation of 5.5%. If 10 million counts were collected, then the standard deviation would be 1.7%.

In three dimensions, the problem is perhaps only more difficult to illustrate, but not to understand. Consider first attaching a flood source to the camera head and rotating it while acquiring data into a SPECT matrix. Acquire 10 M total counts into a 64 × 64 matrix at 64 angular intervals; this is the equivalent of 10M/(64 × π × 32 × 32) = 48.6 counts per pixel for each of the pixels in each of the 64 projections. The standard deviation is 7 counts, or 14% of the count-per-pixel value. If there were no other errors or uncertainties, even those of the combination of the pixel uncertainties, in the reconstruction process, the number we have arrived at gives us a rough estimate of the uncertainty in the resulting transaxial voxels. A simple consideration of the distribution of 10 M counts into the transaxial voxels would give 11.7% standard deviation, but the final results cannot be more precise than the acquired data from which they were calculated.

To illustrate the effect of fewer counts on this thought experiment, consider 1 M total counts. The counts per projection pixel become 4.86 with a standard deviation equal to 2.2, or 45.3%. It is easy to see why low count densities result in noisy transaxial images.

For a more realistic thought experiment, let us turn to a liver-spleen image. The liver and spleen have about 1,100 cc of tissue; for purposes of this example, consider the liver to be a cube 10 cm on a side and the spleen another cube, 4.62 cm on a side. If 10 M total counts are collected in a 64 × 64 matrix at 64 angular intervals, and the average projection of the two cubic organs has 150 square cm or 150/(0.625 × 0.625) = 384 (rounded up to 400) pixels containing counts, then 10M/(64 × 400) = 390 counts per pixel are contained in the average acquired projection image. The uncertainty of 390 counts is 20 counts, or 5.1%.

To extend the liver-spleen illustration, consider trying to achieve better resolution by using a finer-grained matrix and angular interval. If 10 M counts are acquired at 128 angles into a 128 × 128 matrix and reconstructed with the same voxel size, there are 150/(0.3125 × 0.3125), or about 1,600 pixels containing counts in each projection. Therefore 10M/(128 × 1,600) is 48.8 counts per projection pixel with an uncertainty of 7 counts, or 14%. Thus an attempt at better resolution significantly worsens statistical precision.

To the extent that the reconstruction process also degrades the statistical quality of the transaxial images, uncertainties will be larger than those illustrated above.

To test the effect of SPECT reconstruction on statistical precision, Budinger and co-workers (1978) used a set of computer simulations. One of the simulations or computer "phantoms" was a uniform disk with Poisson noise (the uncertainty of radioactive decay). The reconstruction methods used were better than the usual ones employed in commercially available software. For a simulated 1 M total events, the precision was found to be 52% and for 10 M events, 17%. The difference can be accounted for by considering that noisy data have been used to create the transaxial image; errors in noisy data do not cancel out but propagate, so that results from calculations of many steps have large errors. The following formula was proposed (Budinger et al. 1978; Budinger, Gullberg, and Huesman 1979) to treat errors from SPECT imaging of a uniform source:

root mean square (rms) % uncertainty
$$= (120)(number\ of\ resolution\ elements)^{3/4}$$
$$\times (total\ number\ of\ events)^{-1/2}.$$

For a 64 × 64 matrix with an inner circle, about 3,200 pixels have activity, so call these the "resolution elements." The calculated uncertainty for 1 M counts is 51% and for 10 M counts it is 16%, making the formula give results close to the measured values.

Most of our problems do not involve a flood source, however. For the more lifelike problem, Budinger and associates (1978) carried out a series of computer simulations using lifelike situations and created another equation to describe the results. Many of the real imaging situations involve filling only part of the camera area with activity. Under such conditions, the contrast and the numbers of filled and unfilled pixels must be taken into account. The reason is that the information density in the radioactive areas is much higher in the case of a small organ because the counts are packed into fewer pixels. Budinger's formulation of the experimental results included the concept of an effective number of resolution cells that is equal to the number of target cells plus the number of background cells, divided by the contrast or ratio between the target activity and the background activity. The effective number of resolution cells is substituted for the number of resolution elements in the above expression. The results are more encouraging. For a simulated kidney, which occupied 20% of the active area of the matrix and had a contrast of 11:1, and for which the collection of 1 M counts was simulated, a standard deviation of 18% was found. A substitution relates the rms % uncertainty to the number of counts in a resolution cell:

$$rms\ \% = 120\ (N)^{1/4}\ (counts\ in\ resolution\ cell)^{-3/4}.$$

If instead the number of counts in a pixel is substituted, there is an extra factor of the square of the pixel size divided by the resolution cell size, so the formula becomes:

rms % = 120 (total counts)$^{1/4}$
 × (average counts/pixel)$^{-3/4}$ (resolution/pixel)$^{3/2}$,

relating the uncertainty to the total counts, the average counts per pixel observed in the transaxial image, and the ratio of the resolution cell size to the size of the pixel.

This has not been an easy area to study. MacIntyre and colleagues (1983; personal communication 1984) found that the form of the Budinger equation was useful but that a different constant was needed to fit their experimental data. Also, what was meant by the effective number of resolution cells might well be different, since Budinger's group used a computer simulation and one reconstruction method and the MacIntyre group used others. More important, the MacIntyre group also found that uncertainty reaches an asymptotic value around 7% by 10 M total counts, so that no further increase in the numbers of counts has any effect on precision. Thus the system is itself noisy, either because of imprecision in the camera and gantry or because of noise introduced in the reconstruction process. Ramp filters have been used in this work to permit comparisons more easily, but other filtration processes implicit in the back-projection algorithms may have an effect on the uncertainty and resolution.

Attenuation has not been considered in the preceding discussion. Previous work by the same authors (Budinger et al. 1977) suggests that the uncertainty is increased by a factor of 1.3 when attenuation is compensated for.

Jaszczak, Coleman, and Whitehead (1981) also treated the question of accuracy in a paper that discussed resolution, precision, and accuracy. Naturally, their point of view differed from Budinger's, because the effects of attenuation and the filter function were to be included; their formula is cast in different terms:

$$\text{rms \%} = \frac{100 \ (1.8)^{3/2} \ \pi \ R_{eff} \ R_s^{1/2} \ A_{body} \ C_{avg}(FF)^{1/2}}{2^{1/2} \ N^{1/2}}$$

where R_{eff} is the effective radius of the source, R_s is the actual radius of the source, A_{body} is the attenuation factor for nonsource body material, C_{avg} is the average attenuation factor for the center of the source, N is the total number of counts, and FF is the algorithm filter factor and is equal to the integral of the square of the spatial frequency filter function. For the uniform source of 22 cm, the root mean square percent uncertainties calculated for the various filters agreed well with the formula's estimate for a 128 × 128 matrix. This analysis relates the effective radius, the attenuation factor of the non-source body material, and the average attenuation factor for the center of the source all to the attenuation factor in the medium. The results actually are obvious: filters passing only lower frequencies have smaller root mean square percent uncertainty. Thus smooth data have less variation, which is a tautology. Figure 2–14 relates the resolution and precision for the three filters considered.

There are several lessons in this discussion. The first is that neither the angular nor the statistical considerations limit SPECT too seriously unless the examination is time limited by amount of radioactivity administered, physiology, or the patient's condition. The second is that when uniform disks or other really large sources that cover a large percentage of the available pixels are being imaged, much larger numbers of counts must be acquired so that the statistics will be nearly equivalent to those of the patient imaging situation. Otherwise the very experiments meant to test the equipment or to provide it with a flood uniformity correction will only be displaying a lack of experimental design sense. A third lesson is that experiments must be designed very carefully.

ACCURACY OR QUANTIFICATION AND SPECT

A discussion of accuracy is a discussion of quantification: can the numbers of counts in the pixels be taken seriously? There are at least

Fig 2–14.—The resolution of an image is inversely correlated with the uncertainty in the image through the use of filters. The highest-frequency filter is 1, having the best resolution but the poorest statistical precision. As the filters smooth the data more, the noise becomes less and the resolution worse (Jaszczak, Coleman, and Whitehead 1981).

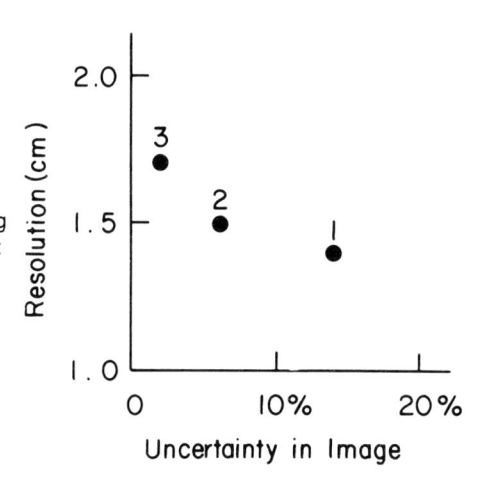

two ways in which the numbers might be used. The first is to delineate structures so that volume could be measured by drawing around the outside of a structure in three dimensions; the second is to correlate the numbers of counts in a voxel or three-dimensional region with an external standard or with numbers of counts in a voxel or three-dimensional region in another part of the image. The numbers of counts per voxel in turn could be used to create functional images to display yet other physiologic information.

Quantification must be approached first from a theoretical point of view, leaving aside all questions such as radioactive decay, patient motion, and patient physiology. Statistics, pixel size, collimator resolution at the surface and at depth in an attenuator, and system resolution must be taken into account. A look at SPECT images again causes us to note that the technique does give images in which structures known to be more radioactive actually are that way on the images, and that the size and shape of structures seems to be preserved even when compared with results of other kinds of examinations such as x-ray–transmission CT. There is a perception that quantitative SPECT is possible. Quantification should be examined in terms of degree, not absolutes: to what extent can the values of counts in a particular voxel be taken to represent the actual amount of radioactivity in that volume in the patient or object, and just how precise are these results?

From the foregoing discussion of precision it is possible to see that if the number of counts acquired is low, there will not be great precision in the results unless numbers of voxels are added together, which means an increase in the size of the resolution cell, or unless the results are highly smoothed, which also means a loss of resolution.

The theoretical idea of quantification, whether volumetric or radiometric, is to be able to measure from outside the patient the actual situation inside the patient. The Issues of quantification of SPECT images were nicely outlined in the introduction of Jaszczak, Coleman, and Whitehead (1981). Quantification can be thought of on several levels: (1) the certainty of detecting a lesion of a certain size in a human body of a particular size and shape, with given radioactive distribution; (2) determining the volume of a portion of the human body; (3) relative or absolute mapping of distribution of radioactivity in three dimensions with accuracy relating to the resolution and to the precision in the quantity of injected radioactivity; and (4) the change of any of these through time, either relatively or absolutely, where intervals may be of the same order as the data acquisition time or longer, up to years. These items describe the kinds of quantification problems SPECT might provide answers to; let it now be said that absolutely every variable and problem of SPECT imaging will have an effect on quantification. This is not to say that numerical results cannot be accurate, but that they will be achieved after much thought, computer programming, and testing. Many of the methods will perforce be pragmatic, tailored to a particular instrument, imaging situation, and reconstruction method, and rigorously tested with appropriate phantoms. Quantification schemes (one hesitates to call them algorithms at this stage) thus devised must be used only under the circumstances for which they were created; this seems obvious, but will have to be reiterated time and again as methods are used inappropriately and found wanting.

There should be nothing wrong with having to cope with each different imaging situation separately except that it is neither so simple nor so intellectually satisfying as the "one-size-fits-all" approach, which does not work in buying clothes, in x ray CT, or in SPECT.

Jaszczak, Coleman, and Whitehead (1981) made some observations on a 30-cm-diameter cylinder containing a series of spheres ranging from 2 to 6 cm in diameter, filled with radioactivity of a concentration ten times that of water in the cylinder. Their first efforts were aimed at accurately presenting the volumes of the spheres. A 75% to 80% threshold value and an automatic edge-detection program gave very good results over the full range of volumes.

Several groups have undertaken to measure organ volume from SPECT sections using computer programs rather than counting squares. The computer programs detect the edges (Kan and Hopkins 1979; Tauxe et al. 1982; Tauxe and Todd-Pokropek 1983), perhaps as a function of the highest count in an operator-selected volume, then count the enclosed pixels. The measurements of known volumes are very accurate and reasonably precise.

Jaszczak, Coleman, and Whitehead's (1981) next experiment was to see if their SPECT system could accurately detect the quantity of activity in a uniform cylinder over a wide range of activities, from 0.009 to 1.08 µCi per ml; the system did admirably, which meant that it was linear over this wide range. Linearity was also tested for a variety of source diameters and was found to hold. Since the measurement of radioactivities over a wide range is one of the strong points of nuclear medicine, SPECT passes this test as a valid technique: it can function accurately over a wide range of activities.

Their final experiment (Jaszczak, Coleman, and Whitehead 1981) was aimed at testing whether SPECT could accurately reproduce the

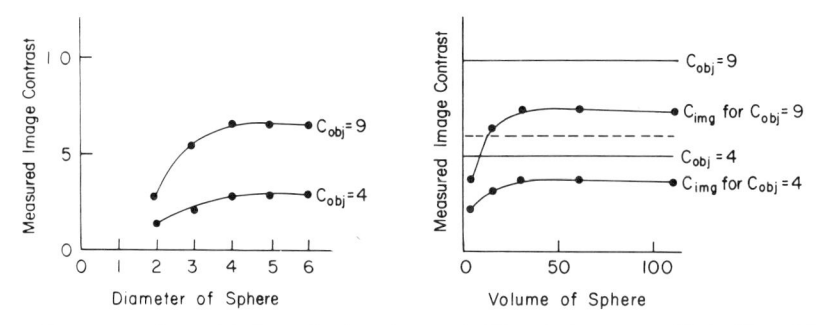

Fig 2–15.—Several hollow plastic spheres of different sizes were filled with activity and imaged in a cylindrical phantom filled with radioactive water. The measured contrast of the spheres is presented on the left as a function of the diameter of the sphere, and on the right as a function of the volume of the sphere. The small spheres show less contrast, but none of the spheres shows the correct contrast (Jaszczak, Coleman, and Whitehead 1981).

contrast of the series of spheres of 2 to 6 cm diameter when they were filled with solutions of 5:1 and 10:1 compared to the activity of the water in the surrounding 30–cm cylinder. Figure 2–15 shows the relationship between the observed contrast and the sphere diameter. Image contrast is defined as the difference between the counts in the image and the counts in the background divided by the counts in the background. Object contrast is the difference between the activities in the small sphere and in the surrounding cylindrical phantom divided by the activity in the cylindrical phantom. Notice that an asymptotic value is approached for each contrast. The authors' answer to this problem was to use a formula that relates the observed contrast to the correct contrast and contains a function that depends on the size of the sphere and the spatial resolution of the system (Whitehead 1977).

It can be seen that the SPECT system should give fairly accurate estimates of the amount of activity in situations in which the activity varies slowly from one part of the image to another; this is an extension of measuring the uniform cylinder. The real problem comes in the very cases that have received so much scrutiny: small "hot" or "cold" lesions with varying contrast. In the general case of masses of tissue of varying sizes with varying function, the size of a particular mass cannot be used to give clues to its contrast because the size cannot be specified. That the accuracy of quantification is related to the spatial resolution of the system is the crux of the problem. It will have to be dealt with in a careful three-dimensional fashion and may call for a re-examination of the filtering process.

More recent work in the area of lesion detection with SPECT (Jaszczak et al. 1982) includes a discussion of the problems and a comparison of SPECT contrast with plane-projection contrast for an Alderson liver phantom. For nonradioactive spheres of 1.0 and 1.5 cm placed centrally in the phantom, contrasts of 0.34 and 0.38 were observed; if they were placed peripherally in the phantom, observed contrasts were 0.32 and 0.54, where a contrast of 1.0 would have been perfect. The planar projection images had a contrast of less than 0.08 in all cases. The spheres were visible with SPECT in spite of the degradation in precision and resolution.

If the amount of activity in a specified volume is the object of the examination, then it may be possible to avoid the reconstruction of images in favor of a process that finds the counts in the volume (Huesman 1984). The advantage of such a technique is that computing time is not expended for image creation. In addition, the statistical uncertainty is easily computed.

Summary

The method in common use today for creation of the transaxial image from SPECT planar projection data is called attenuation-corrected filtered back projection or convolution. A generalized schematic diagram of the computer algorithm is given in Figure 2–16. It should be possible to follow a SPECT reconstruction with this diagram, or a similar one which has put the operations in the correct order. All of the processing is performed in real space, so data may be processed "on the fly," one projection at a time; the computer can therefore arrive at the final results almost as soon as the last planar image is acquired.

Good resolution and accurate, precise quantification are bound up in the design of the instrument and its data acquisition and in the solutions to the problems of interpolation, attenuation, and scattering. There will be more work in these areas. We can expect the investment in computer software to increase as the solutions to specific gamma imaging problems add complication to the concepts of filtered back projection.

THEORETICAL TREATMENT

This discussion of the mathematical theory of back projection owes a debt to the theoreticians of computed tomography, especially Gabor

Theory of Tomography 33

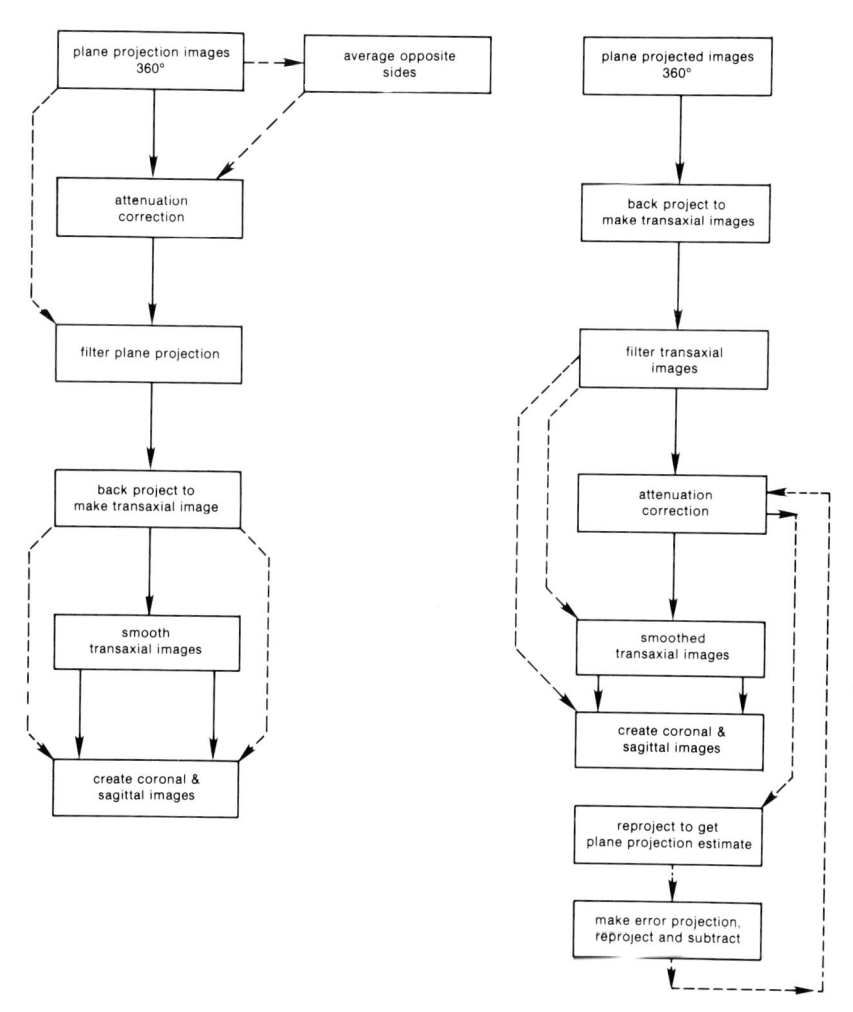

Fig 2-16.—The method in common use today for creation of the transaxial image from SPECT planar projection data is called attenuation-corrected filtered back projection or convolution. Schematic diagrams are shown of two sets of common computer programs used to create SPECT images from projection data.

Herman, who has been especially prolific as both author (1980) and editor (1979). In addition, several articles have discussed SPECT reconstruction theory in careful detail, organizing the various methods into categories (Gordon and Herman 1974; Budinger and Gullberg 1974). The reader is referred to these works and other publications (Rowland 1979; Budinger, Gullberg, and Huesman 1979) for complete discussions. These articles date from an era of great ferment in the field of computed tomography. Mundane considerations of commercial production and secrecy—fast reconstruction, smooth images, and inexpensive computers—have removed a great deal of this discussion from the public arena. Anyone desiring to have rigorous mathematical treatment of the subject should start with Herman's books and follow their leads. The *IEEE Transactions on Nuclear Science* has been a favorite journal of engineers in this field.

Theory was not developed just for SPECT, but for all branches of tomography. One must be able to adapt the generalized discussions to the particular situation and to see intuitively where the difficulties will lie for SPECT: noisy data collected at short range.

We start with the class of solutions that are called analytic because in one form or another they are the solutions of a series of equations of many unknowns. Analytic solutions typically are performed only one time to produce a transaxial image. The other solutions are called iterative because they iterate or repeat a solution method many times until a specified criterion is met, such as least error between the projections of the created solution and the acquired projection data.

Parallel-ray geometry is used in this discussion whenever it is necessary to be specific. Exactly the same solutions cannot be used for fan-beam geometries, unless distortion in the final image is not a problem. The mathematics are entirely similar and have been solved (Herman 1980) because they use one of the regular x-ray CT geometries.

Back-Projection Methods

Simple Back Projection

Many of us have long been familiar with Kuhl's scanner and the idea of back projection. The first of Kuhl's instruments was a scanner on a rotating gantry (Kuhl and Edwards 1963). It could perform all the ordinary rectilinear scanner motions and it could also do longitudinal and transaxial tomography. Because the digital computer of the time was much too expensive and cumbersome to be used in a nuclear medicine laboratory, Kuhl and Edwards (1963) at first used back projection onto an oscilloscope screen to create an image on film (see Fig 2–9). The images thus created, as exemplified in Figure 2–9, were certainly recognizable. Figure 2–17 is an example of a simple arrangement showing the star pattern and extra background that appear when simple back projection is performed.

Simple back projection was examined in a small example earlier

Theory of Tomography 35

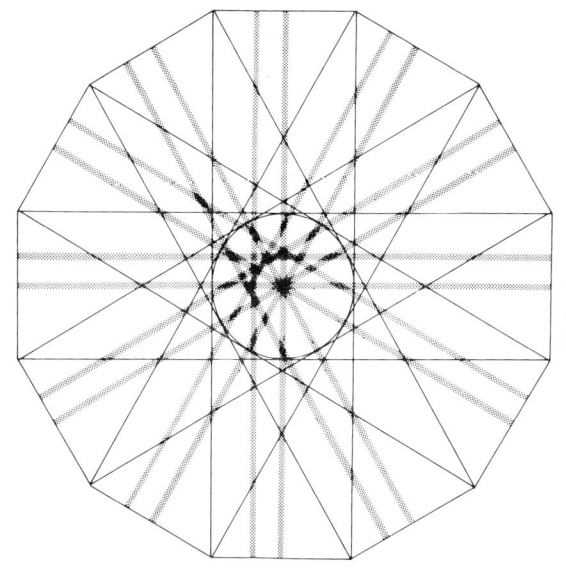

Fig 2–17.—The simple back projection of two points that are back projected from several angles builds a star pattern and extra background.

in the chapter (Fig 2–10). One idea was to subtract the "stars" and add to their centers, which is an iterative procedure. The very high background is actually the result of a difficulty inherent in the simple back-projection method: it inserts an extra twist to the results that the object did not have, and which the mathematical treatment of this whole problem elucidated. In this twist, an extra smoothing is done in the very process of back projection, and unless this is numerically removed, the images will not look sharp.

Filtered Back Projection or Convolution

To vanquish the extra smoothing that the simple back-projection process weaves into the solution, and perhaps to sharpen the results with some extra image enhancement, the following processes are employed in much of the software in use in nuclear medicine:

1. Filtering in real space in the x direction, either before or after back projection. The filter is usually a multiplicative combination in Fourier space of a ramp and another filter (Herman 1980); the most common filters are Hamming, Butterworth, and Shepp-Logan.
2. Back projecting in real space using the principles given below and noting that another filtration is being performed in the back-projection process. This cannot be eliminated because our data are digital and not analog.

Chapter 2

The creation and study of filters is a discipline in itself. Many sources on signal processing discuss filters; Herman (1980) and Hamming (1977) are particularly useful. The whole of the creation of tomographic images really hinges on the creative use of filters and on the knowledge that almost any processing of the data involves filtering, explicitly or implicitly. We have already discovered this, in that simple back projection "accidentally" filters the resulting image to smooth it. It is better that the filtering processes be under control and acknowledged, so it behooves us to become expert with filters.

Filters are most comprehensible in Fourier or frequency space, unfortunately for those who do not feel at home there. Filters are discussed either in terms of what they remove or of what they allow to pass, as in bandpass filtering. In Fourier space, graphs can be drawn to indicate what the filter looks like as a function of frequency. Figure 2–3 shows graphs of several of the most common filters. Note that the ramp passes high frequencies, so it emphasizes high frequencies. Note also that the ramp has not been allowed to continue to infinity. The location of the high-frequency cutoff is very significant. Incorrect choice of cutoff frequency can lead to "aliasing" (the improper appearance of high-frequency information at lower frequencies) when the filter is applied. Strobe methods of matching one rotation speed with another depend on aliasing, in which only the difference between the two speeds is seen, not the rapid rotations or pulsations. For the most part, the filters are not used in frequency or Fourier space but are transformed with an inverse Fourier transform to create a convolution kernel or spatial filter function in real space. Figure 2–4 shows graphs of the spatial filter functions that result from the common filters. Note the depth of the negative part of the filter. As was already noted, because the filters are to be used with digital pixel data, they must be sampled at digital intervals. This leads to distortion, since the effect of the discrete spatial filter on discrete data is not quite the same as its continuous counterpart used on continuous data would be.

Data should be processed with the filter, both to take account of the extra factor that back projection will insert and to do any image enhancement, bandpass filtering, and the like. The ramp filter by itself will exactly cancel out the extra smoothing of back projection, but will also enhance the high-frequency components of the image, so some smoothing or low-frequency bandpass filtration must be employed. One could do these filtration operations one at a time, but mathematics has been kind to us in that the successive application of filters in real space (or in Fourier space) is the equivalent of multiplying the filters together in Fourier space and then applying them. Thus the typical filter in use is a low or medium bandpass filter multiplied by a ramp filter.

New filters are not created for every occasion. A set of standard filters with small adjustments is generally employed. Note that they seem to cover the ground in Fourier space (see Fig 2–3). The closer to the horizontal axis that the line describing the filter comes, the lower the frequency it will pass or the more high frequencies it will filter out. The result is smoother pictures in real space. Planar projection images with good statistics do not need very smooth filters, whereas count-poor images do. Figure 2–5 shows the effect of three of these on actual images. As we have seen, there is some variety of filters usually available to the SPECT user.

It has been noted that some confusion has arisen in the nomenclature of the filters. Since they are named after their inventors, the confusion is worth straightening out. Hamming (1977, p. 89) says the form of the von Hann window is

$$0.5 + 0.5 \cos(\pi k/N)$$

and that the form of the Hamming (or hamming) window is

$$a + (1-2a) \cos(\pi k/N).$$

Herman (1980, p. 124) says the generalized Hamming shape with parameter a $(0.5 \leq a \leq 1)$ is

$$a + (1-a) \cos(2\pi U/A)$$

and is called a hanning window if a = 0.5 and a Hamming window if [i]a[r] = 0.54. Herman's definitions do not match Hanning's. Furthermore, the use of "hanning" seems unnecessary, since von Hann's own name could be used. To give attribution to the inventors, the window with variable coefficients is a Hamming window; if the coefficients are set to 0.5, then it is a von Hann or Hann window.

The spatial filter functions or convolution kernels are applied to the x-directional data for each line of data separately from all the others. Filtering during the reconstruction process is absolutely essential to the production of correct transaxial images.

In some processing, data from opposite sides of the patient are added together, either in an arithmetic fashion (as in an average) or geometric fashion by taking the square root of the product of the values. It is not obvious which of these is preferred. After a series of point source experiments, Larsson (1980) came to the following conclusions: the geometric mean gives more uniform spatial response with depth, as well as less spatial distortion, while the arithmetic mean gives higher spatial resolution. The geometric mean images contain annoying bridges between the more radioactive areas. In a more recent report from the same institution (Axelsson, Msaki, and Israelsson 1984) incorporating a scattering correction into the calculation, the geometric mean is shown to be superior in its quantitative accuracy. The combination of data from opposing sides does not take care of the attenuation problem, because the values are still lower in the centers than where there is less depth of absorber.

During back projection, decisions must be made about how to relate the positions of the pixels at all the different angles to the chosen matrix position for the transaxial slice. It would seem natural that one should make an interpolation between pixels based on the angle the planar image makes with the transaxial image. For a system of 64 × 64 matrices this leads to a large number of calculations of position or the storage of a large matrix of lookup values (having the final matrix size times the number of angular increments for every four values in it) to determine the contribution to the result. It is faster by almost a factor of 2 (Larsson 1980, p. 40) to determine which pixel is nearest and put the whole value into that pixel. This approximation is a low-pass filtering process (Larsson 1980, p. 15), but the linear interpolation emphasizes higher frequencies and seems to contribute to emphasis of noise. Figure 2–12 shows nearest-neighbor filtering. When computer memory becomes more spacious, the interpolation may be looked into again.

Increasing computer speed has made it possible not to have to add data from opposing sides together. Each projection may be treated separately and algorithms developed (such as that of Novak and Eisner (1984)) to take into consideration the properties of the source and detector.

Attenuation-Corrected Filtered Back Projection

The nuclear medicine problem is more complex than that of x-ray-transmission CT, especially in the areas of attenuation and scattering. The difficulty is that the patient's particular anatomy with its distributions of different kinds of tissue—most notably bone, soft tissue, and low-density structures such as lungs and gas-filled bowel—causes a pattern of attenuation that affects the gamma rays on the way to the detector. The effect of attenuation is to make the count densities coming from the center of the patient smaller than they ought to be, so that the reconstructed images have centers that appear less radioactive than they ought to be. Scattering is a second-order effect that slightly offsets the effect of attenuation. Scattered radiation makes the count densities just a bit more than they would be if there were only attenuation and no scatter. The amount of scattered radiation that is detected is a function both of the amount of attenuating material over the source and of the energy window of the detector.

If the exact attenuation coefficents for the whole patient section under consideration were known, it would be possible to use them to correct the planar projection data. Since they are not and cannot be known, ways have been sought to do without them as constructively as possible.

How is this to be accomplished in this less-than-perfect world? The first way is not to correct for attenuation and scatter at all; this works acceptably well in the chest, where a great deal of space is taken up by the lungs, which are not strong attenuators. This tack may be the one to take if there seems to be some problem with the attenuation correction, since an image will always result, albeit with less count density at the center than at the edges. Experiments designed to expose this problem are nearly always performed with a cylindrical phantom of large diameter. This is the worst of all possible cases, simulating a uniform, circular-cylindrical patient of uniform attenuation and uniform activity, of a large diameter (e.g., 20 cm). Figure 2–18 shows the result of attenuation and scattering in the transaxial image of a 20–cm phantom. Using technetium-99m, the intensity at the center is about 15% of what it should be. Note from the graph of intensity as a function of position (Fig 2–18) that the function is flat at the bottom so that the relative densities of a great deal of the image are not seriously affected. Of course the attenuation of thallium-201 is greater and of iodine-131 is less, but even 511–KeV photons are significantly attenuated. Clearly, deep organs containing low-energy gamma emitters are going to give the most problem, but there is no escaping it at any energy.

The simplest correction method is to assume that the patient is a uniform elliptical cylinder (or other simple geometric figure, like the uniform circular cylinder), and that the attenuation is uniform and the activity is uniformly distributed from one side of the body to the other along the voxel's projection path. The patient's major and minor axes are determined either by marking them with sources or by computer calculation from the projection data. An attenuation coefficient for the system, usually a little less than that for the same energy in water because of the entry of scattered radiation into the

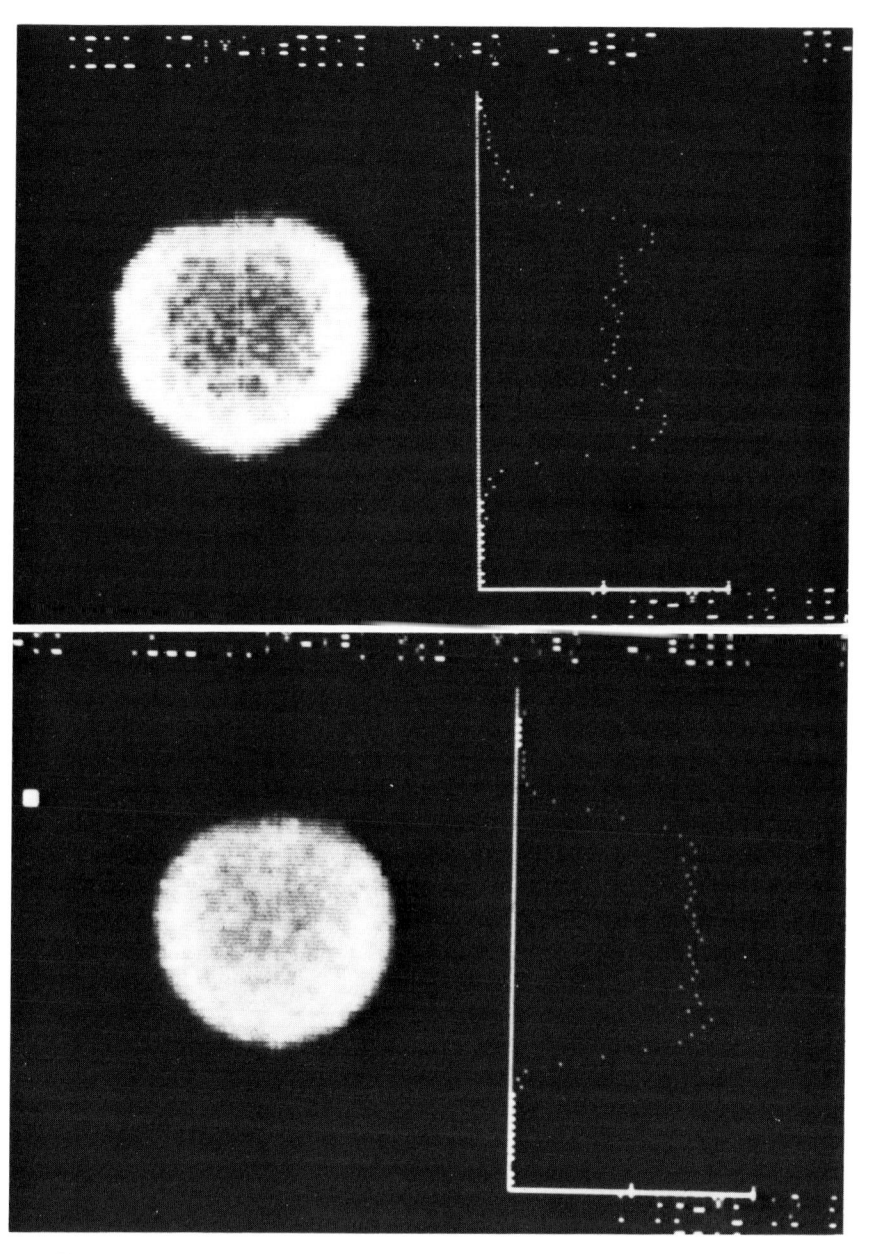

Fig 2–18.—A 20–cm cylinder phantom was filled with 10 mCi in 6.5 liters of water and imaged for 10 seconds per angle for 64 angular increments, using a 64 × 64 matrix. Each image contained 170,000 counts; 10 M counts were accumulated in the complete study. The images were processed with a modified Shepp-Logan filter (same as Figure 2–5) and 1.2–cm-thick slices. The image on the top was created using no attenuation correction, while that on the bottom was corrected with an attenuation coefficient of 0.12 per cm. Profiles through the center of each image are shown beside the images.

window, is applied to each of the rays in each of the projections. This operation combines attenuation and scattering into one correction: rays lost in the attenuation process are partially corrected for by the addition of scattered rays.

Chang (1978) developed an iterative correction as an improvement over the simplest corrections and over the computationally slow iterative methods. The starting point was consideration of the attenuation of a point source. The effect of attenuation for a point source is multiplicative, so a multiplicative correction factor can be developed, of the form

$$c(a,b) = 2 \pi / \int exp(-\mu \, l_\theta) \, d_O,$$

where (a,b) is the position of the point source in the transaxial plane, μ is the attenuation coefficient of the surrounding medium, and l_θ is the distance through the medium at angle θ. When this formula is used for an extended source, some points are overcorrected and some undercorrected, so iteration (see Fig 2–8) is necessary to achieve quantitative results.

The effect of scattering is slightly to offset the attenuation losses in the count densities. Scatter is a three-dimensional effect, having repercussions in planes other than that of the source. Egbert and May (1980) noted that the Chang method could be extended to correct for scattered radiation as well as attenuation. They used operator notation that neatly describes photon interactions in the medium. A photon may be scattered again and again, but to a good approximation only the photons resulting from the first collision will have an effect. The effect of scattering may be found by measuring a point source with and without the presence of scattering medium. In the same fashion as the Chang attenuation correction, a scatter correction that can be used iteratively may be fashioned from the point source information. For other than uniform materials, the form of the correction must be determined. Egbert and May (1980) noted that while attenuation is a phenomenon in the imaging plane for each transaxial image, scattering brings in the effect of all the tissue and activity. The difficulty in applying this method is in devising experiments to measure the effects of scattering for a single case, which can then be generalized to distributed sources and used to describe the behavior of a particular instrument in the clinical situation. The authors suggested that good scatter correction would allow the use of wider windows, giving higher count rates and better statistics.

Axelsson, Msaki, and Israelsson (1984) tackled the scattering problem in much the same way, although with less mathematical formalism. They measured a line spread function at various positions in a large water tank with the Anger camera. The experiments showed that unless the line source was close to the edge of the tank or in the very center, there was not too much variation in the shape of the wings caused by scattering. The scatter function can be approximated by

$$F(x) = A \, exp \, (-Bx),$$

where, from their experiments, $A = 0.035$ and $B = 0.20$ reciprocal centimeters, adequately fitted the data. When the integral of this function is multiplied by the observed line spread function data, the functional form of the scattered part of the data results. When this correction was applied to a liver phantom before the attenuation correction, it produced good results. Among other benefits, contrast and quantitative accuracy were both improved.

This application is actually a simplification of what Egbert and May (1980) proposed. In particular, it is noted that using the same function over the whole scattering medium results in poor corrections at the center and near the edge of the scatterer. The simplification also does not take into account the effect of scattering in planes other than that in which the source is located. There will be more developments in this area as theoreticians sharpen their skills on this problem and as our sense of the three-dimensionality of the problem is heightened.

There is increased realization that scatter corrections may hold the key to quantification of SPECT (Oppenheim 1984). The Duke group (Floyd et al. 1985; Jaszczak et al. 1984) have studied scatter with Monte Carlo simulations and experiments using a dual-window spectrometer to create a scatter correction based upon the subtraction of a portion of the Compton window image. Monte Carlo simulation has also been important in studying the effect of multiple order Compton scattering (Floyd et al. 1984).

Determining body contour from the projection data eliminates a step in which sources are put on the patient and makes it impossible to separate the patient and his ellipse during data acquisition. The algorithms for body-contour determination examine the edges of the planar projection data or the edges of the transaxial image with edge-detection methods to find a body outline in the scattered radiation. A simple linear detection method that detects the first pixel with a value above a certain threshold seems to supply the necessary information. Effort put into this area (Gullberg, Malko, and Eisner 1983) has been paying off in terms of simplifying the clinical examination.

Attenuation correction methods are treated here because they arise here naturally in the course of the discussion of back-projection methods and reflect the current practice in SPECT. Attenuation must be considered in all reconstruction methods.

Filtration of Back-Projected Images

Another mathematical truth about the processes under consideration is that the order in which they are performed does not matter. This is strictly true only in the world of continuous data, but carryovers into the world of discrete pixel data are strong enough to allow us to accomplish the back-projection process before or after filtration. Back projecting the planar data and then filtering is entirely equivalent to filtering the planar data and then back projecting, as just discussed. The filtration in one case is carried out in one dimension, along the line of data, while in the other it is two-dimensional in the transaxial plane. The filters used are the same and the methods are the same. Insofar as one might like to be able to try filtration with different filters, filtration after back projection would allow this conveniently, since back projection would have to be done only once. Filtration is a relatively rapid process, so testing different filters also would be done rapidly.

Fourier Methods

Alternatives to Real Space Operations Already Discussed

For every real-space filtration process, such as that of applying the convolution kernel to the data or to the transaxial image, there is a corresponding Fourier space operation. The spatial data are Fourier transformed into frequency space, processed, then inverse-Fourier transformed back into real space, it is hoped with no losses. Back projection may then be used to create the transaxial images. The rationale for doing this is that the frequency space operations seem more natural to some people—they can "see" what the filters will do.

For example, one group (Budinger, Gullberg, and Huesman 1979) used Fourier transformation in the BKFIL and FILBK algorithms. The BKFIL algorithm involves the following steps: first Fourier transform the planar projection data, then filter in Fourier space, and inverse-Fourier transform the result. The last step is back projection in real space. The FILBK algorithm back projects the planar projection data and then performs the Fourier transformation of the two-dimensional transaxial image and filters it before inverse Fourier transformation. The BKFIL and FILBK algorithms are diagrammed in Figure 2–19.

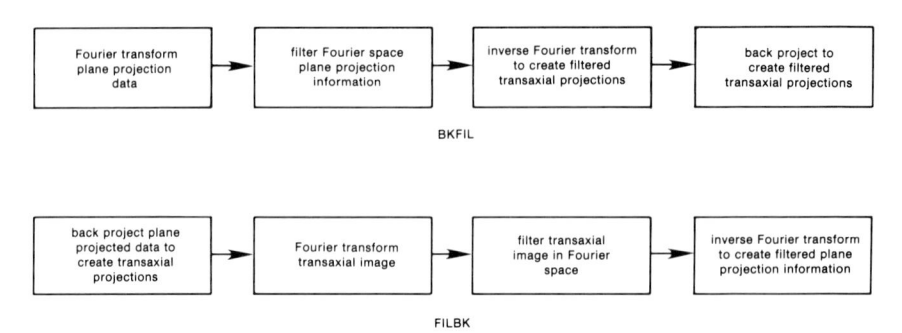

Fig 2–19.—The computer processing of the BKFIL and FILBK operations is shown schematically.

To consider the case of constant attenuation in this formalism, the attenuation is one factor in the equation describing the projection data in terms of the transaxial image and can be separated for treatment during the Fourier transformation part of the calculation. The steps in the calculation are complicated (Budinger, Gullberg, and Huesman 1979, p. 208) and involve a number of calculations equal to twice the sum of the number of angles of data and the number of pixels in a line of planar projection data.

The so-called rho-filtered layergram is an example of a Fourier or frequency-space technique. The transaxial images are Fourier transformed, multiplied by the radial frequency in Fourier space, and then inverse-Fourier transformed. The filtering is by the very ramp filter that is necessary to remove the smoothing effects of simple back projection. Rowland (1979), in a paper that is very elegant in its notational uniformity and very difficult to read only once or just dip into, examined the method closely and compared it to filtered back projection. His conclusions were that the rho-filtered layergram takes four times as much computer time and space as the filtered back-projection method, and that it is less sensitive to the interpolation methods used and more sensitive to filter discontinuities, such as the cutoff frequency of the ramp filter. The large amount of computer time and space required are reasons that this method is not in common use.

Methods for Solving the General Problem

In 1917 Radon considered the question of image projections. From this beginning and from other mathematical treatments of the relationship between the projection data and the object, the whole problem was often cast in terms of a solution in Fourier space. While the experimentalists were solving the problems of creating a SPECT system that would work and learning how to use the computer to produce transaxial slices by back projection in real space, a whole mathematical formalism was developing. Sampling problems, numerical integration, discrete pixel data, and noise all take their toll; the number of equations to be solved may be large. Commercial systems do not use Fourier space methods today because the calculations require computer space and speed and because the transformation interpolations must be carefully done to avoid introducing error.

The major difficulty with Fourier techniques (Herman 1980) is the requirement of interpolation in Fourier space between the Fourier transform of the planar projection data gridded in a spider-web pattern and the Fourier transform of the transaxial data gridded in squares. The interpolation is not very accurate unless the spider-web data are very fine, or, to turn this around, unless the results are to be known only very coarsely.

The discussion of filter functions for the Fourier methods is the same, except that the filters are used in Fourier space, which makes them seem easier.

Other Analytic Solutions

One can approach Radon's equation directly (Herman 1980) and assume that it provides the recipe for producing the transaxial image. If the data are perfect and continuous rather than discrete, this is true; however, since no data are perfect and SPECT data are not continuous, the approximations must begin again. The various approximations are not equivalent and must be tested separately with real data. A series of approximations in one treatment allows the creation of a set of equations to be solved analytically for the transaxial image (Gordon and Herman 1974).

Iterative Solutions

Iterative solutions are the most intuitively obvious. If one starts with a very simple set of projection data, the very first thing one wants to try is to experiment with them until a consistent solution is reached; the problem appeals to the puzzle solver in each of us. Naturally, only an idiot-savant would warm to the kind of problem that is actually presented by SPECT.

The general idea is to start with an estimate of the transaxial image, to reproject it, and then to start to minimize the difference

46 *Chapter 2*

between the experimental projections and the actual data, usually in some squared sense like chi-square or least squares; the process of creating a new guess and taking the differences is repeated until some predetermined level of error is reached. All minimization procedures have their tricks to avoid going around in circles and to achieve the biggest improvement at each step. Overcorrection is a big hazard,

Original Distribution:

2	3
4	5

Projection:

5
9

6	8

Start with first backproj picture:

2.5+3	2.5+4
4.5+3	4.5+4

or

5.5	6.5
7.5	8.5

Then project it:

5.5	6.5
7.5	8.5

12
16

| 13 | 15 |

Take difference along horiz between proj and this value, divide by 2 and add back proj correction

$\frac{(5-12)}{2} = -3.5$

$\frac{(9-16)}{2} = -3.5$

5.5−3.5	6.5−3.5
7.5−3.5	8.5−3.5

or

2	3
4	5

and so we are done

Now suppose we had done both the horizontal and the vertical corrections at once:

5.5−3.5−3.5	6.5−3.5−3.5
7.5−3.5−3.5	8.5−3.5−3.5

or

−1.5	−.5
.5	1.5

or projected

−1.5	−.5
.5	1.5

−2
2

which is overcorrected and so the process must be done again

| −1 | 1 |

−1.5+3.5+3.5	−.5+3.5+3.5
.5+3.5+3.5	1.5+3.5+3.5

or

5.5	6.5
7.5	8.5

and we are stuck in an oscillation

We could ungum the iterative process by halving it at every step

Halve the corrections above:

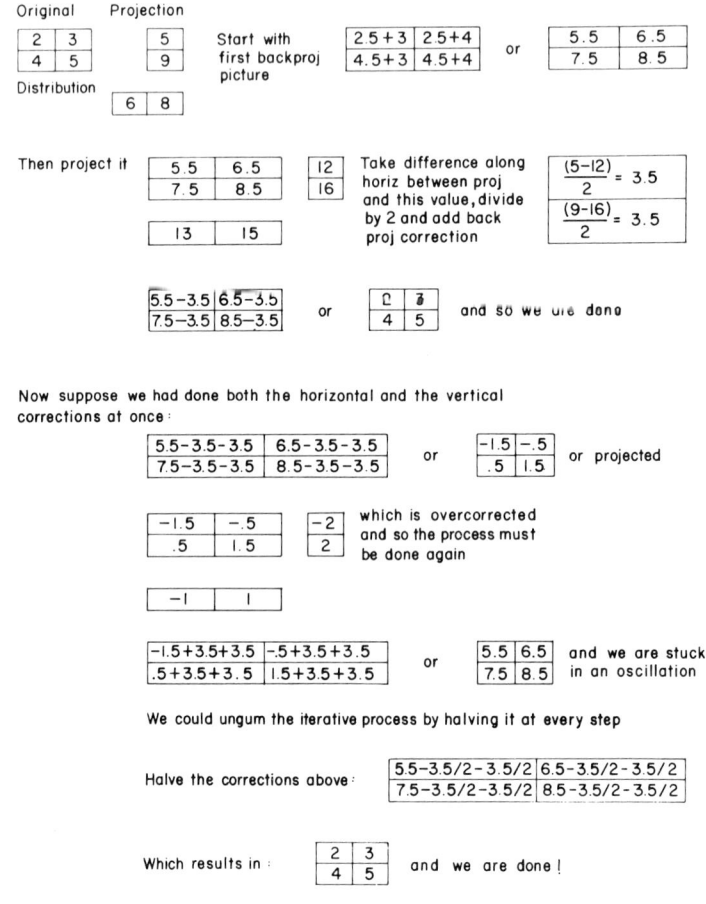

5.5−3.5/2−3.5/2	6.5−3.5/2−3.5/2
7.5−3.5/2−3.5/2	8.5−3.5/2−3.5/2

Which results in:

2	3
4	5

and we are done!

Fig 2–20.—An iterative method for the creation of back-projected images is shown. Once again the original distribution being aimed for (which is unknown in a real processing situation) is shown in the upper left. The starting point is a simple back projection, but it would be possible to start with an average image. In the upper section of the figure only the horizontal corrections to the projections are used, while in the lower section both the horizontal and vertical corrections are incorporated at once. In the lower section we see that halving the correction terms at each step leads to the desired result.

since any method that does not constantly jump back and forth between the planar projections and the transaxial image may very well be overcorrecting (Fig 2-20).

Budinger, Gullberg, and Huesman (1979) described ways to incorporate a priori knowledge about the circumstances into the iterative framework. The general aim is to provide a transaxial image whose projections are within statistical differences of the measured projections. The areas of a priori knowledge are Poisson statistics, assumed or measured attenuation coefficients, and perhaps a model of the part of the body being imaged.

Iterative Real Space Methods

As has already been suggested at several points, it might make good sense to go all the way through the real space methods of the attenuation-corrected, filtered back projection and compare projections of the transaxial result with the initial planar projection data and iterate until a suitable level of error has been attained. As computers become faster, it will be possible to perform the iterative calculations in short times.

Algebraic Reconstruction Techniques

One method, called algebraic reconstruction technique (ART), involves treating one projected point at a time and altering the estimate of the transaxial image around the circle. The alterations may be made additively by adding to or subtracting from each point according to what is called for, or multiplicatively, by applying a factor to all the points. The projection data may be used to set values to zero that are clearly outside the image, for the whole of the calculation. This can be done once and for all. An elaboration of ART is ART3, which allows for noisy data (Gordon and Herman 1974). The procedures may be set up so that the measure of the result goes through a minimum and then gets larger again or so that it will approach an asymptote.

The ART methods may be just as accurate as filtered back projection, provided some tricks (Herman 1980; Herman and Lent 1976) are used. One of these is the application of a nonlinear filter after every so many intervals; another is to assume an upper and lower limit for the values of the results. The starting image may be the result of simple back projection or a uniformly gray image. Since each iteration takes about the same amount of computer time and space as filtered back projection, and since several to many iterations may be required, the methods are not used in nuclear medicine practice.

Simultaneous Iterative Reconstruction Technique

In the simultaneous iterative reconstruction technique (SIRT), all the transaxial picture elements are altered at once, using data from all the projections simultaneously. This may be done in an additive or multiplicative way (Gordon and Herman 1974; Oppenheim 1974; Budinger, Gullberg, and Huesman 1979). The results of SIRT methods may not converge at all unless damping factors are used.

Least-Square Iterative Technique

The least-square iterative technique (Budinger and Gullberg 1974, p. 8) is based on minimizing the difference between the measured and calculated projections in a least-squares fashion. This is done by setting the partial derivatives of the difference with respect to the variables equal to zero. An adjustment, called "underdamping," must be made in the method to cause the results to converge rather than oscillate. The terms contain an expression for the noise of the data that was set equal to the square root of the number of counts for each pixel. The algorithm for the least-square iterative technique, including uniform attenuation, is as follows: add together opposing-side data using the geometric mean, and do five iterations of the least-square method, using the result to find the outline of the object. Now determine the position of each pixel for attenuation correction; that is, locate the pixel with respect to the boundary at each angle. Calculate the attenuation factor for each pixel. Now use the least-square method with all the projections (no geometric means) and the attenuation factors to iterate eight or ten times, which should produce a result within statistical accuracy. A large computer is needed to perform this calculation rapidly, since each iteration takes about as much time as the back-projection process, and ten to 15 iterations must be performed.

Maximum Likelihood Technique

The maximum likelihood technique (Shepp and Vardi 1982; Lange and Carson 1984) is based on statistical methods. The technique is often referred to as EM reconstruction, where "E" stands for expectation and "M" for maximization, describing the two major steps of the technique. Calculations of EM algorithms are similar to those of other iterative techniques. At the heart of minimization and maximization methods is a derivative set equal to zero that produces a series of equations defining the latest approximation to the values in question. The methods are all iterative and require a great deal of computer space and time.

Proponents of EM (Lange and Carson 1984) have shown that the equations are constrained to approach a maximum, however slowly, and to yield positive values for the back-projected image. The EM algorithm does take the Poisson statistics of radioactive decay into account, so it may be very useful for data of poor statistical quality. Approach to a maximum has been accelerated in the computer processing by raising the multipliers to powers, but the algorithm's always tending to a maximum is sacrificed, since the results oscillate (Visampayan et al. 1985).

Comparison of Results

The quality assurance of the implementations of SPECT theories is difficult and time consuming. Gordon and Herman (1974) undertook to discuss the issues involved. Clearly the comparison of methods may be either theoretical or experimental. The theoretical grounds for decision between methods may rest on questions of a shortage of firm theoretical underpinnings or discontinuity in a sensitive part of the theory. To date, the difficulties posed by the addition of Poisson noise to the theoretical framework have been so great that no one has really tackled the problem at this level. In addition, the mental fortitude for considering the effects of every mechanical uncertainty, or every approximation made expedient by shortcomings in computer speed or storage capacity, on the implementation of theory has been in short supply. It is only when one is in the midst of solving these problems that one must ask questions about the desirability of such and such an approximation. Theoreticians rarely have to consider what the effect will be because they do not come close to the implementation.

Gordon and Herman (1974) repeat Herman and Rowland's (1973) complaint about the deficiency of a unifying mathematical foundation for the reconstruction algorithms. Naturally each author cast his discussion in a way that appealed to him and was appropriate to his discipline. Rowland (1979) attempted to address this problem, but the formalism that he used is not very comprehensible to the average mortal.

Experimental comparisons are often much more to the point because they can incorporate all the nuances of the actual situation, often almost unwittingly; they are also very time consuming because of the computer programming involved and the vast number of trials to be made. Evidence of the difficulties is found in a number of papers (and more PhD theses than one cares to consider) in which the authors confess to previous errors in programs and give their new results. The public reporting of such errors is surely but the tip of the iceberg and serves as a warning to all who would essay to turn Radon's equations into transaxial images. Gordon and Herman (1974) suggested measures to be considered in the exhaustive comparisons of algorithms:

1. Test patterns to represent all possible situations; include the obviously idealized, the poorest statistics, the large (so large that it goes outside the field of view of the instrument) and the small; examine the not-so-obviously idealized test patterns for hints of problems, such as those that cause moire effects between the data and reconstruction algorithms; use computer simulations when their speedy generation will help.
2. Consider a number of modes for acquiring projection data; in SPECT this would include focused, parallel, and fan-beam collimation, as well as coded-aperture methods; over- and under-sample the data with respect to angle and matrix size.
3. Examine the effect of errors in every possible mechanical and imaging instrument variable, one at a time, so that the effects can be determined independently.

The next difficulty to be overcome is the evaluation of the images once a set of experimental comparisons have been made. This is related to the criteria that might be used to evaluate the results of iterative methods. For known test phantoms, one can evaluate the difference between the reconstructed transaxial images and the known activity distribution, using some squared measure of goodness of fit. Both quantitative accuracy and resolution should be kept in mind.

Computer time and storage space are also variables to be minimized, because time and space cost money; SPECT practitioners have voted with their dollars. Efficiency in a computer program is a carefully crafted property. It is possible for an algorithm to be efficient, yet for its programmed version not to be. Comparisons of the numbers of computer operations can be made; Fourier transformation takes time and space.

Gordon and Herman's (1974) final point is that the human eye has no equal in the evaluation of images. What is seen is dependent on the display device and the experience of the beholder, so receiver operating characteristic (ROC) methods should be employed to test the results.

BIBLIOGRAPHY

Axelsson, B.; Msaki, P.; and Israelsson, A. Subtraction of Compton-scattered photons in single-photon emission computerized tomography. *J. Nucl. Med.* 25:490–494, 1984.

Budinger, T. F., et al. Emission computer assisted tomography with single-photon and positron annihilation photon emitters. *J. Comput. Assist. Tomog.* 1:131–145, 1977.

Budinger, T. F., et al. Quantitative potentials of dynamic emission computed tomography. *J. Nucl. Med.* 19:309–315, 1978.

Budinger, T. F., and Gullberg, G. T. Three-dimensional reconstruction in nuclear medicine emission imaging. *IEEE Trans. Nucl. Sci.* 21:2–20, 1974.

Budinger, T. F.; Gullberg, G. T.; and Huesman, R. H. Emission computed tomography. In *Image Reconstruction from Projections: Implementation and Applications*, ed. G. T. Herman. New York: Springer-Verlag, 1979, pp. 147–246.

Chang, L.-T. A method for attenuation correction in radionuclide computed tomography. *IEEE Trans. Nucl. Sci.* 25:638–643, 1978.

Egbert, S. D., and May, R. S. An integral-transport method for Compton-scatter correction in emission computed tomography. *IEEE Trans. Nucl. Sci.* 27:543–548, 1980.

Floyd, C. E., et al. Energy and spatial distribution of multiple order Compton scatter in SPECT: a Monte Carlo investigation. *Phys. Med. Biol.* 29:1217–1230, 1984.

Floyd, C. E., et al. Deconvolution of Compton scatter in SPECT. *J. Nucl. Med.* 26:403–408, 1985.

Gordon, R., and Herman, G. T. Three-dimensional reconstruction from projections: a review of algorithms. *Int. Rev. of Cytol.* 38:111–151, 1974.

Gullberg, G. T.; Malko, J. A.; and Eisner, R. L. Boundary determination methods for attenuation correction in single photon emission computed tomography. In *Emission Computed Tomography: Current Trends*, ed. P. D. Esser. New York: Society of Nuclear Medicine, 1983, pp. 33–53.

Hamming, R. W. *Digital Filters.* Englewood Cliffs, NJ: Prentice-Hall, 1977.

Herman, G. T. *Image Reconstruction from Projections.* New York: Academic Press, 1980.

Herman, G. T., ed. *Image Reconstruction from Projections: Implementation and Applications.* New York: Springer-Verlag, 1979.

Herman, G. T., and Lent, A. Iterative reconstruction algorithms. *Comput. Biol. Med.* 6:273–294, 1976.

Herman, G. T., and Rowland, S. Three methods for reconstructing objects from x-rays: a comparative study. *Comput. Graphics Image Process.* 2:151–178, 1973.

Huesman, R. H. A new fast algorithm for the evaluation of regions of interest and statistical uncertainty in computed tomography (abstract). *J. Nucl. Med.* 25:P89, 1984.

Jaszczak, R. J., et al. Lesion detection with single-photon emission computed tomography (SPECT) compared with conventional imaging. *J. Nucl. Med.* 23:97–102, 1982.

Jaszczak, R. J., et al. Improved SPECT quantification using compensation for scattered photons. *J. Nucl. Med.* 25:893–900, 1984.

Jaszczak, R. J.; Coleman, R. E.; and Whitehead, F. R. Physical factors affecting quantitative measurements using camera-based single photon emission computed tomography (SPECT). *IEEE Trans. Nucl. Sci.* 28:69–80, 1981.

Kan, M. K., and Hopkins, G. B. Measurement of liver volume by emission computed tomography. *J. Nucl. Med.* 20:514–520, 1979.

Kuhl, D. E., and Edwards, R. Q. Image separation radioisotope scanning. *Radiology* 80:653–666, 1963.

Lange, K., and Carson, R. EM reconstruction algorithms for emission and transmission tomography. *J. Comput. Assist. Tomo.* 8:306–316, 1985.

Larsson, S. A. Gamma camera emission tomography. *Acta Radiol.* (Suppl.) 363:1–75, 1980.

MacIntyre, W. J., et al. Application of the Budinger equation to evaluate signal to noise ratios of single photon emission tomographic systems (abstract). *J. Nucl.Med.* 24:P75, 1983.

Nahmias, C., et al. Understanding convolution back projection. In *Single Photon Emission Computed Tomography and Other Selected Computer Topics*. New York: Society of Nuclear Medicine, 1980, pp. 19–29.

Novak, D. J., and Eisner, R. L. Distance weighting for improved tomographic reconstructions. *J. Nucl. Med.* 25:P54–55, 1984.

Oppenheim, B. E. More accurate algorithms for iterative 3– dimensional reconstruction. *IEEE Trans. Nucl. Sci.* 21:72–77, 1974.

Oppenheim, B. E. Scatter correction for SPECT. *J. Nucl. Med.* 25:928–929, 1984.

Radon, J. Über die bestimmung von funktionen durch ihre integralwerte längs gewisser mannigfaltigkeiten. *Sachsisch. Gesellsch. Wissenschaft. Leipzig Math. Phys. Kl.* 69:262–277, 1917.

Rowland, S. W. Computer implementation of image reconstruction formulas. In *Image Reconstruction from Projections: Implementation and Applications*, ed. G. T. Herman. New York: Springer-Verlag, 1979, pp. 9–80.

Shepp, L. A., and Logan, B. F. Reconstructing interior head tissue from x-ray transmissions. *IEEE Trans. Nucl. Sci.* 21:228–236, 1974.

Shepp, L.A., and Vardi, Y. Maximum likelihood reconstruction for emission tomography. *IEEE Trans. Med. Imag.* 1:113–122, 1982.

Tauxe, W. N., et al. Determination of organ volume by single-photon emission tomography. *J. Nucl. Med.* 23:984–987, 1982.

Tauxe, W. N., and Todd-Pokropek, A. E. Reply to re: determination of organ volume by single photon emission tomography (letter to the editor). *J. Nucl. Med.* 24:1198–1199, 1983.

Vishampayan, S., et al. Maximum likelihood image reconstruction for SPECT (abstract). *J. Nucl. Med.* 26:P20, 1985.

Whitehead, F. R. Quantitative analysis of minimum detectable lesion-to-background uptake ratios for nuclear medicine imaging systems. In *Medical Radionuclide Imaging,* Vol. 1. Vienna: International Atomic Energy Agency, 1977, pp. 409–434.

3

Instrumentation

This chapter concentrates on the generic rather than brand name instruments but, of necessity, involves many acronyms and instrument names. Using names makes it much easier to tell the models apart. Specific instruments are used as examples of particular concepts.

ANGER CAMERA SPECT SYSTEMS

The Anger camera system considered here includes the camera head and accompanying electronics (whether they are physically located in the camera head or in an accompanying cabinet) and the gantry and table, which are the mechanical parts of the system (the computer hardware, software, and interface are considered in the next chapter).

The rotating Anger camera has quickly become the standard SPECT device for several reasons, the most important of which is that the equipment is commercially available from several manufacturers. Rotating the Anger camera head was a natural extension of the already available motions (Keyes et al. 1977; Murphy et al. 1979). The camera images are projections of the radioactive distribution in the body; projection images are commonly made in several positions around the patient in order to achieve some three-dimensionality. The SPECT technique goes far beyond a few projection images to have the instrument automatically go around the patient and then synthesize the results in the same format as that of the x-ray–transmission CT scanner. It was originally thought to be very difficult to transport a heavy Anger camera head (or two) around a patient, but x-ray–transmission tomography showed that nothing was impossible.

The first attempts put the camera head on a C-arm and could only image human heads (Keyes et al. 1977; Murphy et al. 1979). The gantry design was further developed to allow a hollow center for whole-body imaging. While the details of camera head transport were being worked out, the software was being perfected. Rotating the patient instead of the camera, as well as performing computer simulations, yielded satisfactory images for testing the software during this period.

Anger Camera Head and Electronics

The basic elements of the Anger camera head have not changed in some time but there have been enough additions to make necessary a thorough discussion of the system's parts.

The basic detector is a thallium-activated sodium iodide [NaI(Tl)], single crystal, 0.375 to 0.5 in. (0.95 to 1.27 cm) thick. The crystal thickness balances the need for a detector with sufficient attenuation for low- to medium-energy (100– to 250–KeV) gamma rays against the need for positional resolution equal to or better than the other elements of the system. Thin crystals have good resolution and poor sensitivity. Thick crystals absorb or attenuate more gamma rays, but exhibit poor resolution. The SPECT crystals are 16 to 21 inches (40 to 53 cm) in diameter to image a field of view equal to the whole width of a patient. A gamma ray is detected when it interacts by photoelectric or Compton scattering with the iodide ions of the crystal, which lose electrons. The electrons interact with the crystal lattice to produce light. The amount of light produced is directly proportional to the amount of energy lost by the absorbed gamma ray. The position of light production corresponds to the site where the gamma ray interacted. The build-up of light in the crystal occurs over a little less than a microsecond. Each 100 KeV of energy produces about 13,000 eV of light, or 4,300 photons of 3 eV each. The light produced quickly disperses because the crystal is transparent to the light; about 9% remains as a long-lived phosphorescence with a 0.15–second decay time. In the presence of radioactivity, the phosphorescence contributes a constant glow, which is basically ignored by the system.

Sodium iodide crystal detectors are used because iodine has a relatively high atomic weight and therefore good gamma-ray absorption properties when compared to low-atomic-weight elements; large crystals can be made reasonably easily. In a single crystal there are no boundaries to limit the resolution.

The crystal is set into a reflective medium, usually white aluminum oxide, that directs light toward its back surface. The crystal is protected from air and water vapor, as well as from stray light. Water vapor would be adsorbed, turning the crystal yellow with molecular iodine, which would ruin the energy resolution and cause the crystal to crack. Stray light would present distracting photons for the detection system.

The NaI(Tl) crystal is backed up by a set of photomultiplier (PM) tubes that detect and amplify the light photons produced in the crystal by gamma-ray interactions. The tubes are normally arranged in a hexagonal closest-packed arrangement. They may be round or hexagonal, and range in size from 2 to 3 in. (5.0 to 7.5 cm), so that a 16–in-(40–cm)-diameter crystal is covered with 37 to 91 PM tubes. The PM tubes are attached to the crystal by a very pure silicone grease, which transmits the light as efficiently as possible. The grease must be applied in such a way that there are no air bubbles or nonuniformities. Hexagonal tubes line up better in neat rows but are harder to attach with a good grease seal, because they cannot be rotated to be squashed into place. The shape of the whole assembly or the shape of the active area of the camera is typically round, hexagonal, or square. A PM tube absorbs the light from the crystal on its photocathode and generates about 1 electron for each seven to ten photons absorbed. The subsequent stages of the PM tube, called dynodes, multiply the electrons by having them collide with the dynodes under the influence of a voltage rise, which produces three to five electrons for each collision because of the special oxide coating of the dynodes. The electrons from the photocathode are multiplied by a factor of one million or more, becoming a small electrical pulse at the anode. The PM tube is tuned and controlled by controlling the voltage applied to the dynodes through the pins on the back of the tube. Typically, 300 to 500 volts are applied to the first dynode and 1000 volts more across the whole set of dynodes, with each of the ten (or twelve) dynodes getting $1/10$ (or $1/12$) of the voltage rise. A typical photomultiplier responds more quickly than the crystal, with a rise time of the order of 15 nanoseconds and a transit time of about 55 nanoseconds. The whole pulse resembles the graph in Figure 3–1. An individual crystal-PM tube unit is not safely operated at count rates above 1 million (M) total counts per minute, because the system is dead for the duration of a pulse.

An Anger camera is capable of a maximum of 20,000 to 100,000 counts per second by virtue of its complex electronic properties. The count rate limitation puts an upper limit on the sensitivity of the system.

The PM tube pulse comes off the last dynode and goes out

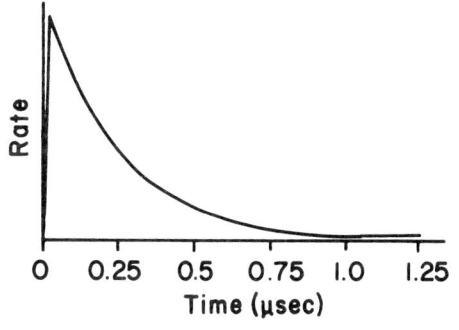

Fig 3-1.—A typical NaI(Tl) crystal-photomultiplier tube combination responds to produce a pulse.

through one of the pins on the back of the tube. The pulse still represents a very small signal, of the order of 10^{-9} volts, and needs further treatment before it can be transmitted out of the area though a wire to the rest of the electronics.

In older cameras, the pulse was preamplified and shaped in the camera head, and sent to the main cabinet for further processing into an image on an oscilloscope screen. Now that it is possible to make miniature microprocessors, all the electronics could be fitted into the camera head. This is not done, however, mostly because the technologist would then be setting switches and pushing buttons on a moving target. At least one manufacturer has located most of the electronics for communicating with the camera head in a small console on a shelf pivoted off the main camera gantry.

The PM tube voltage is maintained by a high-voltage power supply. The voltage from the power supply must be very stable because any shift in voltage means a shift in the peaking of the camera.

Electrical current powers the whole system. If the system is to be stable, the current presented to the instrument modules must be stable in voltage and in frequency. Neither the available power nor the instrument itself should cause or promulgate transients, voltage surges, drops, or spikes. While it is not necessarily up to the instrument manufacturers to protect their instruments from the poor quality of the available power by including safeguards in the design, it is a great deal easier for them to do so than for the users to try to clean up available power in a hospital setting with constant voltage transformers and other devices.

All NaI(Tl)-based detectors must be protected from sudden changes in temperature, because the crystal cannot adjust quickly and may crack if a change amounts to more than 10° F (5° C) per hour, either during shipment or after it is installed. Thus a crystal is carefully protected from temperature extremes and changes during shipment by thick Styrofoam packing and stern warnings against opening its container. After installation, when the camera is not in use, the camera crystal should always be left with the collimator on and must be protected as thoughtfully as possible against temperature change. Modern microprocessors are much less temperature sensitive than their older counterparts, but most computers benefit from a dust-free, controlled atmosphere with regulated humidity. Very dry atmospheres lead to the build-up of electrostatic charge; when this is discharged, effects may ripple through the electronics, tripping switches, burning out components, and causing loss of microprocessor memory.

Because processing the planar projection data to create transaxial images accentuates the difficulties that a camera might have with uniformity and stability, one should particularly examine the causes of the difficulties and determine what is to be done to counteract them. This chapter addresses the electronic remedies, while Chapter 7, on quality assurance, focuses on day-to-day attention to be paid to the instrument to produce good SPECT images.

The problems we see are expressed as differences of sensitivity from one part of the detector to another, from one time to another, and from one part of the rotational circle to another. The effect of sensitivity differences is to produce rings, like the rings of Saturn, on the transaxial images. We know that some of these differences in sensitivity are under the control of certain of the camera's electronic settings; the crystal and the collimator may be responsible for some differences between one part of the detector and another, but they are not under electronic control. Therefore we must correct for the differential sensitivity of the crystal and collimator and seek the causes for the other differences, and correct them either dynamically or once and for all with factory-installed corrections.

Before getting into the details of the problems, let us first consider how the camera is going to be used. It will typically be used to collect patient images of about 10 M total counts in a 64 × 64 matrix at 60 to 100 angles. If this is the case, then corrections with 10 M to 30 M total counts digitized into a 64 × 64 matrix will have sufficient statistical and spatial precision to be used with the clinical examinations. If the instrument is used with a finer matrix grid, such as 128 × 128, or with more total counts, such as one might collect for research purposes, corrections using a 64 × 64 matrix and 10 to 30 M counts will *not* be sufficient. This point is very important, but not easy to remember in practice, because most of the correction matrices and factors are the result of factory designs. There may not be enough microprocessor memory incorporated into the system for a finer grid or the collection of more counts. It takes 14 bits to have storage for more than 10,000 counts per pixel, while 12 bits only allow 4,095 counts per pixel, 10 bits 1,023 counts, and 8 bits 255 counts. The standard deviation of 10,000 is 1%, while that of 4,095 is 1.5%, and of 1,023 is 3.1%. A total of 30 M counts in a 64 × 64 matrix means about 10,000 counts per pixel, while 3 M means about 1,000 counts per pixel.

It might seem possible to correct for any degree of detector nonuniformity, but this borders on the absurd if the differential nonuniformities are too great (Padikal, Ashare, and Kereiakes 1976). There must be a clearly defined limit on the nonuniformities that the system is willing to correct; beyond this, a service call is required.

Since all the current generation of Anger cameras, which are made without light guides between the crystal and the PM tubes, need some sort of correction for the obvious nonuniformities, corrections are built into all of them. A mechanical correction for nonuniformity is the installation of a mask between the crystal and the PM tubes to equalize the response of the system. The simplest of the electronic corrections takes the results of a uniformity flood image and makes a correction matrix from it. The matrix is used to skim or add counts to the image or as a multiplicative correction factor. As we will see in the following discussion, this simplistic approach to a problem with several causes does not solve the difficulties. In addition, the methods, matrices, and/or numbers of counts accepted in the uniformity correction images may be producing results that would not be acceptable for SPECT even if such simple correction were the proper approach. As a result, it is suggested that the computer's multiplicative method of correction, using a count density of the operator's choice and without the possibility of overflow in the pixels, should be used with the older SPECT systems.

At the heart of the variability of the camera's response from one time to the next and from one position to the next are changes and differences in the response of the PM tubes to the gamma radiation. Each PM tube has its own response; the tubes age as they are used, so responses change. In addition, tubes cannot be expected to give the same count rate (have the same sensitivity), even if their spectral response is identical. Figure 3–2 shows the different spectral response of two PM tubes and two PM tubes with identical spectral response but different sensitivities. It is not sufficient to address both of these differences with the same remedy. When there are differential spectral responses, each tube is given its own voltage, so that all the spec-

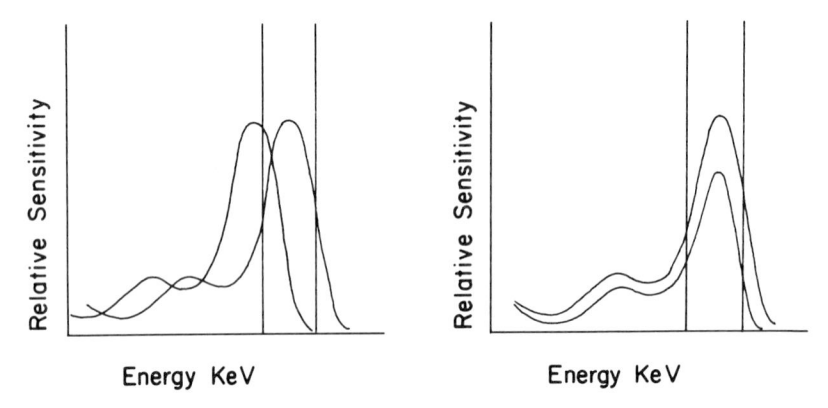

Fig 3–2.—On the left is shown the spectral response of two photomultiplier (PM) tubes that have identical sensitivities but different spectral response; on the right is the spectral response for two PM tubes with identical spectral response but different sensitivities.

tra line up; the voltage for each tube can be made to be an additive correction to the main voltage setting for a particular radionuclide. Since the correction may not be the same for each radionuclide (because the PM tubes' response may not be linear with respect to energy), there may need to be a different correction for each radionuclide or energy range. To make such a correction, the detector system is presented with a source of the desired nuclide; individual PM tube voltage settings are "learned" by a microprocessor and used as corrections when that radionuclide is used. Differential sensitivity is addressed by testing the response of each PM tube to an identical stimulus; some systems do this at the same time that they set the voltage corrections, while others do it continuously by pulsing each tube periodically with an identical tiny light flash and using the response to calibrate the system.

Some systems deal not with individual tubes but with a matrix of points representing the detector surface. If the corrections are more than very subtle and slowly varying over the surface of the detector, there must be some attempt to make the count densities and gridding of the correction matrix match or be higher and finer than those for the situation in which the camera is used.

The window width selected at the operator's console may not actually produce identical results when applied to the output from the PM tubes. Compared to most of the other sources of nonuniformities, this one has been found to be minor, so long as the window levels are not absolute but depend on the already-set peak voltage for each tube or detector area.

Early Anger cameras could not rely on electronic corrections, so their response had to be uniform. To build uniformity into the system, a plastic light guide was placed between the crystal and the PM tubes to guide the light emitted in the crystal into one of the tubes. The light guide did help produce a uniform image, but its imposition between the crystal and the PM tubes decreased the sensitivity and worsened the resolution of the system. When it was removed from the design, electronic corrections had to be substituted, because the uncorrected uniformity image was very nonuniform.

Correcting the energy-dependent spectral response and sensitivity differences of the PM tubes only begins to address the problems; it does not correct difficulties that occurred when the light guide was removed from the camera design. If a phantom consisting of lead bars (or of radioactive lines) is imaged, the image of the lines is wavy, in a pattern that reflects the position of the PM tubes. This is called nonlinearity, since the lines should be straight. Investigations of linearity call for careful computer programming to discover where the centers of the lines are. If the energy peak is set correctly, the lines seem to bend toward the tubes. The same effect makes the tubes appear more active than the spaces between them on a uniformity image. Because nonlinearity is an intrinsic property of the crystal-PM tube coupling arrangement, it must be attacked directly in the correction. The most common way is to present the camera with a pattern of point sources in a square grid (orthogonal hole pattern) or a pattern of lead bars lying first in one direction and then at 90 degrees to that direction, and make an image. A microprocessor "learns" the image and makes correction factors from it. This may be done at the factory for one or several radionuclides or energy ranges, or in the user's laboratory for one or several radionuclides. Again, the fineness of the grid is important, as well as the count density of the correction. A poorly done correction may be worse than no correction at all.

Finally, after all of the above corrections have been made, there may still be nonuniformities that are truly the result of differences in sensitivity of the crystal and collimator. It is fair to address these with count skimming or adding, or with a multiplicative factor, because they do not result from the displacement of counts or of the energy spectrum. When a correction matrix for these nonuniformities is collected, it is particular to that collimator in that position. A new correction must be made for every collimator. Since this correction depends on coordinates in the outside world, it is important to have it match the situation in use; the computer or microprocessor acquiring and applying this correction must take into account the settings of the position switches. Of course, such a correction cannot be expected to cure gross collimator or crystal problems such as crushed lead septa or a cracked crystal, any more than the other corrections can provide function for a nonfunctioning PM tube.

At this time there seems to be no danger of difficulties of image distortion and loss of counts due to dead time in SPECT examinations, because the amounts of radioactivity administered and the distribution of the radiopharmaceuticals at the time of imaging do not present such high count rates. It is possible to put large amounts of activity into a phantom and effectively "bomb" the camera; this is to be avoided. Some cameras have circuits that are designed to sense several kinds of dead-time distortions and to correct for them. The distortions may be the outright loss of counts in high-count areas, the adding of scattered sum-peak counts to the image between two highly radioactive areas, and the distortion of the energy peak by addition of one energy on top of another that produces an extra count. In cameras with dead-time correction, each PM tube is tested for dead-time losses and the losses are corrected for. In the face of all the other corrections and difficulties outlined above, it may be risky to expect this correction to operate properly during rotation. Before making such a correction to a patient examination, it should be performed with a phantom, simulating the patient, imaging nuclide, and situation. Under no conditions should routine uniformity images be acquired at count rates above the limit at which dead time becomes an issue, unless such a uniformity image is to be used with patient examinations for which routine images are acquired at these high count rates.

Ideally most of the above corrections could be made once, very carefully, at the factory, and the correction factors burned into a series of PROMs (programmable read-only memory) and shipped with the instrument. The PM tubes do change with time, so any correction that depends on their characteristics must be able to be changed. One alternative to correction in the user's laboratory is switching Anger camera heads. This operation is not to be performed casually, but the equipment for making such corrections accurately may be less transportable than the camera head.

In addition to stability, some means are necessary to inform the technologist when the correct energy peak has been selected for a particular radionuclide. Otherwise, the daily setting of the energy peak becomes the greatest variable in the operation of the system; what seems like a daily varying system may be nothing more than imprecise peaking from day to day. Older Anger cameras had a count-rate meter to aid in the selection; newer instruments are equipped with a spectrum image, either a gray wedge or a spectrum and a digital count-rate meter. To use either a spectrum or a count-rate meter for peaking, the energy peak and PM tube sensitivity corrections must be operating so that the spectrum or count rate observed is representative of all the tubes, not a few that happen to have a high count rate at the particular setting.

The SPECT system has an added problem that was not apparent before the advent of rotating tomography (although it was an Anger camera problem): there may be changes in the system as the camera head is rotated (Woronowicz et al. 1982; Jahangir et al. 1983). Obviously, the crystal and collimator will not change, but the PM tubes are not immune to outside influences such as gravitational and magnetic fields. The most obvious symptom of trouble is a change in the uniformity of the image with rotational angle, which is relatively easy to measure. The major effect will be a shift in the peak energy, so that the PM tubes are no longer all set on the same peak; this in turn affects the sensitivity as discussed in the preceding paragraphs. With most Anger camera systems it is much more difficult to measure the energy spectra of the individual PM tubes than it is to measure uniformity or linearity, but we really need to have an idea of the spectral shifts. All PM tubes should be extensively tested before they are installed, including tests to prove that gravity does not affect the performance of the tube; motion of the delicate dynodes inside the tube significantly affects the camera's performance. Gravitational effects cannot be shielded against, but magnetic effects can be. Jahangir and co-workers (1983) showed that magnetic shielding was effective in preventing most, but not all, of the changes in the uniformity of a camera as a function of angle of rotation.

Yet other influences may be at work, such as changes in the coupling between the PM tubes and the crystal, which cause changes in linearity (Johnson et al. 1983). The linearity changes observed were not simple functions of position but exhibited relaxation and hysteresis. This topic needs further examination because the effects have not been explained.

The elements of the Anger camera head must be fitted into a housing and shielded from gamma rays, except on the front, which is the active surface. Many of the components are themselves sensitive to gamma rays so everything must be shielded, not just the crystal. Of course, the crystal must not be exposed to radiation from the back or sides.

The common gamma-ray–shielding materials are iron and lead. Iron is much more dimensionally stable than lead, but lead has more

64 Chapter 3

shielding value, so the two materials are usually used together. This has the added advantage of a bimetallic system in which characteristic x-rays generated in one material are absorbed by the other. Magnetic shielding of some kind may also be incorporated inside the enclosure; its purpose is to prevent exterior magnetic fields from influencing the path of the electrons in the PM tubes and thus the energy spectrum of the tubes. The housing typically adds a ring 3 to 5 in. (7.5 to 12.7 cm) in width to the camera head, so that a camera with an active area of 16 in. (40 cm) will be 22 to 26 in. (55 to 64 cm) in total diameter and will weigh 3,000 lb (1,350 kg) or more with its supporting gantry.

The latest innovation is a camera head shaped to accommodate the human shoulders (Larsson et al. 1984), allowing the camera to come close to the human head without losing the base of the skull and neck from the SPECT image (Fig 3–3). The shielding and camera design allow a rim of only 7 cm, so that the base of the skull can be imaged from a short distance instead of out beyond the shoulders.

The camera's active surface is the front of the crystal, because the rest is shielded. A naked crystal is incredibly sensitive, but has no directional resolution. The collimator is a pattern of holes through

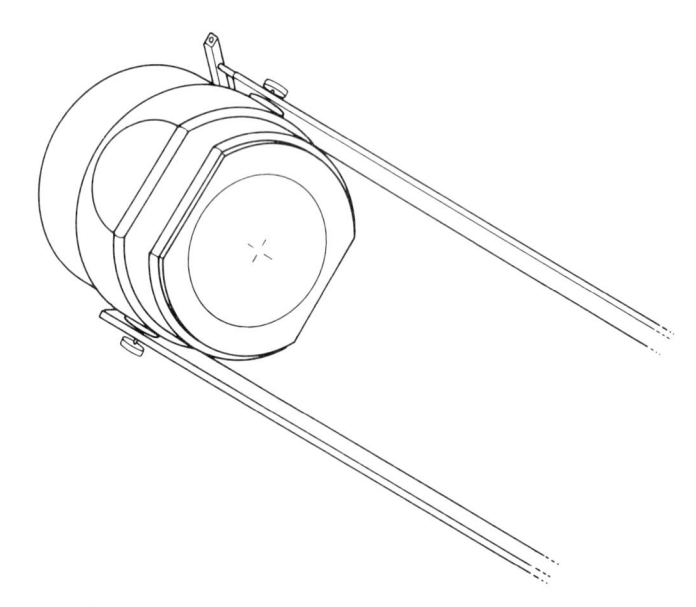

Fig 3–3.—One way to deal with the sudden change in size between the human body and the head is to flatten the sides of the Anger camera so that it can easily pass the shoulders (Larsson et al. 1984).

gamma-ray–absorbing material, usually lead or tungsten, which allows the camera a limited view of a gamma-ray source so that it has directional resolution by limiting the camera's field of view. Of course, the collimator also limits the camera's sensitivity. A general rule is that the more lead there is in the collimator the poorer its sensitivity will be. (It is also possible to make a light collimator for low energies that has poor sensitivity.) More lead is used for higher energies or higher resolution. The active part of the collimator is contained in a steel ring and is covered, usually on both sides, to prevent damage and contamination. While it is interesting to be able to see the pattern of holes in a collimator, leaving the holes unprotected can lead to damage.

The Anger camera in use today will typically be intended to detect a range of energies from the 60– to 80–KeV mercury x-rays of thallium-201 decay to the 364–KeV gamma rays of iodine-131. One collimator cannot deal efficiently with all energies, so collimators are usually designed for one of two different energy ranges and for various purposes. Low-energy collimators should cover energies up to about 200 KeV and medium-energy collimators to about 380 KeV. A collimator designed for gallium-67, with its maximum appreciable energy of 300 KeV, could be useful in some laboratories. Low-energy collimators may be all-purpose, high-sensitivity, or high-resolution; medium-energy collimators are usually not specialized. One must collimate for the highest appreciable energy emitted by the nuclide (or its contaminants), whether that energy is actually used in the image or not.

Most collimators have straight, parallel holes, usually round or square. There is also a low-energy converging collimator that makes small organs larger and is useful for pediatric imaging, thyroid glands, and so on. It is not useful for SPECT, however, because it does not yield parallel rays; a special converging fan-beam collimator (Jaszczak, Chang, and Murphy 1979), which is only fanned in the transaxial (x direction) plane and has parallel holes in the y direction (Fig 3–4), maintains the parallel rows of data for SPECT, but uses more of the crystal surface for smaller parts of the body such as the head. It should give better sensitivity and resolution when used with special software.

Another low-energy collimator that may prove useful for SPECT is a 30–degree angulated collimator. The holes are parallel but angled at 30 degrees. Such a collimator has been used in planar imaging of the heart to allow a close approach to the skin surface and an oblique view of the heart. In SPECT work it is useful for imaging heads, per-

66   *Chapter 3*

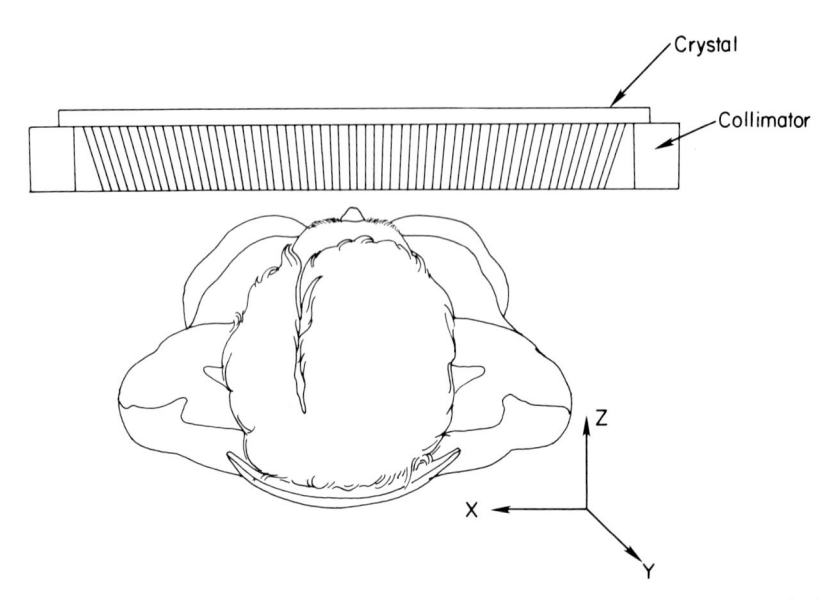

Fig 3-4.—The SPECT fan-beam collimator is flared in the x direction but the holes are parallel in the y direction.

mitting the close approach of a round camera head to the human head without coming into conflict with the shoulders (Esser et al. 1983, 1984; King et al. 1983). In SPECT use, the 30–degree angle of the collimator holes is matched by a 30–degree angle of the collimator face (Fig 3–5) to the axis of rotation so that the data will be taken from transaxial planes. It is to be expected that the resolution and sensitivity of each transaxial slice might be different. Another advantage of collimator angulation is that there is an apparent increase in crystal thickness by a factor of 1.15 because of the 30–degree angle.

Using a collimator with long holes is another way to solve the problem presented by shoulders (Budinger and Gullberg 1974). Such a collimator has poor sensitivity when compared with any of the thinner ones (Kircos, Leonard, and Keyes 1978). The hole size may be increased as the collimator is lengthened, for equivalent resolution (Mueller et al. 1984).

Performing SPECT with other than low-energy collimators (and therefore with radionuclides other than thallium-201, technetium-99m, and pure (p,5n) iodine-123) is a special problem because the modern camera has such exquisite resolution that it is able to resolve the pattern of holes in the collimator. The punctate nature of the plane projection images adds more noise to the transaxial images. Of

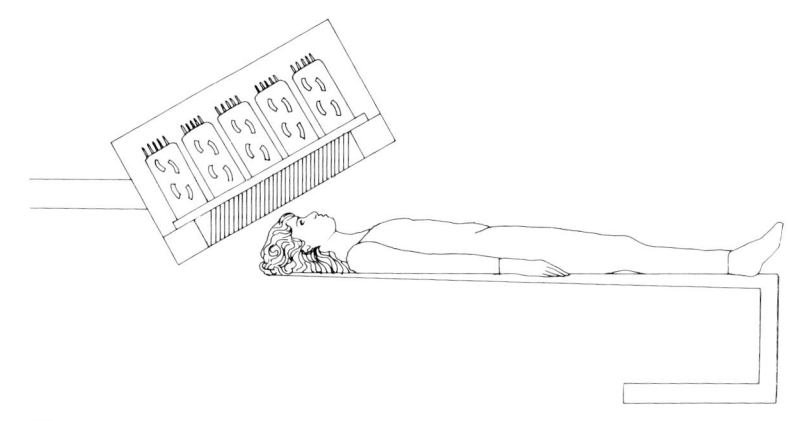

Fig 3–5.—Another way to image the human head effectively is to use a collimator with parallel 30–degree angulated holes. It is rotated with its face at a 30–degree angle to the axis of rotation (Esser et al. 1984).

course, the Anger camera is really tuned to perform with the best efficiency and resolution at about 150 KeV, so SPECT at higher energies does not use it to best advantage.

Iodine-123 occasions special discussion of collimator suitability (Coleman et al. 1983) because of its special emissions. Pure I-123, produced by a (p,5n) reaction, has 1% of 529–KeV gamma rays, which are probably not a problem because they are present in such small numbers. Impure I-123, however, is contaminated with I-124, which is a positron emitter and becomes more dominant as the I-123 decays. The collimator should be tuned to the purity of the I-123 used, although it is hoped—for other considerations such as patient radiation dose and examination statistics—that pure I-123 becomes the only available form of I-123.

The electronics in the Anger camera control cabinet allow the selection of the energy peak setting, energy window width, numbers of energy windows, and viewing of information that the system makes available. Position switches put the patient in the image correctly; these should be used thoughtfully in connection with SPECT, because the software expects to find the patient image data in a particular orientation. For a planar-projection static or dynamic examination the parameters of total counts or total time may be chosen; these are not used for SPECT. There is usually a count-rate meter and an elapsed-time clock. An attached formatter permits direct images to be made from the system at the time of patient imaging. Some systems perform zoom operations, centering on a particular part of the field.

Gantry and Table—Mechanical Operations

The gantry and table together make up the mechanical part of the SPECT system, permitting imaging at 360 degrees around the patient. Considering the weight of both patients and Anger camera heads and the desired precision of movements, the engineering requirements are strict. In addition, some kinds of motion of the gantry and table must be under computer control or at least computer surveillance, requiring interfacing to the computer. X-ray CT instruments have led the way in many of these design areas, but are not too helpful in camera head movement.

The gantry and table are, or could be, expected to be able to move in various directions depending on the examination. All of the motions and actions described may not be available on any one system. We begin with the gantry, continue with the table, and finish with their combination into a system.

At one end, the gantry holds the Anger camera head or heads in position and comprises the mechanics for rotating the camera(s) around the patient. At the other end, it is attached to the floor. For the gantry, which is a static system, strength and rigidity are essential. The bulk and weight must be kept to a minimum, and maximum flexibility should be maintained so that it is easy to use both as a planar imaging instrument and as a SPECT instrument.

The crystal, PM tubes, and attendant electronics must be held rigidly in the housing-shielding as the gantry rotates. The tubes will slide sideways on the grease when the camera head is left at an angle if they are not constrained by a series of spacers around the inside of the assembly. One must not assume that the plate that holds the backs of the PM tubes will be enough to prevent the tubes from slipping.

The camera head should swivel about its gantry connection (Fig 3–6, motion A) under either motor or manual control. The angle that the face of the collimator makes with the ground (also assumed to be the angle it makes with the axis of rotation) should be measurable. It should be possible to maintain this position while raising and lowering the head, or to lock the angle at a particular position. The head should have a wide range of motion, even being capable of being turned over.

The gantry arms should be rigid and not droop or flex. Drooping arms cause an unintended elliptical orbit, and flexing or springiness introduces motion into the planar projection images and destroys resolution. Gantry arms may be attached to the circle of rotation in several ways. One way is with a pivot (Fig 3–6, motion B), so that the

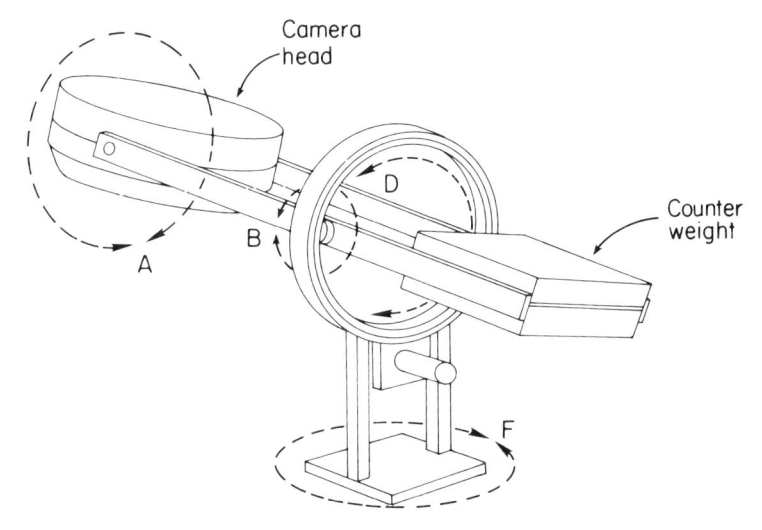

Fig 3–6.—When the gantry arms pivot at their connection to the circle of rotation, several motions should be possible. The camera head pivots on the gantry arms **(A)**, the gantry arm pivots on the circle of rotation **(B)**, the gantry rotates in a circle **(D)**, which should permit more than 360–degree rotation, and the whole system pivots on the floor **(F)**.

head is balanced by counterweights on the other side of the circle, like two people on a seesaw. Different counterweights must be attached for different collimators; the no-collimator situation is difficult to allow for. The pivot should allow for a wide range of motion (motion B in Figure 3–6) to allow the camera to clear obese patients and to image patients on stretchers for planar imaging. The camera head should be able to pass the imaging table, permitting certain movements and quality-control procedures. This pivoting motion may be under manual or computer control or surveillance. Since the camera head rides on the arc of a circle, it does not travel straight up and down. This may necessitate certain adjustments in the case of changes of the angle the camera is making on this pivot, to keep the patient planes in the same y level in the matrix. One possible adjustment is for the gantry arms to lengthen or shorten, with a compensated change in length on the counterweight side of the circle of rotation (Fig 3–7, motion C). General Electric and Picker have used counterweighted cameras of this kind.

Another mode is to have the counterweight and the camera head in the same plane, on the same side of the circle of rotation (Fig 3–8), as one Technicare instrument does. The patient fits between them.

If the camera head is not counterbalanced, there are several pos-

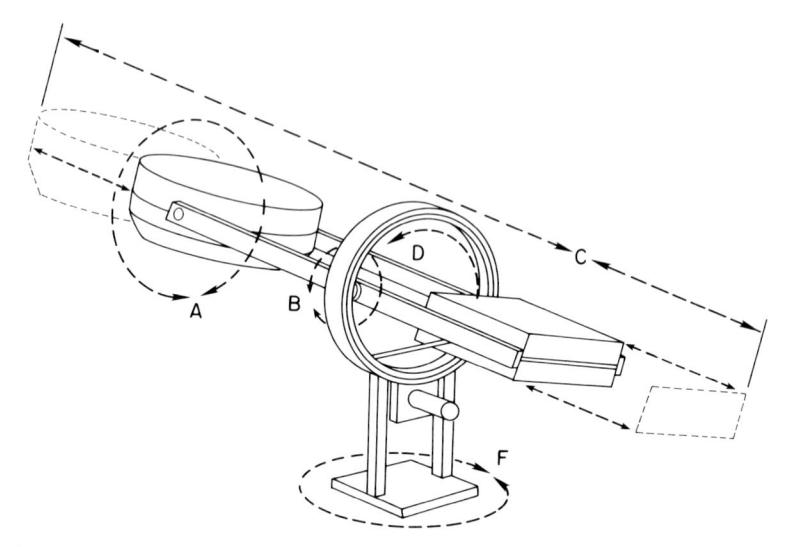

Fig 3–7.—Motion C allows the gantry arms to lengthen and shorten, both for the camera head and for the counterweights. The camera head pivots on the gantry arms **(A)**, the gantry arm pivots on the circle of rotation **(B)**, gantry arm length expands and contracts **(C)**, the gantry rotates in a circle **(D)**, which should permit more than 360–degree rotation, and the whole system pivots on the floor **(F)**.

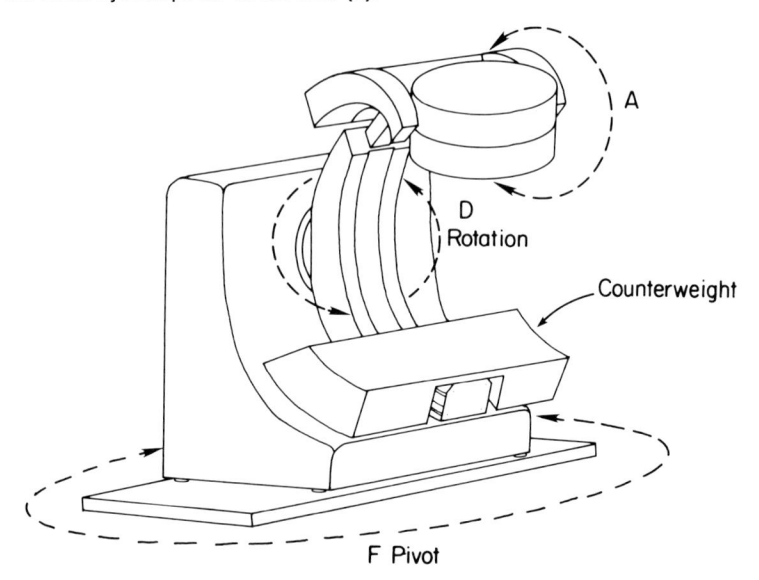

Fig 3–8.—The counterweight and the camera head are on the same side of the gantry. The camera head pivots on the gantry arms **(A)**, the gantry rotates in a circle **(D)**, which should permit more than 360–degree rotation, and the whole system pivots on the floor **(F)**.

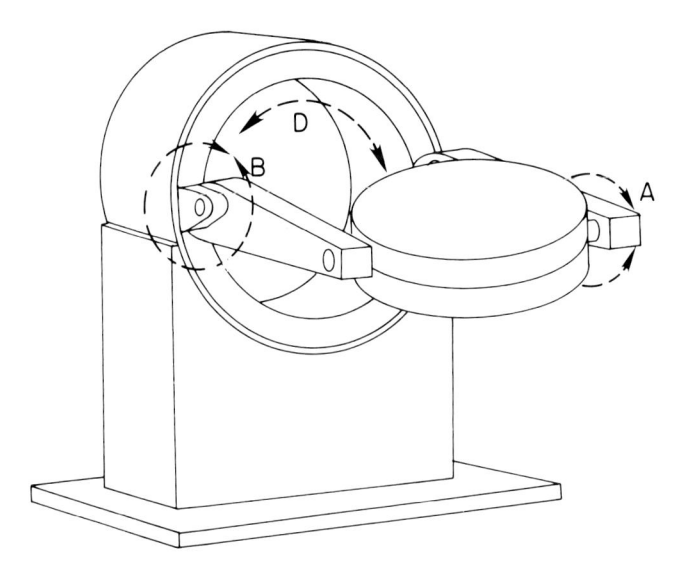

Fig 3–9.—In a camera that is not counterweighted, the gantry arms may pivot on the circle of rotation. The camera head pivots on the gantry arms **(A)**, the gantry arm pivots on the circle of rotation **(B)**, and the gantry rotates in a circle **(D)**, which should permit more than 360–degree rotation.

sible ways to attach the gantry arms to the circle of rotation. One is, again, on arms, which pivot to raise the camera head up and down. In such a case, the same kinds of motions as in the counterbalanced case must be possible to maintain the relationship between the patient and the computer's data-acquisition matrix (Fig 3–9, motions A and B). The Elscint camera has such motion, without the possibility for motion around a pivot in the floor, because the patient couch moves away from the gantry when it is not in use.

Another possibility is for the gantry arms to travel up and down on an elevator to change the distance between the collimator face and the patient (Fig 3–10), as the Raytheon SPECT system does. The up-and-down motion is motor driven. This rigid motion, with no pivots in the attachment of the gantry arms to the circle of rotation, simplifies the computer interactions and minimizes chances for difficulties with the electromechanical connections.

The circle of rotation may itself move up and down to achieve a patient-contour orbit. The gantry arms are held at 90 degrees to the circle of rotation. The up-and-down movement causes camera head motion in the z direction only (Fig 3–11).

The camera head may be suspended between two fixed piers (Fig

Fig 3–10.—The gantry arms may have an up-and-down motion **(E)** to maintain the short distance between the collimator face and the patient that is necessary for the best functioning of the Anger camera. A 90–degree angle is maintained between the camera face and the circle of rotation. The camera head pivots on the gantry arms **(A)**, the gantry rotates in a circle **(D)**, which should permit more than 360–degree rotation, and the gantry arm moves in and out along a radius **(E)**. A concentric-circles orbit is produced (see Fig 3–16).

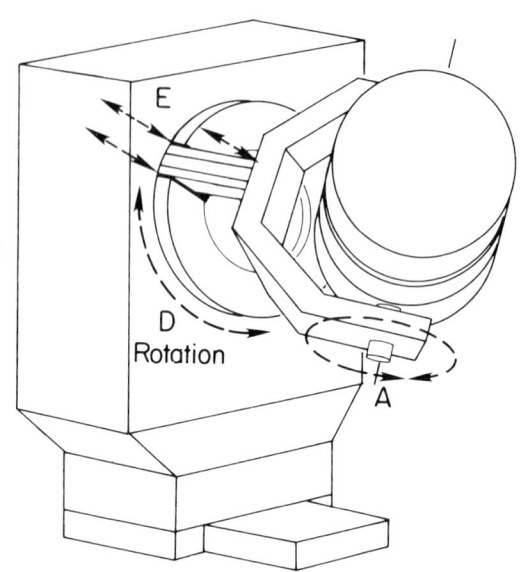

3–12), allowing travel along the suspending beam and rotation around the patient bed. The instrument looks bulky and takes more room space than the others. Technicare is making such a unit.

All of the cameras will go around in a circle. They should be permitted more than just 360 degrees of rotation for ease of patient positioning. The limiting factor is usually the twisting of the cable that

Fig 3–11.—The circle of rotation may have an up-and-down motion **(G)** to maintain the short distance between the collimator face and the patient. Note the pivot of the camera head on the gantry arms **(A)**, the rotation around the circle **(D)**; observe also that the circle of rotation motion **(G)** is up and down only. Such an up-and-down motion of the whole circle produces a circular-elliptical orbit (see Fig 3–18).

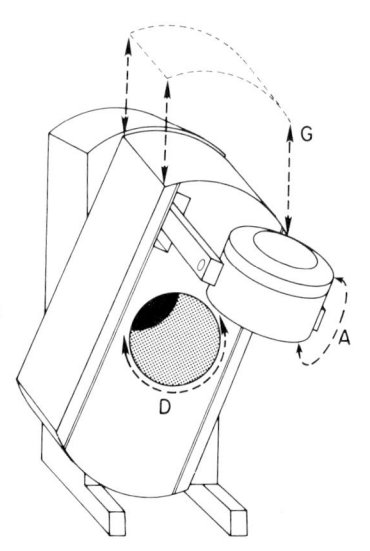

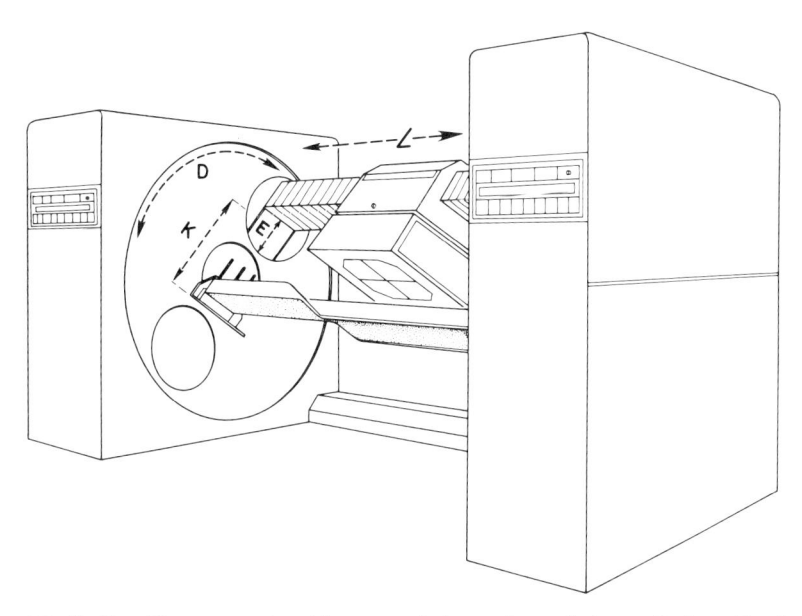

Fig 3–12.—The camera head is suspended on a beam between 2 piers. The head may move along the patient **(L)** for positioning, and toward and away from the patient **(E)** to create a concentric-circles orbit (see Fig 3–16). It rotates around the circle **(D)**. The table may be positioned to put the patient in the center of rotation **(K)**.

connects the camera head to the rest of the electronics. The instrument should not be constrained to begin and end at particular angles, because there are many possible 180-degree images, as for the heart from right anterior oblique to left posterior oblique. A motor and brakes should permit both continuous motion at a number of speeds and start-and-stop motion (called step-and-shoot) with a choice of angular increment sizes. There may be individual position sensors inside the circle of rotation, or the position may be completely relative to the position at the start and the elapsed time or number of angular increments since the start. Continuous motion must be controlled by a motor that will not cause electrical noise and thus disturb the camera electronics. Step-and-shoot motion must stop accurately, not jiggle, and have adequate brakes to hold the gantry at the correct position. The motor and brakes may also be sources of magnetic fields, which may influence the camera energy settings.

A cable connects the Anger camera head with the outside world: it carries voltage to the PM tubes; the energy window and peak selections to the camera head; and the x,y, and z signals from the camera head to the rest of the electronics. The cable is a delicate part of the system since it must twist and untwist. Copper wire will do this only so many times before work-hardening causes it to break, usually in some place that makes finding the break difficult, and necessitates cable replacement. It is wise to keep an extra cable on hand for speedy repair. Simple currents and signals may be transmitted through slip-ring systems, but nothing short of a small telemetry system would be a suitable replacement for the cable; such a solution would open the system to interference from many sources, most notably its own motors. Perhaps fiberoptics could be used in this application.

The gantry may be firmly attached to the floor facing in a convenient direction or it can pivot on a plate in the floor. Which of these makes better sense depends on the method of attachment that has been chosen for the table, since the camera is generally more useful if it is able to image a patient on a stretcher as well as on its own imaging table (see Fig 3–6, motion F). If the table is only hooked to the gantry and can be unhooked and rolled away, the gantry may be fixed to the floor. If the table is fixed to the floor, the gantry should pivot, so that it can "escape" from the table.

There is no part of the human body that we would not like to image with SPECT. The abdomen is about 3 ft (1 m) from the head or feet. Thus, it must be possible for this much of the patient to be stretched out while his liver, for example, is being imaged. For most of the systems, the center of the circle of rotation is open so that the patient can approach it or even go through it. It is also possible to have the gantry arms extend about a meter from the gantry, which means a long lever arm for the heavy camera head.

The table may be an active or passive part of the SPECT system. In either case, it should be strong and unobtrusive. The table surface should be made of some low-atomic-weight material that does not significantly attenuate gamma rays, and be as thin as possible to allow a close approach of the camera head to the patient. It should be rigid enough so the movements of the patient do not cause the table to bounce up and down. In addition, its width should closely approximate that of the patient, so that it does not prevent the lateral approach of the camera head to the patient. The table must be cantilevered to allow the camera head to pass all the way around the patient. There should be a head-holder of a suitable width for the head. With all of this, it would be helpful to remember patient comfort, which is not easily achieved in the midst of these requirements. Straps to restrain and hold the patient should be firm but minimal to avoid their interfering with the examination. Velcro is helpful in this regard.

A table that is not rigid enough may benefit from the addition of a monopod or tripod to help stabilize it, especially when the patient is far from the point of table support, as for head imaging. Beware of parts of the table that may have greater attenuation by reason of reinforcement. These may or may not be marked; suspicious areas may be examined with a portable x-ray unit.

The gantry and table are connected into a system. The one point about this system that sets it apart from x-ray CT imaging is that SPECT should provide somehow for a circle of rotation that follows the contour of the patient's body to get the best resolution from the Anger camera. It is worth emphasizing that a significant space separating the patient and the collimator causes degradation in the resolution of the system (Croft, Teates, and Honeyman 1983; King et al. 1983; Gottschalk et al. 1983). Quite a number of methods have been proposed for patient-contour following (Blum 1983) and some of them are being tried. One should use the simplest system that closes this gap well, with the fewest motions of the parts and the least concomitant adjustment of the information in the computer matrices, since it will have the smallest number of components and function to test and to go wrong.

Since the table is part of a system with many possible adjustments, it should have several motions (Fig 3–13). It should move in and out of the gantry's circle of rotation so that the organ of interest can be positioned easily in the field of view. It should move up and down so that the organ will be located close to the axis of rotation.

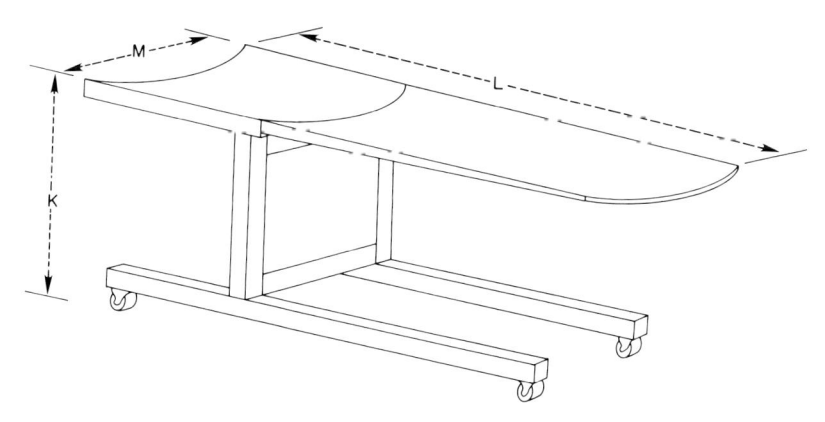

Fig 3–13.—The table is cantilevered to allow the camera head to pass under the patient. The table should have manual motions up and down **(K)**, and in and out of the gantry circle **(L)**. These motions may also be motor driven and interfaced to the computer. A side-to-side motion **(M)** may also be part of the computer-interfaced motions.

76 Chapter 3

In some SPECT systems the table is a passive part of the system, positioned at the beginning of the examination. In others, table motion is used to achieve a patient-contour orbit; this is only practical for single-head SPECT units. For a dual-headed unit, only the camera head motion is practical because it enables the two camera heads to move closer to or farther from the patient in concert. This motion creates a "patient sandwich." The orbit could be called a concentric-circles orbit (Fig 3–14), since the axis of rotation always stays in the center of the computer matrix and the face of the collimator is tangent to a series of concentric circles. This orbit occurs when the change to accommodate patient contour takes place along the radius of a circle whose center is on the axis of rotation. The camera head remains tangent to any one of a set of circles centered at B in Figure 3–14. The equation for a circle is

$$x^2 + y^2 = r^2$$

and its tangent has a slope of $-(x/y)$. The computer only needs to store the angle at which data were acquired, but does not need any information about the position of the camera head or the table, unless it is controlling the action that causes this motion.

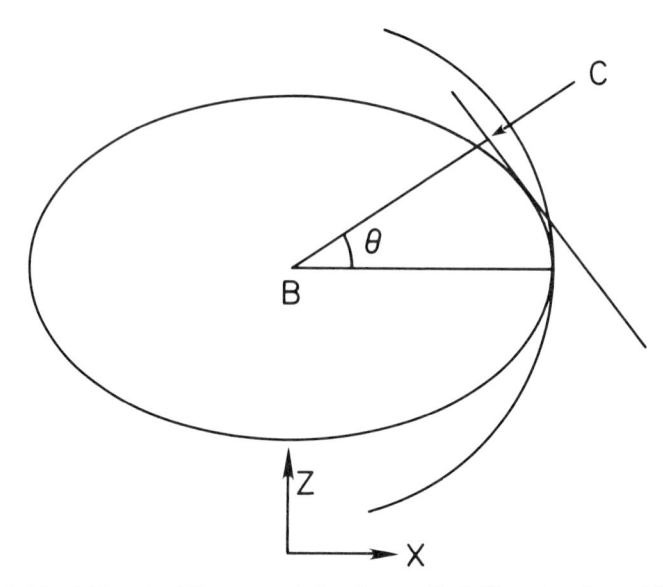

Fig 3–14.—Different orbits are created as the result of different motions of the camera head. In each of the three drawings, data are being acquired at the same angle θ; the location of the center of the computer's matrix is at **C**. The "center" of the patient is at **B**, assumed to be on the axis of rotation. The x direction is horizontal and the z direction is vertical.

Instrumentation 77

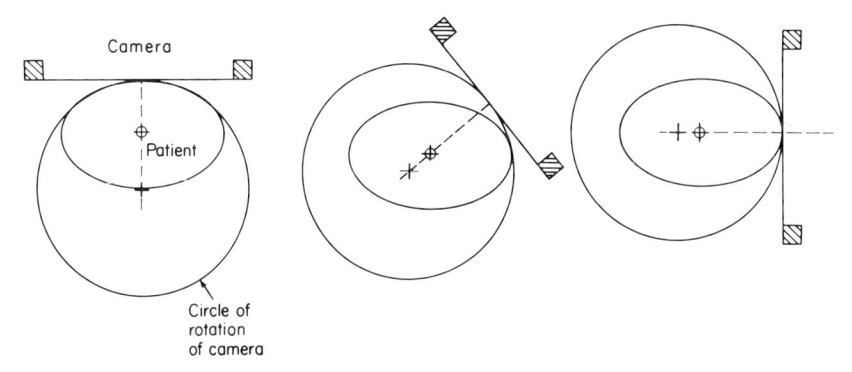

Fig 3–15.—If the table has full two-dimensional motion, it may be caused to move in a complementary ellipse to the patient shape, with the x and z axes reversed. The effect will be to keep one particular point inside the patient at the center of rotation at all angles, creating the concentric-circles orbit (see Fig 3–14), which needs no computer processing because the center of rotation is always in the middle of the computer matrix.

In single-head SPECT systems, if the correct combination of table motion in both the x and z directions is used, it is possible to achieve an orbit that will require no image manipulation by the computer. Otherwise, the motion of the table must be coupled with the computer so the patient information is correctly placed in the matrix when data acquisition is finished.

Two of the possible motions do not require any computer matrix adjustments. One is the table motion of Figure 3–15, in which the table moves in a complementary ellipse to the patient outline. The other is the gantry motion of Figure 3–10 and 3–12, in which the

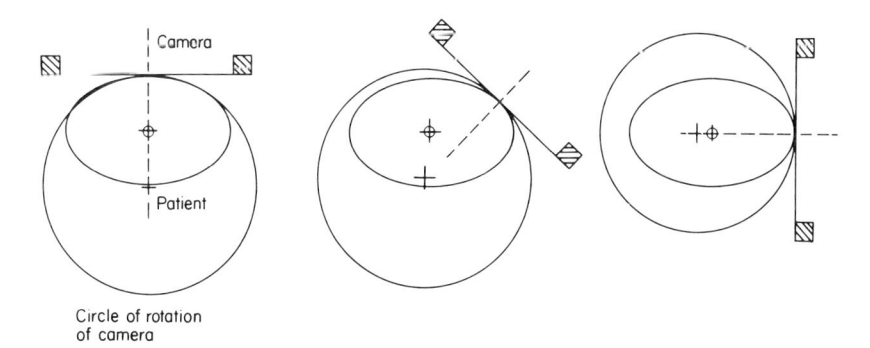

Fig 3–16.—Up-and-down motion of the table causes the center of rotation to move up and down in the patient, necessitating a computer correction to replace the information in the computer's matrix. This is another form of the circular-elliptical orbit (see Fig 3–18). Again, the patient may fall outside the field of view at some angles.

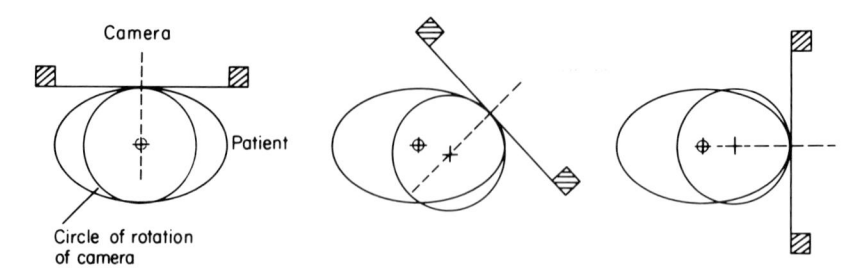

Fig 3–17.—Lateral motion of the table causes the center of rotation to move laterally in the patient, necessitating a computer correction to place the information in the proper place in the matrix. This is a circular-elliptical orbit (see Fig 3–18). Note also that the patient may be outside the field of view on some of the projections.

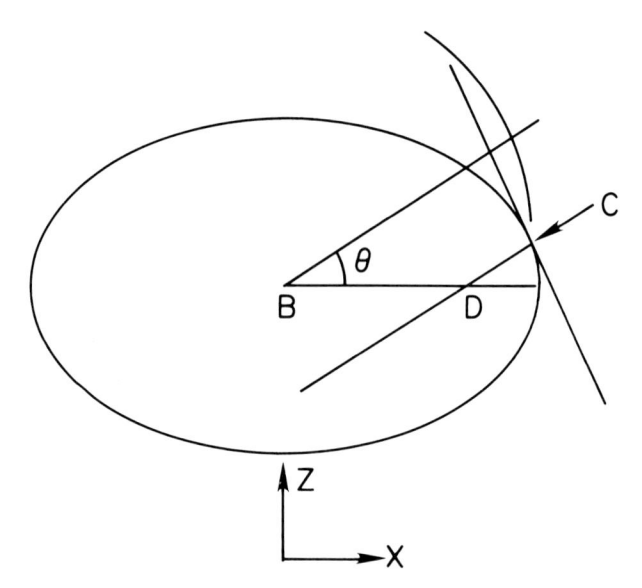

Fig 3–18.—A circular-elliptical orbit results when the circle of rotation is enabled to move in the z direction (up and down). The camera face remains tangent to any one of a set of circles centered at **B,** but the z motion means that the center of the computer's matrix is not directed (by the collimator septa) at the axis of rotation **B,** but at a point **D** along the major axis of the patient (Gottschalk et al. 1983). The computer must store the angular position and z position information in order for it to "know" the position of the center of the matrix relative to the axis of rotation.

camera head moves up and down on an elevator. These two motions, of table and of camera head, are in fact really the same motion, performed by two different parts of the system.

Up-and-down motion of the table (Fig 3–16) is the equivalent of up-and-down motion of the circle of rotation (Fig 3–11). It may be easier to create this motion mechanically and harder to interface it to the computer. Lateral motion of the table (Fig 3–17) is the equivalent of this, but in the other direction. In both of these cases the acquired data must be moved laterally in the matrix to bring the axis of rotation into register in the image; this is called a circular-elliptical orbit. The difference between a circular-elliptical (Fig 3–18) orbit and a concentric-circles orbit is the position of the circle to which the camera collimator face is tangent. It is possible to reconstruct the data acquired from any angle, providing that angle is known. The circular-elliptical orbit has been proposed by Gottschalk and co-workers (1983), who called it an "elliptical" orbit. A true elliptical orbit (Fig 3–19) is difficult to achieve and is not desirable.

After the motion of a particular system has been analyzed, the means for achieving that motion should be examined both from the viewpoint of the possibility for mechanical failure or error and from the viewpoint of patient safety. Engineering questions concern what

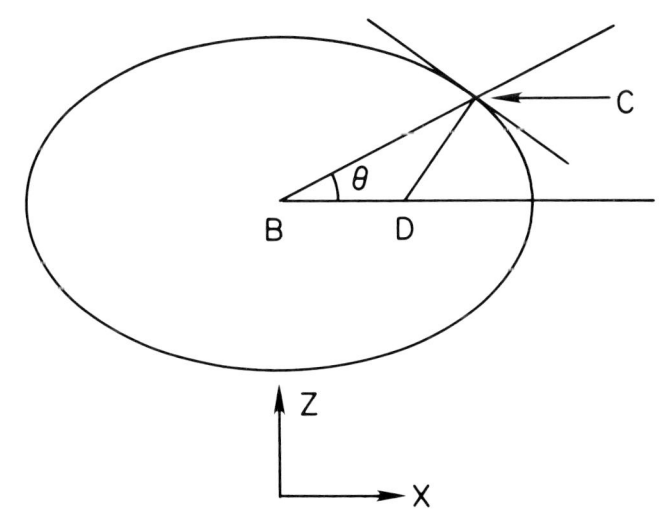

Fig 3–19.—If a true elliptical orbit were used, it would require a complex motion of the camera head to follow the tangent to an ellipse. The equation for an ellipse is $b^2 x^2 + a^2 y^2 = (ab)^2$, and its tangent has a slope of $-(b/a)^2 (x/y)$. The computer needs to know what the ellipse is. This motion is quite unlikely because it means twisting the camera head to allow a tangent to an ellipse.

surfaces are likely to wear or what drive belts to become stretched. Safety questions are those such as whether the patient is safe if he moves or the instrument is misdirected and whether the system prevents errors that could endanger the patient.

In one adaptation for a yet more complex motion involving both the camera and the table, the gantry arms pivot, the camera head pivots on the gantry to stay level, and the table moves in or out (Fig 3–20) to create a concentric-circles orbit. This method has been used manually (Croft, Teates, and Honeyman 1982) and is illustrated in Figure 3–21.

Issues—Sensitivity and Speed

The real issues for the Anger camera in SPECT are sensitivity and speed, which are coupled in the sense that a more sensitive system could be used to achieve either better counting statistics or faster imaging. The Anger camera substitutes sensitivity over a large area for the greater sensitivity that a probe system has in a single slice or a few slices. Sensitivity may be enhanced by using more camera heads.

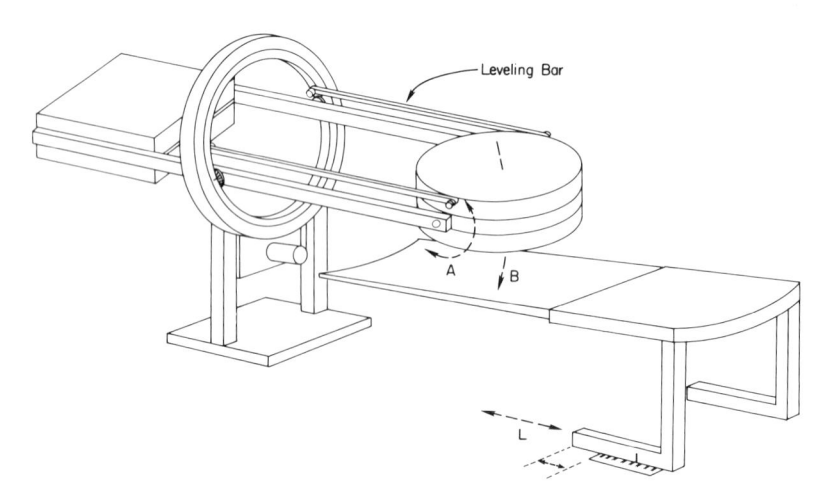

Fig 3–20.—On an older camera, the addition of a leveling bar between the camera head and the gantry keeps the head level at any gantry arm angle and allows manual readjustment of the orbit to fit the patient. As the camera head is brought closer to the patient (motion **B**), the leveling bar readjusts the camera head angle (motion **A**). The technologist moves the table (motion **L**) to the correct position to have the patient data in the correct location in the computer matrix in the y direction (Croft, Teates, and Honeyman 1982). The alignment between the axis of rotation and the computer matrix is maintained, so a concentric-circles orbit is produced.

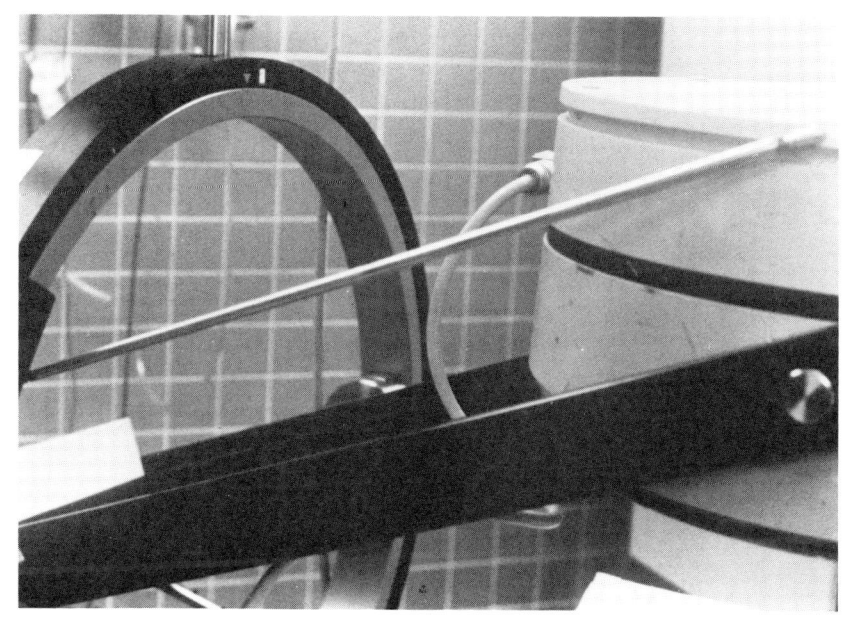

Fig 3–21.—The system described in Figure 3–20 in place in the laboratory.

The use of dual-head systems is in the testing phases now. While the second head doubles the sensitivity or halves the examination time, it does have some drawbacks: the weight means a more ponderous gantry and the electronic balancing of the two cameras is critical to the quality of the images. In addition, since the system is acquiring twice as many data, the computer hardware and software must accommodate it and keep continuous account of which camera is sending which bit of information so that corrections are made according to the proper camera. The computer problems have been solved by x-ray CT systems. The engineering problems are soluble, but their solution could result in a system with a price tag more like that of x-ray CT than like that of Anger cameras of old.

It would seem that more than three camera heads, of a size to image the whole cross-section at once and surrounded by reasonable shielding thickness, would not be productive because they would interfere with each other, preventing a close approach to the patient. Lim and co-workers (1984, 1985) discussed the use of a triangular three-camera arrangement.

Speed is made up of two components. One of these is having good counting statistics by virtue of imaging the patient from a large solid angle at once, which was addressed in the preceding paragraphs. The other is being able to move the system rapidly from one angle to the next to create one set of plane projection images and be able to go on to the next. None of the current Anger camera–based systems can rotate quickly or continuously around and around. They move ponderously and their cords get hopelessly snarled or broken. The latter problem is also an engineering problem and can be solved.

COMPTON SCATTERING DEVICES

There are other ways to use the Anger camera to produce tomographic information. Compton-scattering devices focus radiation from a linear source such as iridium-192 or mercury-203 onto a particular plane in the body and image that plane with an Anger camera placed at 90 degrees to the path of the radiation (Pistolesi et al. 1978) (Fig 3–22). The system has been used in lung imaging, creating coronal slices that can easily be rearranged by the computer into transaxial slices. In practice, the images suffer from multiple scattering. Comp-

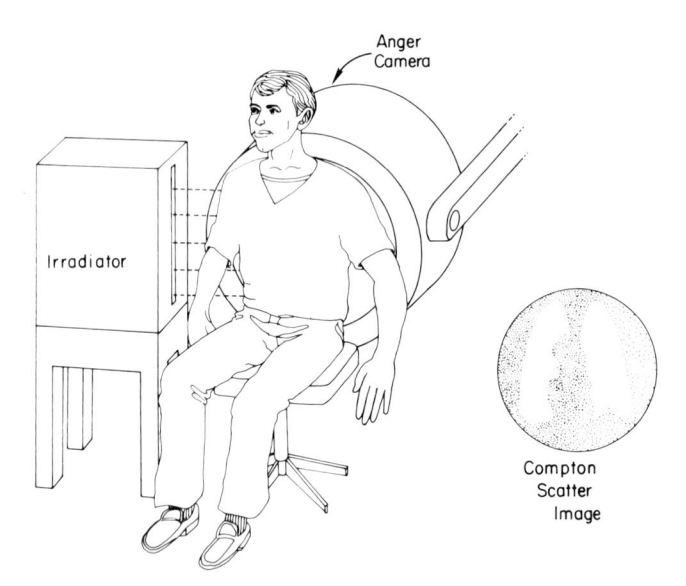

Fig 3–22.—The patient is bombarded with radiation in the same area as the Anger camera face, but several inches in front of it. The camera senses Compton-scattered radiation in the direction perpendicular to the plane of radiation. Because of attenuation in the patient, either two irradiators must be used or corrections must be made to the intensity of the acquired image (Pistolesi et al. 1978).

ton scattering could also be used to help in determining attenuation coefficients for 360-degree SPECT.

This technique has also been used to image heads (Mirell, Anderson, and Blahd 1977). The Compton scatter image was followed by a perfusion image in the same position for correlation.

OTHER 360-DEGREE TOMOGRAPHIC DEVICES

Depending on the design, it is possible for a scanner or set of detectors in a ring to image the patient tomographically much more quickly than is possible for a heavy Anger camera. Many versions of these devices have been created, most of them having in common the use of small detectors moving more rapidly to achieve images. The devices have greater sensitivity than the camera, mostly because they can look at more angles at one time. All of them can only image one or a few slices at a time, rather than a whole area. This is really the discussion of the differences between cameras and scanners all over again, but with a new twist: the scanner may be the device capable of more rapid dynamic imaging, if only in one slice at a time. Table 3–1 gives a number of salient facts about the instruments. To show the full range of instruments, several have been chosen for more discussion.

Mark IV

The generations of Kuhl's scanners first appeared in the literature in a classic paper (Kuhl and Edwards 1963) that described rectilinear and stereoscopic scanning, as well as longitudinal and transverse section scanning. All of these types of images could be produced by a very versatile dual-probe rectilinear scanner that had a circular motion to complement its rectilinear motion (Fig 3–23). The computers of the age were not up to the task of dealing with such data, so all the images were created on film directly, with any manipulation being made with the intensity knob of the oscilloscope. Many present-day nuclear medicine procedures were mentioned as possibilities in the article. By 1966 (Kuhl et al. 1966) data from the scanner were being stored on paper tape for computer processing into a rectilinear format that displayed the transverse image on an oscilloscope screen so that image contrast could be adjusted before photography. The early Kuhl instruments rotated 7.5 degrees between images, so there were 24 sets of linear data around the patient. Kuhl's Mark III (Kuhl and Edwards

84 Chapter 3

TABLE 3–1.—PROPERTIES OF VARIOUS SCANNER-TYPE DEVICES

NAME, NUMBER OF DETECTOR HEADS, NUMBER OF DETECTORS PER HEAD, AND DESCRIPTION OF MOTION

Kuhl's first scanners—2 detectors—opposed. 3–in. diameter × 2–in. detectors scan, then rotate 7.5°, rescan, rotate, etc; each 0.25–cm displacement is recorded, over 25–cm path; transverse section scanning was only 1 of several motions available.

Mark III—4 arrays of 1 detector each, 2–in. diameter x ½ in. with focused collimators; FWHM about 1.3 cm; detectors scan sideways; assembly rotates, then patient is indexed through scanner; 140 KeV; rectilinear scan patient to decide on best sections to get.

Mark IV—4 arrays of 8 detectors, 3 × 1 × 1 in.; detectors with focused collimators slightly displaced; arrays rotate constantly on axle collecting data in 2.5° samples, batched in 7.5° increments; 1 revolution every 50 seconds; linear sample interval, 0.8 cm; made into positron instrument later.

Aberdeen Sectional Scanner (ASS)—2 detectors, with conventional rectilinear scanner heads; capable of conventional rectilinear scanning, arc scanning, transverse section scanning (6–degree increment or 30 double-headed profiles per examination), and longitudinal scanning, a combination of rectilinear approach and x- ray planar tomographic approach; 8.9–cm-diameter detectors with 20–in. focal length.

Aberdeen Sectional Scanner II (ASSII)—Information on this instrument not readily available.

Tomoscanner, Tomogscanner II (J&P Engineering)—2 probe, dual 5–in. (this may vary) detectors, 180° rotation; scans 30 lines; focal length of collimators 13 cm, with detectors 32 cm apart.

Tomogscanner IIS (J&P Engineering)—2 heads with 3 detectors in each; each detector 5–in. diameter × 2 in. NaI(Tl), with focused collimator, 18.5–cm depth of focus; detectors ganged with center-to-center spacing of 14 cm; scans and rotates 6° to go 180° around; 6 minutes per slice for brains and 4 min per slice for livers.

Cleon 710—12 detectors, evenly spaced, each a 20 × 12.5 × 2.5 cm NaI(Tl) crystal and a focused (15–cm focal length) collimator, all with effective 20–cm field; detectors scan across 20 cm, index ⅜ × 2.54 cm toward (one set of 6) or away from (alternate set of 6) center, for a complete travel of 4 ⅛ × 2.54 cm distance toward center from the outside; each line has 128 elements; spacing between slices is controlled by patient couch movement; gantry can be angled ± 20°; instrument does not rotate.

Harvard Head Scanner (improved Cleon 710)—Rotational motion added; 10° rotation; decreased image noise by a factor of 1.7 and removed streak artifacts; number of tangential lines was lowered to 6 because of data storage limitations.

Harvard Body Scanner (10 detectors, for body; modified Cleon 711)—10 detectors, 20 × 12.5 × 2.5 cm, with focused collimators of focal length of 42 cm; each detector scans circular field 51 cm in diameter, using same in-out motion as Cleon 710; entire ring rotates in 18° steps, yielding 20 projections over 5 minutes; does not work very well for positrons because of collimator penetration.

SPRINT (University of Michigan)—Aperture ring of slits in lead cylinder that rotates; surrounding ring of 78 detectors; tilting gantry, 2 collimators: 8 slits, or multiple pseudorandom slits; fan-beam geometry; cylinder rotates ⅛ of circle; only 30% of detector positions filled in prototype.

BODY PART	ENERGY RANGE	TIME/REV OR IMAGE SENSITIVITY (cps/μCi/ml)	NO. OF SLICES OR LONGITUDINAL SPACING	ANGULAR SAMPLE OR FWHM	SOURCE
Body and head	Wide	30–50 min for gold-198	. . .	7.5°, usually 15°	Kuhl and Edwards 1964
Head	Same as Mark IV	5–20 min	4/head, 1 at a time	15°, 13 mm	Kuhl and Edwards 1970, Kuhl et al. 1977a
Head	Used for low to medium energies	50 sec/rev 5 revs per study; 15,400	. . .	7.5° 17 mm 3-D	Kuhl et al. 1976, 1977b
Body and head	Tc-99m collimator	8–15 min per image; 700 to 1200	13 mm	6°, 10–20 mm	Bowley et al. 1973, Dendy et al. 1981, Flower et al. 1981
Body	. . .	. . .	. . .	. . .	. . .
Body and head	Used for <200 KeV	~10 min	. . .	6°, 20 mm	Dworkin 1981, Maublant et al. 1979, Maeda et al. 1981
Body and head	<200 KeV	4–6 min 13,700	14 cm	6°, 13–20 mm	Elliott, Hanson, and Britton 1981
Head	<300 KeV	4 min/slice 12–30K 3.6K or 10,000 17,000	Multiples of 3mm 8 slices, but 1 at once	10.1 mm transverse, 15 mm coronal, or 20 mm coronal	Zimmerman et al. 1979, 1980, Jarritt et al. 1979, Flower et al. 1979, 1981
Head	<300 KeV	. . .	. . .	. . .	Moore et al. 1984
Body	Can go up to 511 KeV	5 min per slice	1 slice at once	18°, 26 mm transverse, 33 mm coronal	Kirsch et al. 1981
Head	140 Kev, 1–123	820–1,330	1 slice at once	8 mm transverse, 10 mm coronal	Williams and Knoll 1979, Rogers et al. 1984

Continued

86   *Chapter 3*

TABLE 3–1.—*Continued*

NAME, NUMBER OF DETECTOR HEADS, NUMBER OF DETECTORS PER HEAD,
AND DESCRIPTION OF MOTION

Tomomatic 64 (Medimatic)—Rapidly rotating detector ring; 4 groups of 16 detectors each, 1.3 × 14 × 2 cm NaI(Tl); focused rectangular-hole collimators, with 115 mm focal length; continuous rotation, covering 180° in 5 seconds; each crystal collects 3 slices; angular sample of 4.5°.
Improvement for Tomomatic 64—Alternate detectors and collimators to get 6 slices with separation of 2 cm, rather than the 4 cm of the original instrument.

HEADTOME—Hybrid single-photon-positron scanner has 64 16 mm wide × 28 mm high × 70 mm long NaI(Tl) crystals in a ring; lead wedges between crystals; detector ring in gantry; rotates in 5.6° steps and wobbles (for PET); SPECT collimator is 64 sets of tungsten fins driven by big wheel gear, which makes fins wave up to 30° in either direction; also has positron collimator.

HEADTOME II—hybrid single photon-positron scanner for heads; 3 detector rings, each with 64 16 × 28 × 70 mm crystals, separated by tapered lead septa; ring diameter, 42 cm; 10 cm longitudinal coverage; detector and collimator rotation; choice of collimators; patient aperture size 240 mm and imaging field 210 mm; does not swing collimator fins; both collimator and detector rings rotate in SPECT mode; has 4 collimators, 1 for positron, 3 for single-photon.
Gammatom-1—Has 36 2-cm diameter × 3.8-cm long crystals in 4 banks or arcs; focused collimator; continuous movement with 1.8° sampling; some horizontal movements may collect more than 1 slice.

MUMPI—Hollow cylindrical single crystal; rotating collimator; acquires 4 orthogonal two-dimensional images simultaneously, 8 slices at once.

1970; Kuhl et al. 1977a) scanner, designed for imaging heads with Tc-99m, permitted automatic selection of the slice to be imaged from the rectilinear scan views. It rotated the four 2–in. diameter by ½ in. thick NaI(Tl) crystal detector heads 15 degrees between views. Three to five minutes were required for each slice. Collimators were optimized to provide a nearly even resolution at the surface and in the middle of the head. This instrument was in everyday use in 1970, with the average examination consisting of four rectilinear views and one or two transverse sections, all taking about an hour.

The Mark IV system (Kuhl et al. 1976, 1977a) was designed to be ten times as sensitive as the Mark III. Each of the four detectors of the Mark III was replaced by a linear array of eight crystals, each 3 in. high by 1 in. wide by 1 in. thick. Thus, a square box of detectors surrounds the patient's head. The crystals are 3.2 cm center-to-center

BODY PART	ENERGY RANGE	TIME/REV OR IMAGE SENSITIVITY (cps/μCi/ml)	NO. OF SLICES OR LONGITUDINAL SPACING	ANGULAR SAMPLE OR FWHM	SOURCE
Head	<200 KeV	5 sec; running 30–60 sec, 170,000 and up	3 slices, 4-cm space	4.5 or 9°, 12.5–17 mm transverse, 19–23 mm coronal	Lassen, Henriksen, and Paulson 1981, Stokely et al. 1980
Head	. . .	. . .	6 slices, 2-cm space	. . .	Stokely 1982
Head	Including positrons, multiple collimators	3–40 sec per revolution, 16,000 to 26,000	. . .	5.6° 10–25 mm transverse, 20–30 mm coronal	Uemura et al. 1981
Head	Same as HEADTOME	10,000 to 60,000	1 at a time	6.5–11.5 mm, 18–37 mm coronal	Hirose et al. 1982
Head	. . .	10,000 to 15,000	. . .	1.8°, 7 mm	Cho et al. 1982
Head	Tc-99m	1 sec	8 (2-cm slices)	. . .	Logan and Holmes 1984

distance apart. Each array is offset so that data from opposing arrays will interlace, producing a uniform FWHM of 17 mm. The whole box of detectors rotates, stopping every 2.5 degrees. Data from successive 7.5–degree increments are stored for processing. A full 360 degrees' worth of data is acquired in 50 seconds and processed in the next 30 seconds. Successive 50–second images are acquired until the statistics are satisfactory; five revolutions or 4.2 minutes are normally required for a slice of a single-photon study. More recently, the Mark IV has been fitted with a second set of collimators for positron imaging (Kuhl et al. 1977b), giving the same resolution as for single-photon work, but with only one-third the sensitivity because of the greater amount of lead that must be used in the collimators. Sensitivity could be doubled by increasing the crystal thickness from 1 in. to 3 in. Kuhl points out numerous advantages to using a single-photon

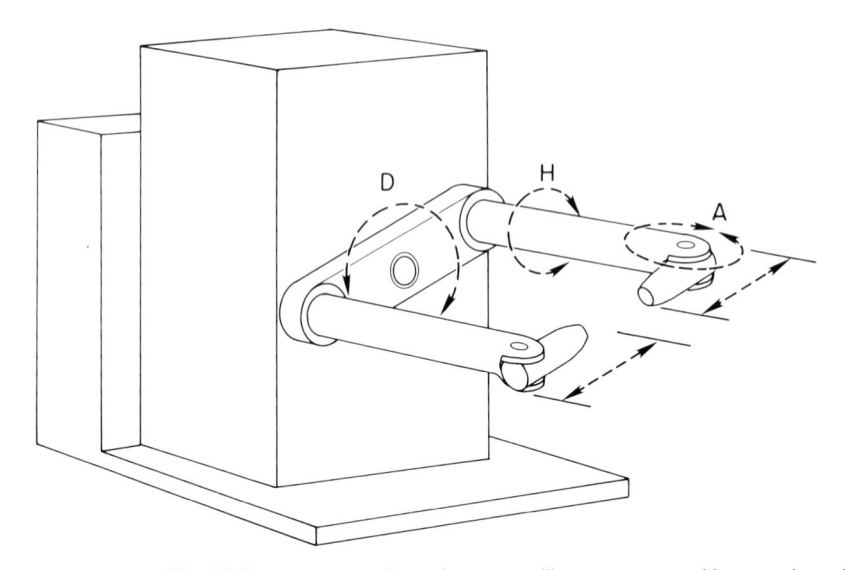

Fig 3–23.—The Kuhl scanner was based on a rectilinear scanner with a number of added motions. The dual detectors could each go up and down on their elevators (a manual motion) and could pivot around the gantry arm (motion **A**). The gantry arms swiveled (motion **H**), which in fact created the ordinary rectilinear motion. The gantry rotated (motion **D**) to create transaxial images (Kuhl and Edwards 1964).

mode for detecting even positrons. One can differentiate two radionuclides from each other by pulse-height analysis, allowing serial examinations without making it necessary to wait for radioactive decay of the positron emitter. Also, of course, the instrument maintains its versatility for performing both PET and SPECT examinations. With its 50–second rotation time, however, the instrument is not capable of really rapid dynamic imaging.

Aberdeen Sectional Scanner

The Aberdeen sectional scanner (ASS) (Bowley et al. 1973) was inspired by Kuhl's success with the improved rectilinear scanner. It has two detector heads and is capable of rectilinear and arc scanning, as well as longitudinal and transverse section scanning, with dual probes, moving in a circle in 6–degree increments. A slice can be imaged in 12 minutes. Data were originally collected on paper tape and reconstructed by a PDP 8I computer. This instrument continues to be used, both at Aberdeen (Flower et al. 1981) and elsewhere, in a commercialized form (Maublant et al. 1979; Maeda et al. 1981).

Cleon 710

The Cleon 710 (Stoddart and Stoddart 1979; Zimmerman et al. 1979, 1980; Jarritt et al. 1979; Flower et al. 1979, 1981; Hill et al. 1982) was designed to take advantage of the focused collimator and its depth resolution by putting a set of 12 detectors with such focused collimators all around a gantry and having them scan in and out, as well as back and forth (Fig 3–24). Each detector is expected to cover half the distance to the middle, while its opposite covers the other half. Adjacent detectors move in opposite directions to avoid getting in each other's way. The gantry originally did not rotate, but the Harvard group-redesigned instrument does (Moore et al. 1984). The image of a slice, a composite of 12 (now six with rotation) individual scans, can be made in four minutes. The short time for an individual scan makes possible dynamic studies in which each image is a running average of a series of individual scans. The Cleon 710 has a high, even sensitivity because of its large number of detectors and the collimator design. Great variations in reported sensitivity figures for this instru-

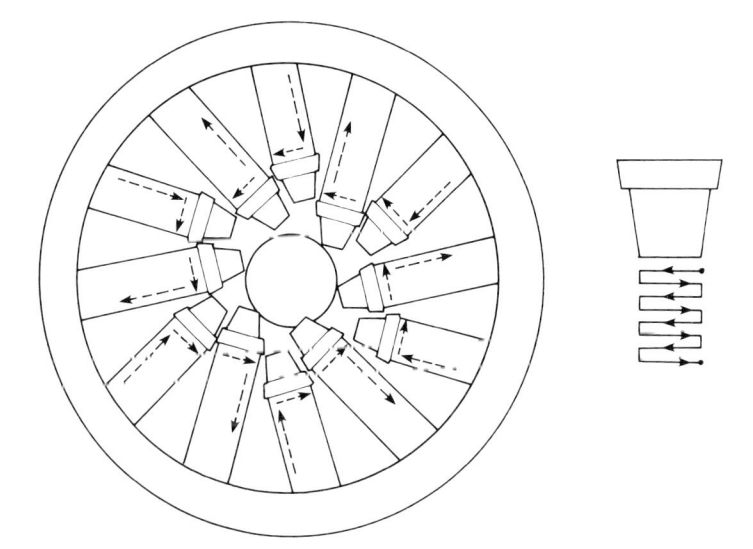

Fig 3–24.—The Cleon 710 has 12 detectors around the patient's head. The detectors are large (20 × 12.5 × 2.5 cm) crystals with a large photomultiplier tube (8.7 cm) and a short-focus collimator. The motion of the detectors is coupled so that six are scanning from side to side and in, while six are scanning from side to side and out. There are 128 data elements per scanning line and six scan lines 1 cm apart for each detector; the whole assembly rotates through two angles of 10 degrees each (Zimmerman et al. 1980; Moore et al. 1984).

ment are caused by software errors (Zimmerman et al. 1980). The instrument was designed to image heads and to work with energies of less than 300 KeV.

Harvard Body Scanner

The Harvard body scanner (Kirsch et al. 1981) is an elaboration on the Cleon 710; the differences are that it has ten probes instead of 12, the collimators have longer focal length, and the scanner has a large opening so that bodies as well as heads can be accommodated. The individual detector motion is the same, but to cover the patient thoroughly the gantry rotates through 18–degree steps, yielding 20 projections in five minutes. Collimators were designed for a wide energy range, but do not perform well at 511 KeV because of septal penetration. A few units of this type were available commercially as the Cleon 711 (Johnston, Bindseil, and Jones 1981).

Tomomatic 64

The Tomomatic 64 (Stokely et al. 1980; Lassen, Henriksen, and Paulson 1981; Stokely 1982) was specifically designed to add speed to the list of things that a ring of detectors could do. Speed is required to study the brain's blood flow with noble gases such as xenon-133 and xenon-127. The Tomomatic 64, designed to image heads at radionuclide energies of less than 200 KeV, is commercially produced by Medimatic (Fig 3–25). It has four groups of 16 detectors, each a 1.3 × 14 × 2 cm NaI(Tl) crystal, all backed by 100 PM tubes. Each crystal is collimated to participate in collecting three slices of data. The whole assembly rotates through 180 degrees in five seconds, with data sampling every 4.5 degrees. Dynamic images are running averages of speedily collected data.

A new collimator has been designed with alternating staggered centerlines to give six slices per pass, each 2.0 cm apart (Stokely 1982); of course, this change adversely affects sensitivity, because the detected photons are split among six slices instead of three. Clinically, the trade-off is worth while, because the new collimator makes it possible to see lesions that would have fallen between the slices of the old collimator.

Medimatic has added to the Tomomatic product line a number of other instruments with the capability of imaging the body as well as the head. The largest instrument can accumulate data from eight slices simultaneously and changes its aperture size to accommodate

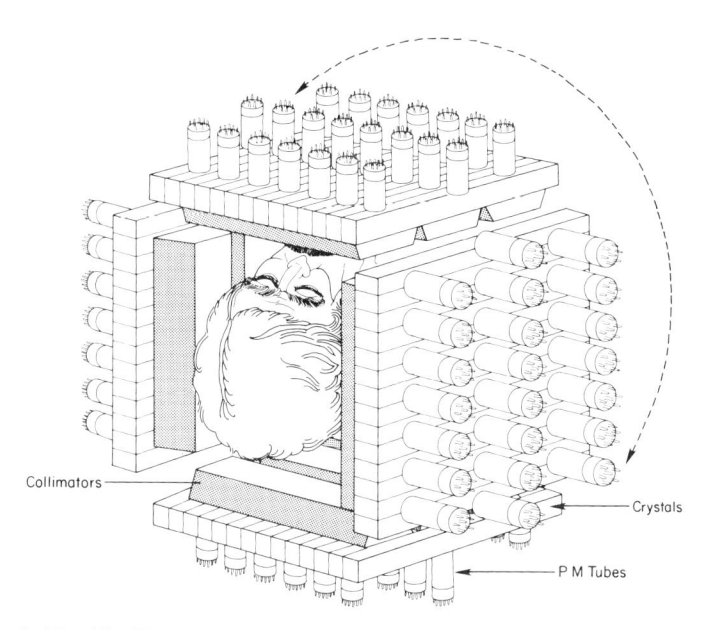

Fig 3–25.—The Tomomatic 64 has four groups of 16 detectors. It rotates through 180 degrees to collect rapid dynamic images of three slices of a patient's head (Stokely et al. 1980).

the shape and size of the part of the body being imaged. There should be more development in this area as larger institutions perceive a need for dynamic data acquisition.

SPRINT

The single photon ring tomograph (Williams and Knoll 1979; Rogers et al. 1982a, 1982b, 1984) is made up of a lead cylinder ring surrounded by as many as 78 detectors, each equipped with a converging collimator. (The prototypes have not filled all the detector positions.) The instrument is designed to image technetium-99m and iodine-123. The lead cylinder collimators designed for use with the instrument are a set of eight slits and a multiple pseudorandomly coded aperture; both collimators are designed for complete data collection with a revolution of one-eighth of a circle. The lead cylinder rotates continuously, while the detectors are stationary. Resolution is 8 mm FWHM in the transverse direction and 10 mm axially. The gantry tilts for more clinical versatility. Analysis of the properties of this instrument suggests that an improvement of a factor of 4.6 in the sensitivity could be achieved by installing three complete sets of detectors, using parallel-hole collimators, and increasing the number of slits in the lead ring to 14. The coded-aperture lead ring has no great advantage over the ring with slits unless the background is high.

HEADTOME II

The HEADTOME II (Hirose et al. 1982; Uemura et al. 1981) is the second instrument of its type, designed in Japan as a hybrid emission-computed tomographic instrument (for more on hybrids, see following). As its name implies, the HEADTOME II is designed to image the brain (Fig 3–26). The detectors are arrayed in three 42–cm-diameter rings, each separated from its neighbors by lead septa. For positron imaging, the detector rings wobble and rotate for adequate sampling; in the single-photon mode, the collimator also rotates. Four collimators, two each for single-photon and positron modes, were designed for the instrument and are all attached together for easy changing. The rotating collimator for single-photon work has tungsten fins whose angle to the radial direction varies from 0 to 35.2 degrees. The

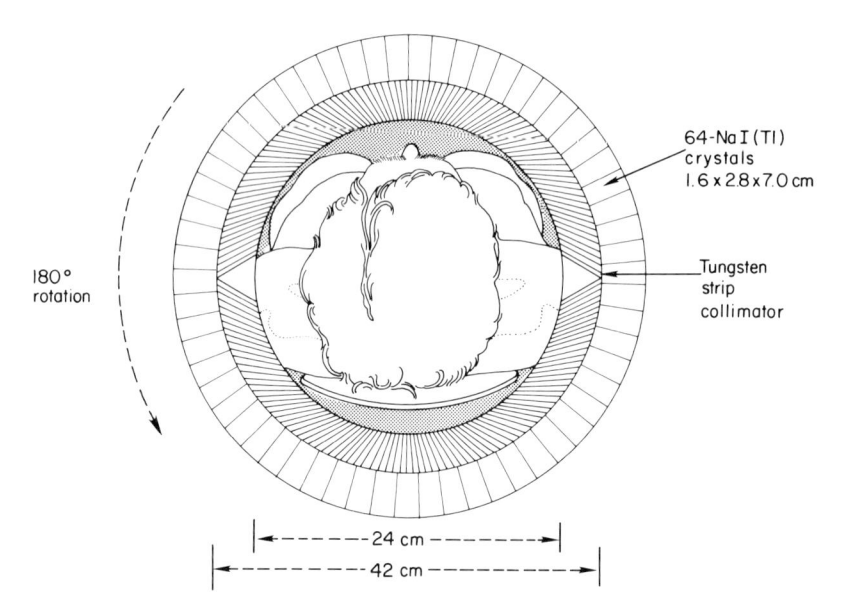

Fig 3–26.—The HEADTOME II is a ring of detectors around a specially designed tungsten collimator. The collimator rotates 180 degrees around a patient's head. It can rotate rapidly for dynamic studies or in a step-and-shoot fashion for higher resolution (Hirose et al. 1982).

collimator designed for the HEADTOME II was considered to be a great improvement over the one for the original model, which had moving tungsten fins. The movement caused both mechanical and software problems.

HYBRID POSITRON-SPECT INSTRUMENTS

It would seem a matter of common sense that to get the most mileage out of a tomographic imaging instrument, the unit should image positron-emitting nuclides as well as single-photon emitters. One instrument should be designed so that it would serve for all energies. Certainly one computer and one computer program might reasonably be expected to do this, no matter what the source of emissions or the detecting device.

This makes good sense until one considers the niceties of design that each class of nuclides requires. The 511–KeV emission of positron annihilation requires a detector of substantial thickness for sensitivity and suggests the use of coincidence detection for the two emitted photons, necessitating the use of dual detectors. Coincidence detection of annihilation photons takes the place of the extremely cumbersome, insensitive, poorly resolving high-energy collimator.

The most exciting positron emitters, carbon-11, nitrogen-13, and oxygen-15, have short half-lives and must be imaged quickly or in steady state. There is true necessity for great speed. These nuclides are not universally available, inexpensive, or of wide utility in the general practice of nuclear medicine.

There are generator designs that could make positron-emitting gallium-68 as common as technetium-99m, but there is really no reason for this in the face of the universal acceptance of technetium-99m, especially since gallium's chemistry has not been shown to be any more transparent than technetium's. On the other hand, technetium-99m and even iodine-123, as typical single-photon gamma emitters, do not require thick detectors or coincidence detection, but instead need lead collimation. Single-photon emitters enjoy wide acceptance and the instruments to use them are generally available, while the positron emitters are still tools of research and limited to those institutions with large research support. For these reasons, most developers and manufacturers of SPECT equipment have not taken seriously any need to make the instruments versatile enough to image positron emitters as well.

As for using the same computer for single-photon- and positron-emission tomography, it is certainly possible, but probably not desirable, because one tomographic system, perhaps in combination with a planar imaging device or two, is all one minicomputer should reasonably be expected to handle. A large computer could certainly handle the output of more than one kind of imaging device, but the nuclear medicine minicomputer is not a large computer. It is not reasonable to expect one minicomputer to handle all the data processing needs of a busy nuclear medicine department. It thus makes very good sense to dedicate a minicomputer to each tomographic imaging instrument.

The imaging of both single-photon emitters and positron emitters with the same instrument has not been ignored by everyone, however. Kuhl's Mark IV (Kuhl et al. 1977a, 1977b) has been converted for positron imaging. Kuhl has defended the use of lead collimation rather than coincidence detection and claims sensitivity of twice that of the PETT III under conditions of equal counts emitted by the source. Of course, the approach of the Mark IV does not permit rapid dynamic detection. The HEADTOME and its successor the HEADTOME II are dual-range instruments, using tungsten and lead collimation. Any instrument designed for both gamma and positron-annihilation photons must use collimation, because gamma rays cannot be detected by coincidence. Positron imaging is a demanding discipline in its own right and should not be asked to play second fiddle to SPECT. Instruments with dual purpose should be created only if they can truly serve both energy ranges effectively and without compromise.

LIMITED-ANGLE TOMOGRAPHY

Because truly 360–degree tomography is now being successfully carried out with a number of commercially available instruments and because it is so much better than limited-angle tomography, this discussion of limited-angle tomography is minimal.

Limited-angle tomography means that imaging is carried out from one or a few angles, using maneuvers other than 360–degree rotation or a ring of detectors to produce images at different depths. Because limited-angle instruments stay on one side of the body, they are usually confined to producing sagittal or coronal rather than transaxial slices. The planes are too widely separated to allow the fabrication of transaxial slices from the data. In addition, no matter what attention is paid to computer algorithms for reconstruction, deblurring, and image enhancement, ambiguities remain that cannot be resolved by calculations based on limited-angle data. Worse still, most such devices are unable accurately to image a uniform source or to reconstruct large sources correctly (Price, Patton, and Rollo 1980). Suetens and associates (1983) considered the question of limited-angle x-ray tomography and proved that blood vessels cannot be reconstructed from only two orthogonal views unless other a priori knowledge is used.

A great many devices have been designed for limited-angle tomography. Each seems to accentuate a certain problem, but overall it remains impossible to separate information according to plane of origin in order to produce an image of a particular plane.

The rectilinear scanner is a limited tomographic device because the focused collimator gives the sharpest image of activity in its plane of focus. It seemed reasonable to think of ways in which the instrument might be extended to provide truly tomographic data without scanning many times. The Searle-Siemens Pho-Con is a hybrid camera-scanner that allows this by using focused collimators and rectilinear motion together with a seven-PM-tube Anger camera head to separate one plane from another. In addition, computer programs have been written to process the data further to remove the counts from interfering planes. They have been minimally successful because of the limited view.

Several attempts have been made to use the Anger camera to create tomographic images without moving the camera head (or the patient, if possible). Angled collimators, for seeing under structures, have been employed. In one development, an angled collimator was attached to a motor drive. As the collimator rotated in the plane of the crystal face, the imaging table moved parallel to it to keep the patient always in the camera's field of view. A computer algorithm was then used to sort out the data to achieve tomographic images. This device with all its moving parts was hard to maintain in working order. Again, data from the planes could not be unambiguously separated.

Angled collimators have been used in original ways to image smaller organs, such as the thyroid and heart. A four-quadrant, moving, angled collimator required two separate views of the patient for reconstruction of tomographic images from eight separate images. It could be used only for normal-sized hearts and other small organs (Chang, Lin, and Henkin 1980).

The seven-pinhole collimator (Vogel et al. 1978) has been the most popular example of limited-angle tomographic devices. Other pinhole devices have been tried but have not enjoyed the wide use of this one. The seven-pinhole collimator was developed and used for heart imaging. It has the flaw of reconstructing the center of the field with fewer counts than are actually present; this was not so much of a problem using Tl-201 because the center of the heart is not radioactive. Because of this artifact, however, patients must be very carefully positioned so that their heart does not accidentally lie in the region of less sensitivity, thus creating false-positive results.

Coded-aperture instruments were an attempt to make the Anger camera receive data in Fourier space, which could be deconvoluted by laser light, as a hologram, to yield three-dimensional data as holograms do. The coded aperture is a special collimator with a pattern of rings of absorber alternating with nonabsorbent material or a pattern of holes in absorber material. The reconstruction of real Poisson-distributed data was discovered to be much more difficult than the theoretical reconstructions of data that are not statistically limited; it still had the problem that even in holographic images, one cannot truly get around behind an object. Small organs were imaged best.

The difficulty with all limited-angle tomographic devices is their inability to resolve the ambiguity of the position of radioactivity without data from both sides of the source. The difficulties of attenuation and scattering (which are discussed later for SPECT) are compounded. It is not necessary to use limited-angle methods now that the development of 360–degree tomography has advanced to its current level.

BIBLIOGRAPHY

Blum, A. S. Improving SPECT image quality by body contour following. In *Emission Computed Tomography: Current Trends*, ed. P. D. Esser. New York: Society of Nuclear Medicine, 1983, pp. 163–173.

Bowley, A. R., et al. A radioisotope scanner for rectilinear, arc, transverse section and longitudinal section scanning: (ASS—the Aberdeen Section Scanner). *Br. J. Radiol.* 46: 262–271, 1973.

Budinger, T. F., and Gullberg, G. T. Three-dimensional reconstruction in nuclear medicine emission imaging. *IEEE Trans. Nucl. Sci.* 21:2–20, 1974.

Chang, W.; Lin, S. L.; and Henkin, R. E. A comparison of the performance parameters of the 7–pinhole collimator and the quadrant slant hole collimator (QSH). In *Single Photon Emission Computed Tomography and Other Selected Computer Topics*. New York: Society of Nuclear Medicine, 1980, pp. 113–125.

Cho, Z. H., et al. Performance of single photon tomographic system—GAMMATOM-1. *IEEE Trans. Nucl. Sci.* 29:484–487, 1982.

Coleman, R. E., et al. Collimation for I-123 imaging with SPECT. In *Emission Computed Tomography: Current Trends*, ed. P. D. Esser. New York: Society of Nuclear Medicine, 1983, pp. 135–145.

Croft, B. Y.; Teates, C. D.; and Honeyman, J. C. Single-photon emission computed tomography of the liver. In *Digital Imaging: Clincal Advances in Nuclear Medicine*, ed. P. D. Esser. New York: Society of Nuclear Medicine, 1982, pp. 271–282.

Croft, B. Y.; Teates, C. D.; and Honeyman, J. C. Single-photon emission computed tomography and albumin colloid imaging of the liver. In *Diagnostic Imaging in Medicine*, ed. R. C. Reba, D. J. Goodenough, and H. F. Davidson. The Hague: Martinus Nijhoff, 1983, pp. 590–600.

Dendy, P. P., et al. A clinical trial of the value of a tomographic section view to identify liver abnormalities by radionuclide imaging, with special reference to metastatic disease. *Eur. J. Nucl. Med.* 6:51–55, 1981.

Dworkin, H. J. Initial clinical impression of whole body tomographic scanning. In *Emission Computed Tomography: The Single Photon Approach*, ed. P. Paras and E. A. Eikman. Washington D.C.: U. S. Government Printing Office, HHS Pub. FDA 81–8177, 1981, pp. 199–210.

Elliott, A. T.; Hanson, M. E.; and Britton, K. E. Tomogscanner 2S—technical evaluation. In *Emission Computed Tomography: The Single Photon Approach*, ed. P. Paras and E. A. Eikman. Washington, D.C.: U. S. Government Printing Office, HHS Pub. FDA 81–8177, 1981, pp. 211–214.

Esser, P. D., et al. Initial experience with an intelligent gantry system for single photon emission computed tomography. In *Emission Computed Tomography: Current Trends*, ed. P. D. Esser. New York: Society of Nuclear Medicine, 1983, pp. 105–119.

Esser, P. D., et al. Angled-collimator SPECT (A-SPECT): an improved approach to cranial single photon emission tomography. *J. Nucl. Med.* 25:805–809, 1984.

Flower, M. A., et al. Feasibility of absolute activity measurements using the Cleon emission tomography system. *Radiology* 133:497–500, 1979.

Flower, M. A., et al. A comparison of three systems for performing single-photon emission tomography. *Phys. Med. Biol.* 26:671–691, 1981.

Gottschalk, S., et al. SPECT resolution and uniformity improvements by noncircular orbit. *J. Nucl. Med.* 24:822–828, 1983.

Hill, T. C., et al. Initial experience with SPECT (single- photon computerized tomography) of the brain using N-isopropyl I-123 p-iodoamphetamine: concise communication. *J. Nucl. Med.* 23:191–195, 1982.

Hirose, Y., et al. A hybrid emission CT—HEADTOME II. *IEEE Trans. Nucl. Sci.* 29:520–523, 1982.

Jahangir, S. M., et al. Count-rate variations with orientation of camera detector. *J. Nucl. Med.* 24:356–359, 1983.

Jarritt, P. H., et al. A new transverse-section brain imager for single-gamma emitters. *J. Nucl. Med.* 20:319–327, 1979.

Jaszczak, R. J.; Chang, L.-T.; and Murphy, P. H. Single photon emission computed tomography using multi-slice fan beam collimators. *IEEE Trans. Nucl. Sci.* 26:610–618, 1979.

Johnson, T. K., et al. Spatial/temporal/energy dependency of scintillation camera nonlinearities. In *Emission Computed Tomography: Current Trends*, ed. P. D. Esser. New York: Society of Nuclear Medicine, 1983, pp. 71–80.

Johnston, G. S.; Bindseil, L. A.; and Jones, A. E. Single photon emission transaxial computed tomography. In *Emission Computed Tomography: The Single Photon Approach*, ed. P. Paras and E. A. Eikman. Washington D.C.: U. S. Government Printing Office, HHS Pub. FDA 81–8177, 1981, pp. 268–273.

Keyes, J. W., Jr., et al. The Humongotron—a scintillation-camera transaxial tomograph. *J. Nucl. Med.* 18:381–387, 1977.

King, M. A., et al. Preliminary characterization of the properties of a new rotating SPECT imaging system. In *Emission Computed Tomography: Current Trends*, ed. P. D. Esser. New York: Society of Nuclear Medicine, 1983, pp. 91–104.

Kircos, L. T.; Leonard, P. F.; and Keyes, J. W., Jr. An optimized collimator for single-photon computed tomography with a scintillation camera. *J. Nucl. Med.* 19:322–323, 1978.

Kirsch, C.-M., et al. Characteristics of a scanning, multidetector, single-photon ECT body imager. *J. Nucl. Med.* 22:726–731, 1981.

Kuhl, D. E., et al. Perforated tape recorder for digital scan data store with grey shade and numeric readout. *J. Nucl. Med.* 7:269–280, 1966.

Kuhl, D. E., et al. The Mark IV system for radionuclide computed tomography of the brain. *Radiology* 121:405–413, 1976.

Kuhl, D. E., et al. Design and application of Mark IV scanning system for radionuclide computed tomography of the brain. In *Medical Radionuclide Imaging*, Vol. 1. Vienna: International Atomic Energy Agency, 1977a, pp. 309–320.

Kuhl, D. E., et al. Radionuclide computerized tomography for brain study. In *Reconstruction Tomography in Diagnostic Radiology and Nuclear Medicine*, ed. M. M. Ter-Pogossian. Baltimore: University Park Press, 1977b, pp. 281–291.

Kuhl, D. E., and Edwards, R. Q. Image separation radioisotope scanning. *Radiology* 80:653–666, 1963.

Kuhl, D. E., and Edwards, R. Q. Cylindrical and section radioisotope scanning of the liver and brain. *Radiology* 83:926–936, 1964.

Kuhl, D. E., and Edwards, R. Q. The Mark III scanner: a compact device for multiple-view and section scanning of the brain. *Radiology* 96:563–570, 1970.

Larsson, S. A., et al. A special cut-off gamma camera for high-resolution SPECT of the head. *J. Nucl. Med.* 25:1023–1030, 1984.

Lassen, N. A.; Henriksen, L.; and Paulson, O. Regional cerebral blood flow in stroke by Xe-133 inhalation and emission tomography. *Stroke* 12:284–288, 1981.

Lim, C., et al. Triangular SPECT system for brain and body organ 3–D imaging: design concept and preliminary imaging result (abstract). *J. Nucl. Med.* 25:P6, 1984.

Lim, C. B., et al. Triangular SPECT system for 3–D organ volume imaging: clinical prototype and dynamic imaging potential. *J. Nucl. Med.* 26:P11, 1985.

Logan, K. W., and Holmes, R. A. Missouri University multi-plane imager (MUMPI): a high sensitivity rapid dynamic ECT brain imager (abstract). *J. Nucl. Med.* 25:P105, 1984.

Maeda, T., et al. Three-dimensional regional cerebral blood perfusion images with single-photon emission computed tomography. *Radiology* 140:817–822, 1981.

Maublant, J., et al. Transverse CAT of the myocardium with Tl- 201. *Eur. J. Nucl. Med.* 4:457–459, 1979.

Mirell, S. G.; Anderson, G. W.; and Blahd, W. H. A tomographic brain-imaging system using Compton-scattered gamma rays. In *Medical Radionuclide Imaging.* Vienna: International Atomic Energy Agency, 1977, pp. 255–262.

Moore, S. C., et al. Improved performance from modifications to the multidetector SPECT brain scanner. *J. Nucl. Med.* 25:688–691, 1984.

Mueller, S., et al. SPECT imaging with the long bore collimator: loss in sensitivity vs. improved contrast resolution (abstract). *J. Nucl. Med.* 25:P106, 1984.

Murphy, P. H., et al. Radionuclide computed tomography of the body using routine radiopharmaceuticals. I. System characterization. *J. Nucl. Med.* 20:102–107, 1979.

Padikal, T. N.; Ashare, A. B.; and Kereiakes, J. G. Field flood uniformity correction: benefits or pitfalls? *J. Nucl. Med.* 17:653–656, 1976.

Pistolesi, M., et al. Chest tomography by gamma camera and external gamma source: concise communication. *J. Nucl. Med.* 19:94–97, 1978.

Price, R. R.; Patton, J. A.; and Rollo, F. D. Single photon emission computed tomography: an overview. In *Single Photon Emission Computed Tomography and Other Selected Computer Topics.* New York: Society of Nuclear Medicine, 1980, pp. 1–17.

Rogers, W. L., et al. SPRINT: a single photon ring tomograph (abstract). *J. Nucl. Med.* 23:P59, 1982a.

Rogers, W. L., et al. SPRINT: a stationary detector single photon ring tomograph for brain imaging. *IEEE Trans. Med. Imag.* 1:63–68, 1982b.

Rogers, W. L., et al. Performance evaluation of SPRINT, a single photon ring tomograph for brain imaging. *J. Nucl. Med.* 25:1013–1018, 1984.

Stoddart, H. F., and Stoddart, H. A. A new development in single gamma transaxial tomography—Union Carbide focused collimator scanner. *IEEE Trans. Nucl. Sci.* 26:2710–2712, 1979.

Stokely, E. M., et al. A single photon dynamic computer assisted tomograph (DCAT) for imaging brain function in multiple cross sections. *J. Comput. Assist. Tomog.* 4:230–240, 1980.

Stokely, E. M. A contiguous-slice design for single photon emission tomography (SPECT). *J. Nucl. Med.* 23:355–356, 1982.

Suetens, P., et al. An attempt to reconstruct the cerebral blood vessels from a lateral and a frontal angiogram. *Pattern Recog.* 16:517–524, 1983.

Uemura, K., et al. The headtome: a hybrid emission tomographic system description and applications. In *Emission Computed Tomography: The Single Photon Approach,* ed. P. Paras and E. A. Eikman. Washington, D.C.: U. S. Government Printing Office, HHS Pub. FDA 81–8177, 1981, pp. 181–198.

Vogel, R. A., et al. A new method of multiplanar emission tomography using a seven-pinhole collimator and an Anger scintillation camera. *J. Nucl. Med.* 19:648–654, 1978.

Williams, J. J., and Knoll, G. F. Initial performance of SPRINT: a single photon system for emission tomography. *IEEE Trans. Nucl. Sci.* 26:2732–2735, 1979.

Woronowicz, E. M., et al. Factors affecting single photon emission computed tomography image quality and recommended QC procedures. Milwaukee: General Electric, 1982.

Zimmerman, R. E., et al. Performance measurements of an emission tomographic brain scanner (abstract). *J. Nucl. Med.* 20:628, 1979.

Zimmerman, R. E., et al. Single photon emission computed tomography with short focal length detectors. In *Single Photon Emission Computed Tomography and Other Selected Computer Topics.* New York: Society of Nuclear Medicine, 1980, pp. 147–157.

4

Computer Needs for SPECT

The computer has become an accepted part of the nuclear medicine laboratory for data acquisition and processing, largely as the result of the development of nuclear cardiology. Gated cardiac studies cannot be performed without a computer. Many dynamic studies have been put on a quantitative basis using the computer. The advent of SPECT has meant yet one more type of examination that cannot be performed without this tool.

The computer is a device that rapidly acquires and processes numeric information. It does what it is programmed or wired to do with great speed and accuracy. It cannot think, write its own programs, or misbehave. It differs from a calculator in being able to send to and receive information from a number of auxiliary devices or peripherals. The basic operation of a computer uses a large number of on-off switches to perform calculations, and has not changed since the concept was first introduced and developed; what have changed are the kinds of on-off switches that are used and therefore their speed and cost.

This chapter reviews the parts of the computer (Fig 4–1) in light of what is required for acquiring, processing, and storing SPECT examinations. Certain trade-offs among time, space, and money must be explored so that each user can determine the optimum point. The decision is based on the normal operation of the laboratory in terms of number and complexity of examinations and level of skill of the technologists, the method of reading and archiving examinations, the need for recall of computer information, and the availability of other assistance with the computer.

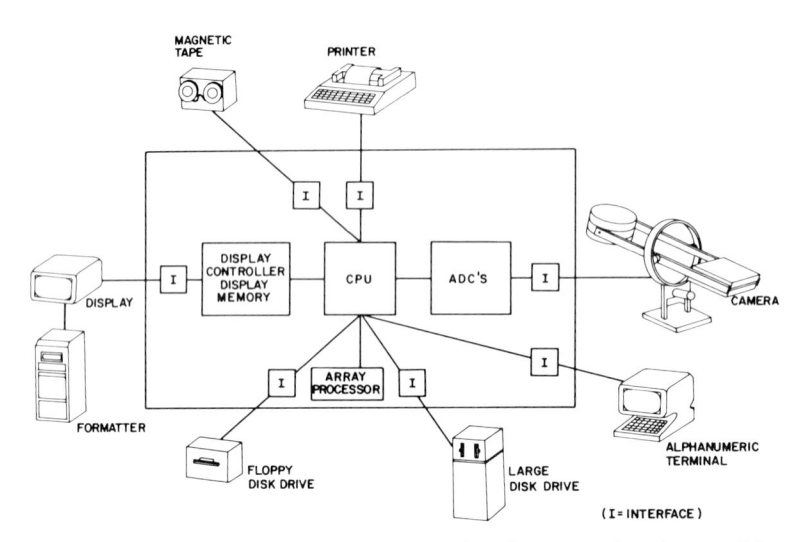

Fig 4–1.—The parts of a computer system designed for general nuclear medicine use and SPECT acquisition and processing. Pictures of computers would have been included if they were either interesting to look at or instructive, but one large metal cabinet looks like another.

A computer system is made up of hardware (the part you can kick) and software (the part you relate to). Each of the major developments in nuclear medicine has meant proliferation of software. Producing good software takes a great deal of time and creativity and is more difficult than producing good computer hardware. This chapter should give the reader an appreciation for the importance of effective software.

TYPICAL COMPUTER SYSTEM

Central Processing Unit

The central processing unit (CPU) is what actually does the labor of computing and what directs the traffic for the operations of other devices attached to the computer. It is the most basic part of the hardware; many abilities of the system follow from the choice of CPU, such as word length and cycle time. The CPU typically consists of an arithmetic logic unit to perform mathematical and logical operations, some memory for storing starting information and intermediate results (random-access memory, or RAM), sometimes some memory for the storage of built-in programs that usually cannot be tampered with by the user (read-only memory, or ROM), and a control unit for directing the order of operations (Fig 4–2). Read-only memory may be devoted to the operating system, language interpreters and compilers, peripheral device drivers, and other permanent parts of the software. Random-access memory may be utilized for image storage, temporary program storage, display storage, or any combination of these. Every CPU needs some RAM, but may have some ROM. In addition, the CPU may have the capability of controlling more RAM or ROM installed externally to it, in the case of the microprocessor chips. Included with the arithmetic logic unit may be functional extensions such as array processors, bit-slice processors, or floating-point processors, all designed to speed the processing of large amounts of data over similar paths. Parallel processing of large quantities of data may reduce processing times by a factor of 100, although it is more reasonable to expect a factor of 10. The CPU and its memory are said to be volatile if information is not retained when the power is turned off; RAM is often volatile, while ROM is not.

A computer accepts and stores information in units called words. Words are broken into individual binary numbers called bits. The bits may in turn be combined not only into words but also into parts of words, called bytes.

The choice of CPU decides what word size the computer will consider normal (8–bit words for older microprocessors, 16–bit words for newer microprocessors and older miniprocessors, 32–bit words for yet newer microprocessors and newer miniprocessors, 64–bit words for large main-frame computers). The word is the most basic unit that the CPU processes. The longer the word, the more information that

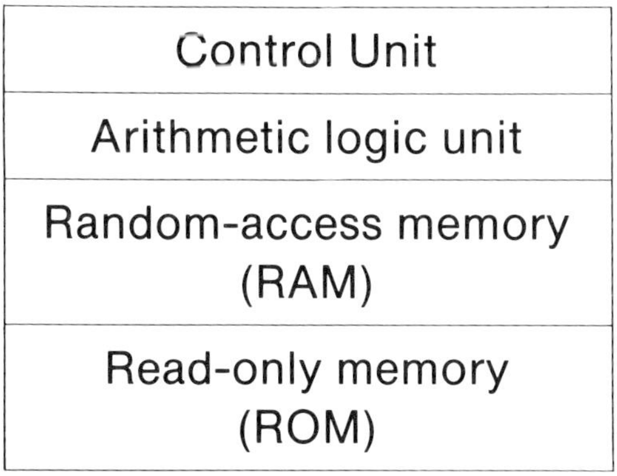

| Control Unit |
| Arithmetic logic unit |
| Random-access memory (RAM) |
| Read-only memory (ROM) |

Fig 4–2.—Schematic diagram of the CPU. The CPU may take up several boards or be integrated onto a little chip, perhaps 2.5 cm × 5 cm × 5 mm.

can be packed into it, either as data or as a programmed instruction. Certain applications are not possible if the word length is too short. Nuclear medical data consist of counts acquired from a small area; these may range from 1 to as many as 10,000 counts or more. The word length should be large enough to treat this information: an 8–bit word can store 255 counts, one 12–bit word 4,095, and a 16–bit word 65,535. If one word will not do, so-called double-precision operations must be resorted to, with attendant lack of speed and doubling of space requirements for the associated operations and storage.

The CPU has a characteristic speed or cycle time between instructions that determines the speed of all of its operations. To give such speeds in microseconds or nanoseconds does not mean much until we know how many operations we want to carry out. The calculations for SPECT require more operations than most other nuclear medicine examinations.

The names of CPUs in use in nuclear medicine today are the PDP 11/34 and Data General Nova 4, which are both minicomputer units, and Intel 8086, Motorola 68000, and LSI 11/23, which are microprocessors. The distinction between mini and micro is as much one of physical size and age as it is of function or speed. The LSI 11/23 addresses 131,072 16–bit words of memory and executes instructions at 1/250,000 second. The M68000 has 16– and 32–bit operations and the Intel 8086 16–bit operations (Wittie 1983).

Once a system has been developed and proved efficient, as several of the commercially available nuclear medicine packages have, there is a natural reluctance to change CPUs. Although a newer unit might offer greater speed or longer word length, the whole software package might very well have to be reprogrammed completely and changed in approach to take advantage of its properties.

Power and Air Conditioning

The CPU is physically anything from one chip to many boards. These are housed in a cabinet. Power is supplied by a regulated power supply and cooling is done by a set of fans. It is important that the power supplied to the unit be of high quality because voltage drops cause the computer to lose information from its memory and surges can burn out delicate parts. Cooling is essential because the instrument generates heat and would burn up without it. The air should be dust free so it will not form a film that could cause a spark or conducting pathway. All this seems obvious, but should be attended to when the computer is installed and in yearly checks afterward.

Machine Language and Operating System

A CPU is distinguished by the instruction set, that is, the machine language to which it responds, and by the operating system, which governs its interactions with the rest of the system and is the software of the control unit of the CPU. A particular CPU may be operated with any one of a number of systems, each for a different procedure, but it has only one machine instruction set; it is analogous to one person having several roles in life. One kind of operation might be to allow only one task at a time, while another might partition the computer into several parts so that several terminals could be active at once.

Software in the form of an operating system keeps track of the various operations the computer is performing and prevents them from coming into conflict. For example, the operating system includes methods for making decisions about whether to accept information from the keyboard first or whether to store information on the disk first. This is usually not obvious to the user, who does not have to participate in any of the decisions, but will have to wait if his use is not the favored one.

Operating systems are written for particular CPUs with a particular kind of operation in mind. In nuclear medicine we see examples of the same CPU programmed in one case to do only one task for one user at a time and in another case to allow one user to set up an acquisition while a second user is processing information gathered previously. Often the manufacturer will supply an operating system; the nuclear medicine computer vendor may decide not to use that operating system but to write his own, because he feels that it would be better suited to the nuclear medicine laboratory. The specialty operating systems are often not nearly as good as the original manufacturer's and make it impossible to use software created for that CPU (with the standard operating system) by other software houses. There have been some attempts to create universal operating systems that would allow standardizing operations and programs. To some extent, UNIX and CP/M represent successes in this area. Differences, designed to exploit the special properties of a CPU, creep into each particular version, however.

The operating system also contains programs called "drivers" for peripheral devices so that the CPU may interact with them. Each device, such as a disk unit or a joystick, must have a driver if it is to be interfaced to the unit.

Programmable computers are those that respond to instructions from outside. The programs, or software, come in several distinct levels. At the most basic level is the machine language or binary-coded instruction set to which the computer actually responds. All instructions to the computer must be translated into this form. Assembly language is a mnemonic form that is translated by an assembler into machine language. The mnemonics may be the same for many CPUs but the machine language instruction set is different for each; assembly language programmers must study the meanings of the mnemonics carefully. The most difficult (for humans to understand) assembly language is used because it can make certain operations much faster or take up less space in the computer. It takes a long time to write programs with this language, however, because every little detail must be spelled out for the computer; in addition, the programs are difficult to decipher. A certain mystique surrounds assembly language programming. Programmers employed by nuclear medicine computer vendors often write in assembly language; most end users do not care to do this.

The higher languages result in software that can be read and understood more easily by human beings because they look and seem more like neat math or algebra. Such languages as BASIC and FORTRAN are in common use today, but we can expect to see Pascal, Ada, and APL in use in the future. The recent trend has been toward languages that force the programmer to structure or modularize the programs, a practice desirable both for ease of reading and alteration and for programming efficiency. All higher languages must be translated into machine language, either by a compiler that translates the whole program and stores the translation for use (FORTRAN) or by an interpreter that translates the program line by line during use (BASIC). Interpreted language programs are easy to write, alter, and use, small to store, but slow to run. Compiled language programs are more cumbersome, may produce more efficient operation, take more storage space, and take longer to get organized and into operation. Computers may be supplied with or without the necessary interpreter or compiler software to allow the end user to program, no matter in what language the applications programs were originally written. Some systems do not even have the means to allow the user to access programs he might write himself.

To avoid obsolescence for as long as possible, the computer's flexibility should be maintained. While special-purpose computer modules designed to acquire data may not ever need to be altered, a nuclear medicine computer should not be purchased unless it has the ability to do different things in each laboratory. This means the computer should be programmable.

What do the particular needs of SPECT imply for the CPU parts and their software? Memory space and processing speed are essential, because SPECT involves the simultaneous use of more numbers than planar imaging. The CPU memory space must be adequate to hold enough of the information so that the system is not seriously restricted by the time it takes to retrieve information from the magnetic disk. For a 12– or 16–bit word, there may be a limit to the amount of memory that can be addressed unless special programming is done. It has already been mentioned that data word size may be a limitation. Processing speed is enhanced by array processors or some other hardware device.

Let us see how much time is involved in preparing transaxial images. The intrinsic speed of the processor, the number of calculations to be made, and the time it takes to shift data in and out (I/O) of the memory from the disk or internal RAM are the factors that make up processing time. It is often possible to streamline software but only up to a certain point. If the calculations must be made serially, they will clearly take longer; an array processor makes it possible to do parallel calculations on images or parts of images, thus speeding up the calculations. Calculations may be made while the images are being acquired or afterward. In a number of circumstances, all of the information is really not known until all the planar projections have been acquired. For example, the whole matrix need not be reconstructed because the organ is only in part of it; uniformity corrections are usually done on all the data at once but could be performed as the computer is acquiring more data; or some quality-control questions about technique should be answered before reconstruction proceeds. Current processing times per transaxial slice image, using array processors, for 64 × 64 matrix images with 64 angles, range from two to five seconds. If the matrix or the number of angles is larger, the processing time will be correspondingly longer. These processing times are commensurate with the times currently required for x-ray CT images (the matrices are larger and the number of angles greater in many cases). If the SPECT examination requires the reconstruction of 32 transaxial images acquired into a 64 × 64 matrix at 64 angles, and if 2.5 seconds are required per image, a total of 80 seconds is required for processing. If 128 angles were used with a 128 × 128 matrix, the time will be eight times as long, or more than ten minutes. If no array processor is used, multiply the time by a factor of 6 or 7. If, in addition, all the calculations are done using an older computer in fixed-point numbers, multiply again by another factor of 10. Human patience allows us the latitude of only one order of magnitude; one to ten minutes for all the processing is acceptable, while 100 minutes is not, in clinical imaging.

There will also be some overhead for processing before the actual reconstruction starts and after it is finished. This is for uniformity correction, filtering, body outline definition, and attenuation correction. Operator intervention and processing set-up time also must be added into the total processing time. The creation of coronal, sagittal, or oblique images should be quite fast because they are all made from the transaxial images, without reference to the acquired data.

Magnetic Storage

Once the computer has acquired data or processed data to create new images, it must have some place to put the information. Also the CPU needs a nonvolatile storage medium for programs, and perhaps intermediate storage. The earliest form of storage was paper tape, but it proved so cumbersome, slow, and perishable that magnetic systems were invented. Various forms of magnetic tape have been used; they are all serial access, meaning that all of the information must be scanned on the way to finding the desired part. Tape drives have been getting faster and the amount of information that can be packed on a length of tape has been increasing, but it is still a slow medium if a great deal of information is involved. Open-reel tapes and cassettes are used for archival data storage.

Magnetic disk storage has been used in nuclear medicine for a number of years. Small floppy disks that hold 1 to 25 million bits of information, up to large fixed disks capable of holding many millions of individual bits of information, have been used. In general the larger the total storage available on a particular device, the more expensive the device and its reader/writer, but the cheaper the storage cost for each individual bit of information and the more rapid the access to the information. Hence, a big investment returns a large amount of rapid storage at a smaller price per unit. Each computer is likely to be equipped with more than one magnetic storage device.

Each of these magnetic storage media has its own format, usually determined by the operating system and by the particular programs in use with it. Because of this individuality, tapes or disks from one vendor's computer cannot be expected to be read by another vendor's computer. Tapes have been more universal, because the placement and number of tracks on tape (either seven or nine) are standard, even if the information format is not. With clever decoding and programming, taped information may be accessible by more than one computer.

All magnetic media must be stored carefully, away from the hazards of magnetic fields and heat. Information is erased by magnetic fields, and heat causes shrinking and stretching and changes the shape of the substrate. Since position on the medium denotes the relative position of the information, the position must be maintained. Floppy disks cannot stand pressure. Hard disks are very sensitive to dust and particles in the air because the read/write head rides on a cushion of air that is smaller than a dust particle. The equipment should be maintained so that it reads and writes the same way all the time, or some of the stored information will become inaccessible. For example, even a minor adjustment during a service call may result in inaccessibility of data.

Nuclear medical data impose certain requirements on the computer storage medium. When data are acquired, they are usually buffered and stored on some rapid random-access medium such as hard disk. The data rate requirements of SPECT are no more than those for ordinary studies, but the quantity of information to be acquired means there must be space to receive it. One frame of data contains between 64 × 64 × 8 (32,768 or 32 K) and 128 × 128 × 16 (262,144 or 256 K in computer jargon) separate bits of information. (Note that we are talking about bits; it may take up to 16 binary bits to represent 1 pixel's worth of counts.) The SPECT data are collected for 60 to 128 angles, so the limits of frame information for one examination are 2 million (M) to 33 M bits. The customary computer information unit is the byte; 8 bits equal 1 byte, so the range just noted is 250 K bytes to 4.2 M bytes. These numbers are still in the realm of those collected during many dynamic nuclear medicine examinations, such as technetium-99m pentetate (DTPA) renal studies. If we also consider dual nuclides, gating, or dynamics, however, the data acquisition requirements become greater.

Suppose for a moment that the acquisition of 64 angles of 64 × 64 matrix information at 16 multigated intervals is required and that we must be prepared for more than 255 counts in each pixel; the data will require 64 × 64 × 64 × 16/8, or 524 K bytes, for acquisition. Or suppose that in 50 minutes we wish to acquire 25 dynamic SPECT images of 32 angles each, in which the information will not contain more than 255 counts per pixel. The data will require 25 × 32 × 64 × 64 × 8/8, or 3.3 M bytes, of storage for acquisition.

The next requirement is that the processed images, as well as the initially acquired information, be stored on a magnetic disk so that they can be referred to quickly for a least some period of time. A typical processed image is contained in a 64 × 64 matrix, 2 bytes deep (which means it can contain counts up to 65,535 counts per pixel). The number of these images ranges from 5 for some small bright lesion to 64 when the whole field is reconstructed with slices 6 mm thick. The system must be prepared to store 64 × 64 × 64 transaxial images and perhaps 32 for each set of coronal and sagittal or oblique images. This adds up to (64 + 64)× 64 × 64 × 2 bytes, or 1 M bytes, of storage for all the processed images, provided there has been no gating, dynamics, or dual nuclide work. Dual nuclides mean double the amount, with perhaps more space for subtracted images. Gating means there may be 8 to 16 times as much information. Some of these estimates are upper limits, but they give an idea of the amounts of immediate storage needed.

Multiply the above requirements by the numbers of such examinations that might be performed in a few days to get the amount of storage needed. It is not satisfactory to delete information immediately after it is processed or even the very next day, because such a practice does not allow time for questions or for changing technique. One must remember that the operating system and the nuclear medicine and SPECT programs also take space, as do other nuclear medical examinations for which the computer is used.

For true flexibility, a disk 20 times the size of one of these examinations will keep most laboratories from data overload, although a large, busy laboratory might prefer to use a 320 M-byte disk, usually in tandem with some smaller disk capable of holding one or two acquisitions. No matter what the disk size is, it is always possible to fill it and to wish that it were larger.

Interface to Camera

The computer must interface to the camera in at least two ways: it receives information from the camera about the position of scintillations and it signals the camera when to rotate and start a new image (in step-and-shoot systems). More complex information about the position of the camera head, patient couch, and gantry angle may also be passed back and forth. In addition, most computers will be programmed to accept a gating signal for cardiac examinations and to control camera acquisition based on that signal.

If the Anger camera is an analog device that puts out voltages to indicate the x and y positions of the scintillations, as well as a triggering signal to indicate a valid pulse, there must be computer hardware to decode the signal and make it digital for the computer. Such a device is called an analog-to-digital converter (ADC); it accepts the analog pulses and creates digital signals for the computer input. These devices are faster than the Anger camera now and pose no special restriction on the flow of information. The ADCs must be checked to be sure they are operating properly and that the information being put into the matrix position corresponds to the position of the scintillation.

Some Anger cameras operate digitally themselves and emit digital signals. The camera's signal may need to be shifted in voltage before the computer can accept it, but should be otherwise ready for digital storage and processing.

When information is sent from the camera to the computer, it may be stored in list mode, in which case it is entered directly into storage with a timing signal, in a static separate frame mode, or in a dynamic framing mode. A great deal of storage space is needed, but after acquisition the data may be reformatted interactively, providing greater accuracy in framing. If the data are stored in static or dynamic frame mode, they are usually piled up in buffer storage on the way into disk storage. The dumping of the buffers is automatic and usually invisible to the user. Data are also buffered on their way between one storage medium and another and for display.

The SPECT data are typically acquired in a dynamic mode. The framing rate corresponds to the time expended for each angular collection or, for the continuously rotating gantry, the time it takes to traverse each angular increment; this time is typically of the order of ten to 20 seconds, so the framing rate is not fast. There is nothing extraordinary about this rate; even gated SPECT does not push the computer to great data acquisition speeds. It is the amount of SPECT data and attendant processed images that stress the ordinary nuclear medicine computer's data storage capacity.

Display Hardware and Software

Display hardware consists of an oscilloscope and the computer controller for it. The oscilloscope is usually responsible for the number of lines or resolution and the ability to show color, while the computer regulates the number of shades of gray and the refresh rate. The computer program control for the display includes all of the contrast enhancement, interpolation, and blow-up programs. There should be at least 64 gray levels available, plus a 512–line display. Gray scale as a function of count density should be under operator control. The screen should be broken up into regions so that several images or cines may be shown at once.

Each vendor has chosen a particular display system. Since the technology changes quickly, one can expect yet further improvements in displays at both the hardware and software levels. The effectiveness of the display depends on an understanding of visual physiology and psychology as well as on the technology available.

Display software, from the use of color and gray scales appropriate to the imaging situation, has been extended to include three-dimensional images with various attributes. Tiling algorithms allow the smooth shading of a surface, while wire structures allow us to see inner structure through the mesh of the outer surface. The images need not be seen from one position only but may be rotated or viewed obliquely. This topic is addressed in the next chapter in the discussion of displaying processed data.

Long-Term Storage—Film and Magnetic Media

Film currently provides the portable medium for diagnosis and display. Typically, a formatter of some kind is used as a slave to the display oscilloscope to provide a photograph of whatever the computer has processed. The formatter should be carefully chosen so that it does not distort the images. Exposure time, trace intensity, and contrast should be adjusted so that as many gray levels as possible are visible. Variables should be tuned to match the image so that the desired details are visible.

Many institutions will also want some long-term magnetic storage to archive SPECT data. Magnetic tape, either open-reel or cassette, or magnetic disks may provide a suitable medium. Decisions as to which to use can be made by examining the economics of space, time, and money involved. The SPECT data that have been uniformity corrected are stored together with any data necessary to reconstruct transaxial images correctly. In time it will be possible to store SPECT data on PACS (picture archiving and communications systems) networks so that they can be called up and manipulated along with other patient images. At that time, storing processed images might well be worth while.

NUCLEAR MEDICINE AND SPECT SOFTWARE

A computer designed for use in nuclear medicine today will come with a basic set of acquisition and processing programs and a number of applications programs usually supplied by users and improved by the vendor. The acquisition programs should allow the full range of dynamic, gated, static, and list mode operations in use today, with matrix dimensions and pixel sizes commensurate with the image information to be acquired. Gated acquisition, with the ability to reject bad beats for a requisite number of frames per beat, should be a routine possibility.

Nuclear medicine processing programs should include easy access to the stored information, all manner of contrast enhancement, and windowing functions in black-and-white and color, with at least 64 shades of gray in the accompanying display. Cine format presentations should be easy to create and to use. Imaging of rectangular and irregularly shaped regions of interest should be possible; their formation can be facilitated with joystick, mouse, or light-pen interaction with the computer. Activity-vs.-time curves should be able to be formed for a number of regions of interest at one time. All of these functions are taken for granted on nuclear medicine systems in operation today, but all of them had to be programmed laboriously and must be programmed again for any new choice of CPU.

All computers should be supplied with the requisite amount of documentation for operations, programming, troubleshooting, and maintenance. Documentation may consist of one very thin booklet or of books and books of instructions and data. Not quantity, however, but quality of the documentation is the important consideration. It is probably more difficult to test the documentation than any other part of the system. "Ask the man who owns one" may still be the best advice.

Acquisition of data for emission tomography should be an extension of other nuclear medicine data acquisition, but it is more complicated, since at very least the computer adds control of the camera's movement to the list of things it must do. The software should permit both step-and-shoot and continuous operations; it should permit stopping the gantry at any angle and continuing the acquisition right there. There should be considerable flexibility as to the choice of numbers of angles, time per angle, acquisition of standard views during the tomographic acquisition, and matrix sizes, as described in the next chapter. The software should permit dual-energy and dual-camera acquisition, as well as gated SPECT. It will be next to impossible for the user to add to or change anything in the acquisition programs, so programs must arrive complete. The user might be able to devise his own, but this is very difficult.

The acquisition process may be controlled by the camera with the computer as a passive observer or it may be controlled by the computer. In either case the only information about the position of the camera head during the examination may be what has been typed in by the operator at the start of the examination. All the other positions are inferred from the starting position and the information about the number of angular increments.

In most extant systems, the camera moves in a circular path around a semielliptical patient. At the present time, the patient contour is observed by the computer either from information given to it on request about the width of the patient or from scatter in the transaxial images. More complex camera hardware will permit automatic patient contour orbits as a result of gantry and/or table movements. The computer should be able to acquire information about the position of the system parts and to direct the movement of the parts, if it is indicated. Probably the SPECT acquisition software should be individualized for each camera system.

Specifics of SPECT processing are treated in the chapters on theory and data acquisition and processing, so the subject is discussed here in general terms only. SPECT processing is derivative processing, more like the distillation of a Fourier transform image from a gated cardiac acquisition than like the activity-vs.-time curves of a radiorenogram. As such, the processing is subject to fashion and new discoveries, which to some extent represent better ways to accomplish a given end. It is therefore necessary that the system be so flexible that it can accept some new and different filter or some new gantry hardware advance without requiring reprogramming or the laboratory's scrapping its computer system and starting over again. The only way to be flexible is to fractionate the processing into its smallest parts so that the programs can be made modular, receiving standard input and delivering standard output. Then new modules can be substituted for old. If programs and the operating system conform to industry standards, it may be possible for the vendor to change CPUs without having to start all over. Equipment-specific software, such as device drivers, would have to be reprogrammed. It is sensible for potential users to inquire into provisions for the future, both as to new software and how it will interdigitate with the old, and as to the ease of upgrading to new hardware when the time comes.

Between the chapters on theory and data processing, the behavior of SPECT software was described. Here, we describe the various SPECT software packages that are available. There are several vendors of computer systems and software as well as of complete systems that include the computer, the Anger camera, and the software.

There are no guarantees that the systems will work the way the advertising literature says they will. One must be especially wary of promises for the future, since programmers are expensive and may not quickly produce what was hoped for. Obviously, SPECT requires a somewhat more sophisticated computer system than those used for ordinary nuclear medicine data acquisition and processing. It requires more integration between the camera and the computer. The SPECT software is more subtle, voluminous, and not as highly developed at this point as that for other nuclear medicine procedures.

Several computer software systems exist for SPECT; however, they become obsolete as the computers are upgraded and as new protocols and algorithms come into common use. The new packages may contain the latest ideas, sometimes even before the programmers are quite finished with them; the more mature products have had the problems worked out and the most obvious flaws removed.

The systems in use today have several roots. The SPETS (Larsson 1980) software package was developed in Sweden for the combination of the General Electric (GE) 400T camera and the Digital Equipment Corporation (DEC) PDP 11/34 computer with the RT-11 operating system and Gamma-11 nuclear medicine software. A SPECT camera-computer interface was provided; software to go with a DEC-supplied video display controller board was available to allow the computer to use the GE formatter. The system requires 92 K of central memory, a floating point processor, and a disk with at least 10 M bytes of storage. Data are stored in a 64 × 64 matrix that is 16 bits deep; a choice of 16, 32, 64, or 128 angles is available in the step-and-shoot mode.

The parts of the system operate well together because the software was written to put them together. The theory and operational choices are very well documented (Larsson 1980). User documentation is more than adequate. The package has been available commercially, and may be still, from Picker. Special adaptations must be made to use the software with other than GE cameras; there is less difficulty with some cameras than with others (King et al. 1983). The Analogic AP400 array processor can be added to this system to accelerate processing.

The PDP 11/34 computer is programmable in FORTRAN and BASIC. The RT-11 operating system is popular among users of DEC computers, so there is a great deal of public domain and proprietary software available.

The University of Michigan software (Rogers and Keyes 1980), until recently commercially available from Medical Data Systems (MDS), can control any one of a number of cameras. The MDS software had been developed to the point where it would acquire and process data from a dual-head SPECT system. The system uses a Data General Nova 4 CPU with 128 K bytes of core memory and a 16–bit word. The operating system was written by MDS for the CPU. There are 2 M bytes of memory in the logic rack and a bit-slice processor for parallel processing. The company was shifting more of the processing into the terminals in the A^3 units. Available disk storage runs from 1.2 M-byte floppy disks through 80 M-byte removable and nonremovable disks to 300 M-byte nonremovable disks. The computer is programmable in FORTRAN, if the FORTRAN compiler was purchased with the system.

The ADAC Laboratories supply SPECT software that controls many of the available cameras; ADAC also sells a SPECT camera. The ADAC CPU is a DEC LSI 11/23 with 11 other attendant microprocessors in the system. It has 25 K bytes or more of program memory and 2 M bytes of display memory. It uses a 16–bit word and the RT-11 operating system, or one that cooperates with RT-11. Disk sizes run from 10 M through 50 to 80 M bytes. The larger model incorporates an array processor. The computer can be programmed in BASIC and FORTRAN and can also use software written for the CP/M microprocessor operating system. The SPECT processing software includes a center of rotation adjustment, even as part of a clinical examination. The operator can choose the filter, which is applied after reconstruction. An iterative attenuation correction is included in the software, but its application takes more time than the standard method and seems to produce no better results. Display software for this system does not allow the user the freedom to adjust the density of the image to allow for the presence of an overly dominant "hot" area.

General Electric developed the Star computer system as a general-purpose nuclear medicine computer with SPECT programs and the GE SPECT unit. The Star has a Data General Nova 4X CPU, with 128 K bytes of core memory and optional Analogic AP400 array processor, which is necessary to have speed for SPECT processing. The CPU uses a 32–bit word, but data words in older versions of the software were not large enough for some nuclear medicine examinations. The operating system is RDOS, which is a Data General product. Disks come in 25 and 80 M-byte sizes. The computer is programmable in FORTRAN. The SPECT software was developed by GE using the SPETS software (Larsson 1980) as a starting point.

More recently, GE has announced its Starcam system, which integrates the computer into the camera. The computer is based on an

Intel 8086 for processing, supported by other computers of the Intel 8000 series for acquisition, floating point processing, display, and keyboard data acceptance. It is assumed that the Intel 8000 series processors, which are faster, will be used when the software is prepared to go with them. There are 512,000 bytes of processing memory. The system supports an 84 M-byte disk. The announced intention is to make the computers network so that computing power and large disk drives can be shared.

Computer Design and Applications, Inc. (CD&A) had been developing SPECT software as part of their nuclear medicine package. The software has now been acquired by Siemens. The CPU is a micro T-11 controlling a 2903 bit-slice processor for parallel processing. It has 256 K bytes of program memory and the same amount of display memory, as well as 500 K bytes of image memory. The system uses the RT-11 operating system, again with the availability of a great deal of nonnuclear-medicine general software. It controls disks from 40 M to 140 M bytes. It can be programmed in FORTRAN and BASIC. The company had been developing a large DEC VAX-based system capable of performing all the processing for a nuclear medicine department, using the VMS operating system, and accepting data from their data acquisition units.

The Siemens ECT processor has been under development. It processes data from Siemens cameras that have been acquired by the Siemens Scintiview system. The CPU is an Intel 8086 microprocessor with a Siemens AP4 array processor. It has 512 K bytes of program memory and 1,024 K bytes of image memory. It uses the Intel RMX-86 operating system and can control an 80 M-byte Winchester disk. It is programmable in FORTRAN. It will have to be seen how the CD&A acquisition will affect Siemens' computer development.

The Elscint APEX computer, based on the Intel 8086 CPU, uses an 8089 chip for input/output and an 8085 chip to control the terminal. It controls 640 K bytes of core memory and an AMD 2901 bit-slice processor. The disks range in size upward from 15 M bytes. The computer is an integral part of the system, permitting acquisition into either 64 × 64 or 128 × 128 matrix sizes in continuous operation, with a choice of angular increment. The FORTRAN compiler is expected to be available for this computer in the future.

The preceding paragraphs do not cover the complete range of computers available with SPECT software, but should be sufficient to indicate the major types of options most recently available.

In addition to the commercially available software packages, others can be acquired. Huesman and co-workers (1977) developed a package of programs at Donner Laboratory that is available to anyone. The programs use Fourier space methods, whereas most of the other programs discussed perform all their calculations in real space. The package was written for use on a large computer, but the small computers have been getting bigger and faster, so its use on nuclear medicine minicomputers is not impossible now.

A complete review of software should not leave out the systems designed for use with the probe-based instruments. The most notable of these are the Cleon 710 and 711, and the Medimatic Tomomatic 64.

The Cleon 710 is controlled by a Data General S/230 Series Eclipse computer with 128 K bytes of core memory. The computer was supplied with a 10 M-byte hard disk drive and dual 600 K-byte floppy disk drives. The computer can acquire or process data. It is programmable in FORTRAN. The Cleon 711 or Harvard Head Scanner remains a research instrument.

The Medimatic Tomomatic 64 was originally controlled by a Univac U77 computer with 64 K of core memory, operating with a 24–bit word. Currently, the smaller instruments still use the Univac, while the larger ones are controlled by a DEC MicroVax II, with 1 M bytes of core memory.

Operations

Under the heading of management come the strategies for operating the system and managing the personnel. It is not possible to foresee the place of SPECT in the nuclear medicine laboratory in five or ten years. Some laboratories are preparing to acquire data from all major imaging examinations in the SPECT mode, while others have made little or no use of it. Given the wide spectrum of applications described in Chapter 8, it is difficult to be more than general about the numbers of cameras and computers that a laboratory should have. Various operating strategies are examined here, so that everyone might find a comfortable model. While studying each of the figures, the reader should notice where compatibility between one instrument and the next must be observed.

On one end of the spectrum is the busy laboratory in which most major examinations are SPECT examinations. In such a milieu, one operating strategy is to have each camera be a law unto itself, with its own computer (see Fig 4–3). Once the processing is finished, the results might well be shifted (either by moving a disk or through electronic means) to an imaging station for diagnosis, thus freeing the

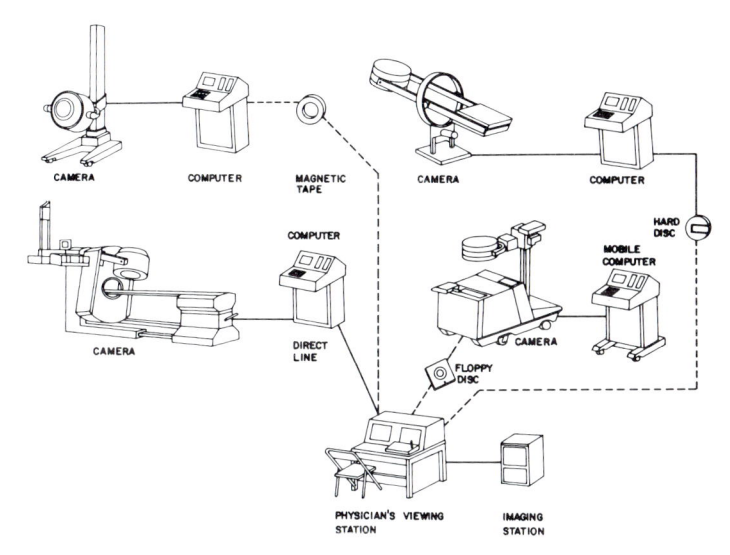

Fig 4–3.—Diagram of a laboratory in which each busy camera has its own computer. The results may be viewed at each computer or taken (often by hand-carrying tapes or floppy disks) to a central viewing station in the physicians' reading area.

system for another examination. Another strategy would be to have only acquisition units attached to each camera and to send all the data to a central computer for processing (see Fig 4–4). The central computer and its operator would have to keep up with the load, accomplishing the processing, film exposures, disk management, and archival storage. If each SPECT examination can be reconstructed in five minutes, it is not unreasonable to expect someone to be able to produce two completed examinations per hour, plus keep abreast of file maintenance and other computer housekeeping duties. Cine and other image presentations for diagnosticians could be handled by an imaging station or a videotape system, unless the central computer could also allow queries from the physicians while processing of SPECT images was taking place. Diagrams rather like those that are made to help decide where to place furniture can be useful in putting together the pieces of a working camera-computer system.

In the smaller laboratory, or one in which SPECT is not much used, the system must perform other duties. In such a case it is possible to treat the SPECT examination just as one would any other procedure that takes a large amount of computer power for processing (Fig 4–5). It is the necessity for computer power that creates the difficulties. The SPECT needs are so great that very often the computer

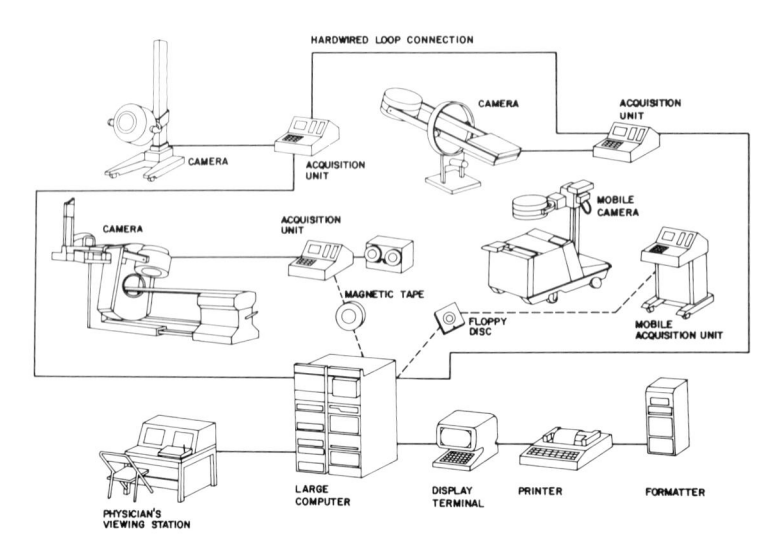

Fig 4–4.—Diagram of a laboratory in which only acquisition units are attached to each camera. The data are sent to a larger central computer for processing and ultimate viewing. The links between the units may be a network, some sort of hardwired connection such as an RS232 connection, or the hand-carrying of a magnetic medium, perhaps directly to the other unit or to some intermediate "translator." This system looks very similar to that shown in Figure 4–3; the difference is that each camera is served by a relatively inexpensive acquisition unit, instead of a full-blown system.

cannot be allowed to perform other duties, such as acquisition, while processing is in progress. This can be a hindrance in a busy laboratory. A way around the problem is to isolate the SPECT system so that the computer and camera work as a unit, and to schedule no other acquisitions during the routine time for SPECT processing. Such an operating strategy may very well make one or two technologists responsible for the whole SPECT operation, which would be very helpful.

Some persons see computers as fearsome creatures; others have no sympathy with the operation of complex instrumentation. These persons should not be put in charge of the computer or the SPECT camera. In its daily operation the computer needs a friend or friends who will stick up for it and guard it against bad conditions. It should be operated sympathetically and gently. The computer behaves according to its programmed logic, but sometimes it takes human cleverness to figure out what the logic might be. The operator should have the patience to do this. A calm, peaceful, orderly setting will contribute to the stable operation of the system, with fewer noticed and unnoticed mistakes and fewer missing data.

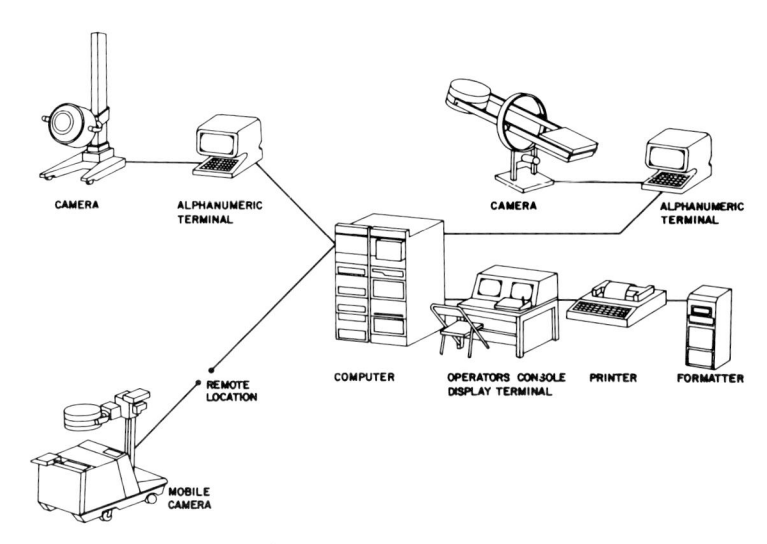

Fig 4-5.—Diagram of a laboratory in which one computer serves several cameras. The cameras need not be all of one brand, as long as they are compatible with the computer. This is the pre-SPECT configuration of most laboratories. Two, three, or four cameras might be served by the one computer, with simultaneity of operation, more or less, for acquisition or processing or both.

Off-line processing and an imaging station have both been mentioned. The implications of off-line processing are several: the computer power for processing may not have to be replicated for each SPECT camera and, indeed, the cameras might be from different manufacturers and still be compatible with the processing hardware and software; and there will always be a short time lag while the data are being transferred, which seems to be handled more efficiently in some laboratories than in others. Once the data have been transferred, they must wait in the processing queue, but the camera and acquisition system are free to acquire another examination. Throughput may be a problem if the processing system handles a variety of examinations; there may be a significant delay, which could be a problem in certain cases. Some laboratories have a special person come in on a second shift to process information collected during the day. The principal objections to this are that such a person does not know what occurred during acquisition and cannot find out, and the results are not produced for diagnosis on the day of the examination.

An imaging station separate from any of the processing computers allows physicians and other interested parties to view the images without disturbing the flow of computer acquisition and processing. It is essential that the images and cine presentations be available to the diagnosticians, and viewing them with an imaging station is often more convenient than doing so in the computer room. Analog video data storage with a video cassette system allows information to be stored according to a protocol and is the least expensive option. It allows no further data manipulation. An imaging station (a small computer), attached to enough disk storage to hold the examinations of several days, allows examination data and reconstructed images to be viewed together, with a number of contrast-enhancement and image-manipulation functions.

Networking is a PACS (picture archiving and communication systems) concept. Standards have not yet been fully developed for passing image data around between one instrument or computer and another. Until standards are promulgated, several vendors and many users will experiment with various methods. For now, compatibility is best achieved by using magnetic tape or possibly a small computer such as an IBM PC or a Macintosh as an intermediary to translate data from one floppy disk format to another for transmission between SPECT computers. Some older systems already have solved various communications problems, so there is a certain amount of compatibility; however, one can never assume that two computers of different makes or of different operating systems will "speak" to each other or read each other's disks.

BIBLIOGRAPHY

Huesman, R. H., et al., eds. *User Manual: Donner Algorithms for Reconstruction Tomography.* Berkeley, Calif.: Lawrence Berkeley Laboratory, University of California, 1977.

King, M. A., et al. Preliminary characterization of the properties of a new rotating SPECT imaging system. In *Emission Computed Tomography: Current Trends,* ed. P. D. Esser. New York: Society of Nuclear Medicine, 1983, pp. 91–104.

Larsson, S. A. Gamma camera emission tomography. *Acta Radiol.* (Suppl.) 363:1–75, 1980.

Rogers, W. L., and Keyes, J. W., Jr. *Michigan Tomographic Reconstruction Program, MTOM—Version M7.* Ann Arbor: University of Michigan, 1980, pp. 1–32.

Wittie, L. D. Microprocessors and microcomputers. In *Encyclopedia of Computer Science and Engineering,* ed. A. Ralston and E. D. Reilly, Jr. New York: Van Nostrand Reinhold, 1983, pp. 969–977.

5

Data Acquisition and Processing

The parts of a working SPECT instrument, its hardware, algorithms, and software, have been treated in the three previous chapters. We now discuss how to use the system in terms of the rationale for the choices to be made in clinical and research laboratory circumstances. Since acquisition and processing make two complementary parts of the total examination, we consider them serially.

The variables of data acquisition and processing and their effects on the resulting images are explored one by one. It is assumed that the SPECT instrument is functioning properly. The consequences of instrument malfunction are discussed in the chapter on quality assurance (Chapter 7).

ACQUISITION VARIABLES

Uniformity, Linearity, and Other Corrections

Before acquisition of SPECT information begins, the system must be quality controlled. Requisite procedures must be performed to make sure the camera acquisition will be satisfactory as far as linearity and uniformity are concerned. As was stressed in Chapter 3, the matrix size and count densities for the quality control procedures must be at least as great as those of a SPECT examination, or the very procedures designed to produce quality will actually ruin the images. The rest of this chapter assumes that the camera is functioning well, with all quality assurance and correction images collected whenever necessary.

Each manufacturer has arrived at a different solution to the problems that create nonuniformities in the Anger camera field and has installed different microprocessor-controlled circuits to eliminate difficulties. The user should try to discover how each of the corrections of his system functions and under what circumstances they will not work correctly. When in doubt about the correction procedures, one should try to make the tests and correction images approximate the clinical situation in count rate, but collect four to ten times as many counts as in the clinical setting. The user must look into the methods for quality assurance for his own systems and be sure that quality control procedures are carried out effectively and efficiently.

Some cameras assume a built-in relationship between different nuclides, so that characteristics "learned" for one energy are automatically related to those at other energies. Other cameras require repeaking and acquiring of new correction factors for each new nuclide. Either method may be acceptable, depending on the care with which all the relationships are built.

The controls of most Anger cameras include switches to change the orientation of the image in the system, so patient images can appear in the correct orientation on film. The position of the switches affects the orientation of data acquired by the computer. Thus it is necessary for correction factors made from data acquired by the computer to be stored in the same orientation as the patient data with which they are to be used. For example, if uniformity is being corrected with a 30 M-count image acquired in a computer file with the switches in the zero position, and then tomography is performed with the patient's feet closest to the gantry, setting the switches to put the patient image upright in the persistence oscilloscope and formatter fields will necessitate two changes from the usual practice. The first is a rotated correction image; the computer software should have built-in protection against using the wrong orientation for correction. The built-in protection will have to be overridden with a special program. The second change is that the transaxial images may not appear in the usual CT orientation for transaxial slices, but may be upside down or backward. Careful use of marker sources for orientation, as discussed later in this chapter, will help.

Center of Rotation and Absolute Pixel Size

In most other uses of the camera and computer together it is sufficient to have the camera image in the computer's matrix; there is no necessary connection between the position of the matrix or the size of the pixels and the image of the camera on that matrix. In SPECT this relationship must be established, and in a particular way. The camera image should be centered in the matrix so that the axis of rotation is in the center of the matrix, and the image must be the same shape as the camera head. In addition, the absolute size of a computer pixel must be defined and checked periodically. The measurement of pixel size provides the absolute distance necessary for the use of the attenuation correction, which is defined in terms of centimeters, not pixels. More is said about this in the quality assurance chapter. Some instruments allow for the computer to adjust the collected matrix data to put the axis of rotation in the center of the matrix. Like uniformity, this correction might better be attended to with a screwdriver than by a computer correction, if possible. Whether the correction is done manually or by the computer, it will be done with reference to information collected using point or line sources.

Collimator

The choice of collimator depends on the radionuclide to be used and the examination to be performed, assuming the gantry is strong enough to rotate any of the collimators available for the camera. The precaution of collimating for the highest energy must be observed. The most trouble comes from a nuclide with a wide range of energies, because it is tempting for the user to ignore the highest energies. Collimating for the highest energy is often difficult, so experiments must be performed to study the effect on resolution of using collimators with lower energy ratings (Polak, English, and Holman 1983). In the case of iodine-123, the collimator should be chosen to match the expected quantity of iodine-124 impurity at the time of imaging (Coleman et al. 1983).

Collimators can be designed to emphasize resolution or sensitivity. Greater sensitivity comes from larger holes, shorter holes, and thinner septa. Better resolution comes from smaller and longer holes. The collimator is tuned to a particular energy with the length of the holes and the thickness of the septa. If the energy is exceeded or the holes are not long enough, a point spread image will have not only the central hole showing, but broad wings (Fig 5–1) caused by septal penetration. The effect of such septal penetration on the modulation transfer function (MTF) is to make the collimator less sensitive to high-frequency changes. Resolution is fuzzed out by septal penetration.

126 Chapter 5

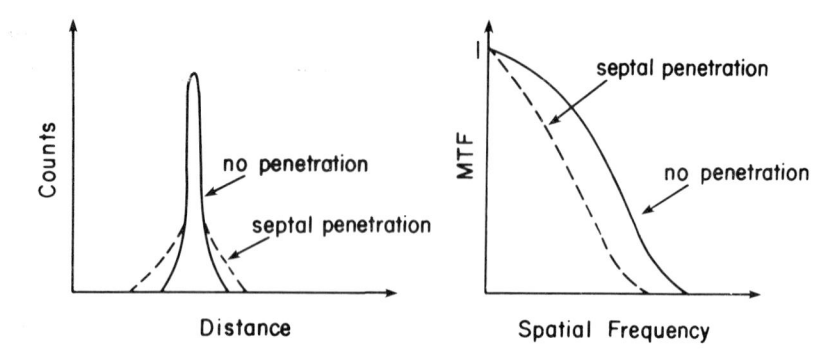

Fig 5–1.—The point-spread function when the collimator septa are penetrated, compared to one when they are not. The modulation transfer functions of the two point-spread functions are compared on the right.

Septal penetration occurs in the collimator and is to be differentiated from scattered radiation in the patient or object, which causes the same general shape of line spread function, but is only found in the presence of a scattering medium, provided there is no collimator septal penetration (Fig 5–2).

Collimators cannot be designed so the septa are uniform in thickness in every direction. Three-, four-, and six-sided figures can be closely packed; when circles are densely packed, it is usually in a hexagonal array, because this is the closest packing possible. The most likely hole pattern for a collimator is a hexagonal array, so if the camera is presented with a very radioactive source or a source of an energy higher than that for which it was designed, septal penetra-

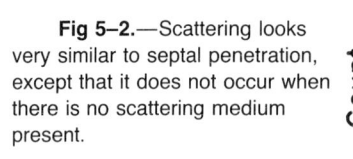

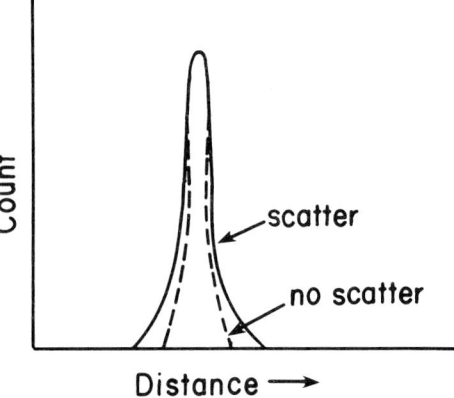

Fig 5–2.—Scattering looks very similar to septal penetration, except that it does not occur when there is no scattering medium present.

tion will cause a six-sided star pattern from the collimator. Figure 5–3 shows such a pattern from a source. Some collimators have square symmetry and a four-sided star pattern.

Collimators may be specially designed for certain parts of the body. For example, the human head is smaller than the camera's field of view, is at the end of the body, and is of a very different size from the shoulders. The angulated collimator (see Chapter 3) allows us to take advantage of the head's being at the end of the body to reduce the radius of rotation. A collimator with long holes achieves the same purpose, but by using the long holes to get around the shoulders (Mueller et al. 1984). A fan-beam collimator (see Fig 3–4) allows the use of more of the camera's crystal for detection (Jaszczak, Chang, and Murphy 1979; Tsui et al. 1984). It can be used for any part of the body that does not fill the field of view, but a check must be made to be sure this is true at all angles. Extremities are especially well imaged by fan-beam collimators. Because the angle the collimator accepts is great, the resolution should be better; the count rates may or may not be better, depending on the collimator design.

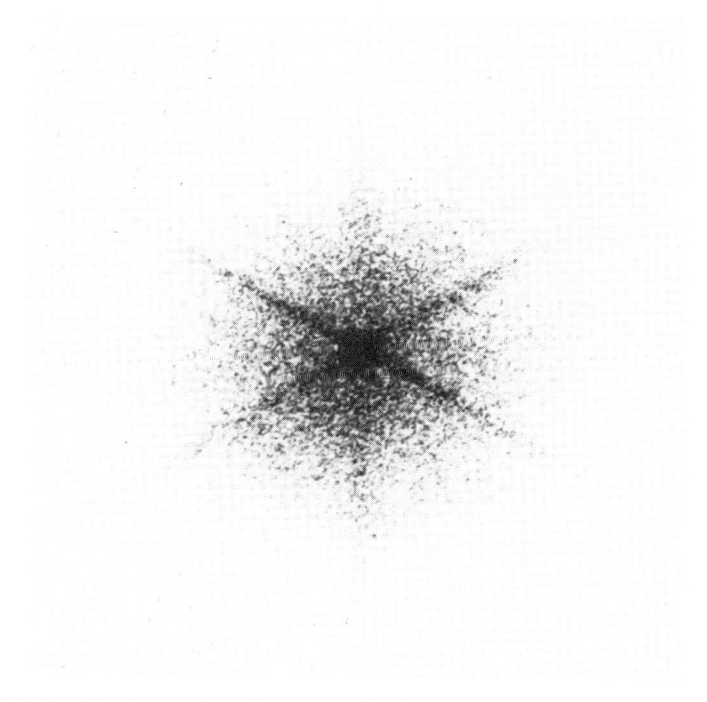

Fig 5–3.—The image of a point source, showing the hexagonal pattern of penetration. This image was made with an iodine-131 source on a technetium-99m collimator.

Energy Setting and Windows

Energy peak settings are selected in the same ways as for planar imaging. Linearity and uniformity depend on setting the energy peak in the same, reproducible way every time a particular radionuclide is imaged. To this end, most cameras incorporate push-button nuclide settings, so the energy peak need not be reselected each time the nuclide is used, or at least the whole process need not begin at the beginning. Energy peaks may be selected automatically by reference to the highest count rate in a narrow window for the correct nuclide, but can also be tuned in by reference to a visible spectrum or a gray wedge. The highest count rate may be used as an aid in peaking, as long as the source is not surrounded by scattering material. The lower-energy peaks, such as for thallium-201, must be found with the source well away from back-scattering medium.

One must be sure that the method of notifying the operator of the camera whether or not the energy selected is on the peak is as sensitive as the instrument. In our experience with an older camera, the spectral display had to be combined with the count rate to achieve a satisfactory, reproducible peak.

Multiple peaks may be desirable. There are several ways they might be used, but many cameras are not versatile enough to take full advantage of these possibilities. First, multiple peaks may allow the camera to collect counts from several energies so the counts can be added together to make an image; this would be useful for work with nuclides such as gallium-67, which has several peaks. (One should look into whether the camera also applies its correction factors for all the energy peaks or just the principal one.) Second, multiple peaks may be used to image two different parts of a single nuclide's energy spectrum, such as the photoelectric and Compton scatter peaks from technetium-99m; in this case, the results must remain separate and be stored separately in the computer. Third, multiple peaks may be used for several nuclides, so that the patient may be imaged simultaneously with two nuclides; these results also must be stored separately by the computer. Each of these modes of operation requires something different from the multichannel analyzers or spectrometers that select the counts to be included in the energy window (Fig 5–4). In Figure 5–4, A, there are questions about corrections for these three peaks; are they all corrected and, if so, how? What does scattered radiation, different for each peak, do to the correction? Looking at Figure 5–4, B, suppose we wish to image the photopeak and Compton scatter separately; the peaks are coupled, but the lower

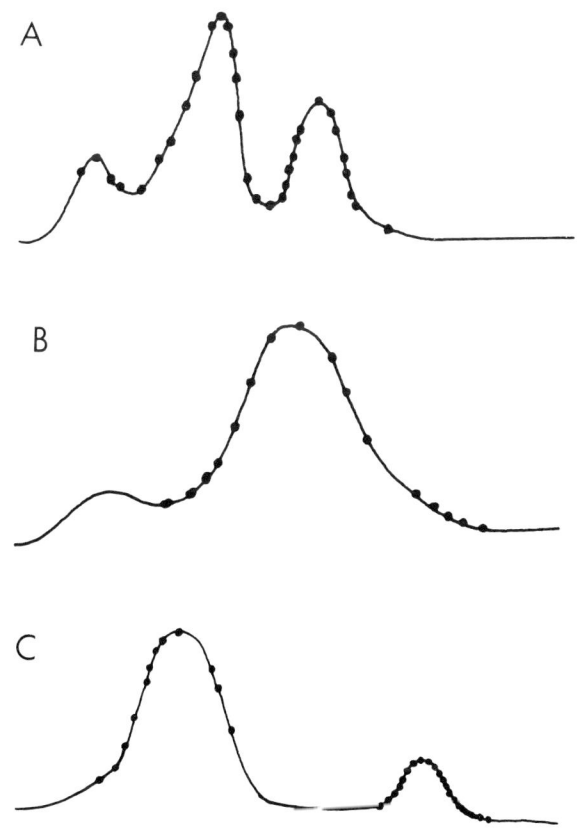

Fig 5–4.—**A,** gallium-67 spectrum. The positions of the other two peaks are usually based on the first one, so they all move as the lowest-energy one moves. **B,** technetium-99m spectrum, showing the photopeak and Compton scattering. **C,** graph shows technetium-99m and iodine-131 simultaneously.

one is not the one on which to base the settings. What happens when scattering medium is used? What kinds of corrections are appropriate for the Compton scatter peak? Further questions arise with Figure 5–4, C: what are the effects of spilldown and spillup, sum peaking, on the images and on the corrections? Interactions in the instrument may mean spectral superposition is not observed. These peaks must be independently set and the instrument must be able to do all of its corrections at both energies regardless of interference from the other nuclide. This is a tall order; scatter from the higher-energy peaks becomes a serious issue (Saw et al. 1984; Floch, Alazraki, and Wooten 1984).

Window setting becomes the next point after the peak is selected, although in many instruments the two are coupled, in the sense that one is telling oneself that the peak lies in the center of the window. Window width allows the capture of as much of the primary radiation as possible, while removing from consideration scattered radiation and radiation from other peaks or nuclides. Only primary radiation contributes to a sharp image of the distribution of radioactivity. For low- to medium-energy radionuclides, the Gaussian shape of the peak and of the scattered radiation overlap, so that there is tension between accepting as much of the primary radiation as possible and eliminating the scattered radiation from consideration. Since the scattered radiation is of lower energy than the primary radiation, it is not symmetrically placed about the peak, but forms a subpeak on the low-energy side. The scatter peak is always present, even in the absence of any scattering medium around the source, because of scatter originating in the collimator and the crystal itself. Because the spectrum of a radionuclide observed without scatter is as pure as it can be, this spectrum is used for peak and window selection. If the window can be chosen independently of the peak, it is soon seen that it should be set slightly asymmetrically to the high-energy side, if the purpose is to avoid as much scattered radiation as possible (Fig 5–5).

The conventional way to operate an Anger camera is to center the window about the peak; before microprocessor nonuniformity corrections, this was the only way to assure a uniform image. The windows might be narrow or wide, but they were always centered. It is now possible to use a microprocessor to correct for the effects of an offset window (King et al. 1983; LaFontaine, Graham, and Stein 1984). It is by no means obvious that this maneuver will work for all

Fig 5–5.—The technetium-99m spectrum in an Anger camera with an asymmetric window indicated.

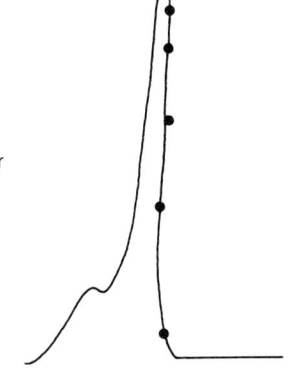

cameras or that the contrast increase is worth some of the nonuniformities introduced (La Fontaine et al. 1984).

If the asymmetric window is not practical, one can try narrowing the window to see if it will improve the instrument's performance (Croft, Teates, and Honeyman 1982). The improvement caused by decreasing the amount of scattered radiation in the image will be balanced by increased uncertainty in the counts because of lower count density.

Each Anger camera is an individual. This is expressed in many ways, including the meaning of "window width." The standard meaning of a percentage window is that it is a percentage of the peak setting; thus a 15% window at 140 KeV is 21 KeV wide, from about 130 to 150 KeV if the window is symmetrically placed. A symmetric 40% window would be 56 KeV wide, from 112 to 168 KeV. The energy resolution of a large flat thallium-activated sodium iodide [NaI(Tl)] crystal should be 15% to 20% at 140 KeV, or 21 to 28 KeV full width at half maximum (FWHM). A window that is narrower than the FWHM must be precisely set to avoid losses of large numbers of counts. As the window width is varied from the narrowest to the widest setting, there should be an increase in the count rate. Figure 5–6 shows the variation in count rate with window width for two cameras from the same manufacturer.

Current practice is to set a narrow window, 10% to 15%, offset to the high-energy side for cameras whose uniformity is adequate when this strategy is used. Every system must be tested to see if it is uniform enough and stable enough to accept a narrow offset window.

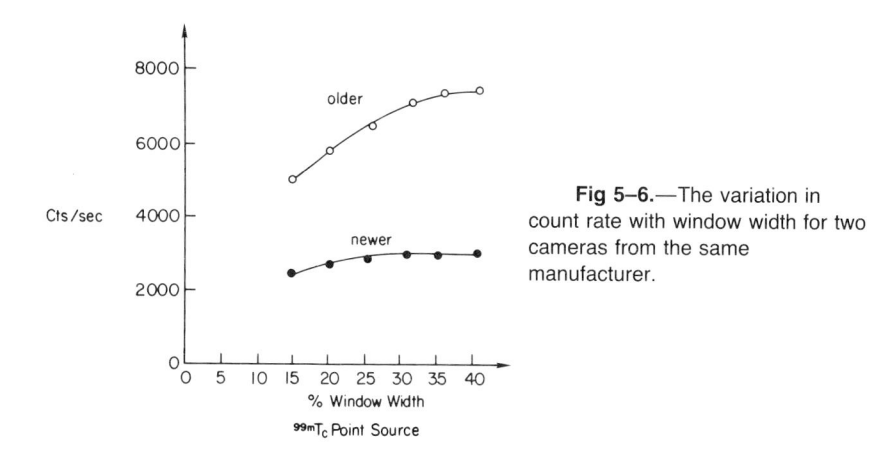

Fig 5–6.—The variation in count rate with window width for two cameras from the same manufacturer.

Another approach to the scattering problem involves the removal of scattered counts by processing, which is treated later in this chapter.

Matrix Size, Angular Increment, and Implications

The choices that need to be made, based on the desired resolution and statistical properties of the information, are those of computer matrix dimensions, number of angles (or angular segments if the motion is continuous), time per angle, patient dose, and whether to image for 180 degrees or 360 degrees around the patient.

The matrix sizes used are typically 64 × 64 or 128 × 128, implying a pixel size of 6 × 6 mm or 3 × 3 mm, respectively, for the camera with a large field of view. In addition, the question of the number of angular intervals to use is related to matrix size, since one would wish to keep the angular resolution consonant with the spatial resolution; for a 30–cm-diameter object, one should use about 180 angles with the 128 × 128 matrix and 90 angles with the 64 × 64 matrix; there is a factor of 8 difference in the amount of computer storage space each requires. The range of choices available commercially may differ, but each system has choices similar to these. Spreading the counts over the larger number of pixels and angles, assuming the same total time for the examination, increases the statistical uncertainty and thus the noise in the final images. The best way to decide which matrix size to use is to look at the planar resolution of the system and the requirements for resolution in the results. Camera resolution, respiratory or other movement of the organ (as in imaging lung, liver, or heart), or count rate limitations may make any more matrix resolution than 64 × 64 unnecessary. In addition, the larger matrix takes eight times as much computer storage, working space, and processing time, so that in older (smaller, slower) systems, computer limitations may make moot the question of which matrix configuration to use.

Step-and-shoot discontinuous motion calls for a choice of a number of angles and dwell time, which determine the total time of the examination; for continuous rotation, the total time for a rotation is chosen, and in some cases the number of angular increments into which the rotational information is collected may be chosen. Collection in list mode, with the time signals being related to the angular position, and a finely gridded matrix would allow reformatting with a range of resolutions and precisions; list mode would require a great deal of disk space for the initial collection.

Larsson (1980) experimented and found that with the GE 400T system, either a 64 × 64 or a 128 × 128 matrix was sufficient because there was an improvement in resolution of less than 1 mm in going from the smaller matrix to the larger. He also found that if point sources were being imaged, the artifacts of a 64-angle acquisition were obvious, but that the noise and statistical inaccuracies of clinical data seemed to make the use of 128 angles unnecessary. His use of 64 angular data increments clinically, which means 32 angular increments in the reconstruction (since opposing data are added together), is a compromise.

180 vs. 360 Degrees of Data Collection

For some organs and some imaging situations, 180 degrees of data collection may be in order. Low-energy photons, such as those of Tl-201, do not penetrate the body well, so there is very little activity to be measured on the other side of the patient; it has been felt by some practitioners that best use could be made of the imaging time by acquiring data from only the more radioactive half of the body (spending twice as long at each angle). Since 180-degree acquisition has been used most extensively in cardiac imaging, the reader is referred to Chapter 8 for a thorough discussion of the two sides of the question.

Time per Angle or Total Examination Time

The amount of time that can be devoted to each angular image depends on the patient's condition and technologist's ingenuity, as well as the practical amount of time to spend on the examination.

The general principles for SPECT are the same as those for the rest of nuclear medicine: while keeping the radiation dose to a minimum, acquire the greatest number of counts consistent with patient comfort and immobility. Preventing patient movement is the task of trained technologists, but the length and conduct of the examination are important too. In deciding on the acquisition variables of matrix size, time per image, and number of angular intervals, one may wish to choose a certain number of total counts or a total length of time for the examination, and optimize the other variables to fit these constraints.

No matter in what light one considers the question of numbers of counts collected, it is always better, all other things being equal, to have more rather than fewer. In nuclear medicine, the other things are never equal: the question is whether to acquire more counts by using more radioactivity and increasing the patient's radiation dose, by increasing the time per image and thus increasing the likelihood that the patient will move and spoil the examination, or by using a different radiopharmaceutical or nuclide. These are hard questions that do not have identical answers in all situations. The SPECT practitioner should always be aware of the numbers of counts per pixel being acquired and be thinking of ways to maximize the counts.

The count rate is directly proportional to the amount of activity of the radionuclide given to the patient, as is the patient's radiation dose. It must be the clinician's decision whether the benefit of more counts will offset the cost in radiation dose. It is not ethical to increase the radiation dose merely for convenience or to reduce the time spent imaging. To improve the images and obtain more information, however, one should consider increased amounts of radionuclide activity, keeping in mind that the uncertainty of the results varies as $1/N^{1/2}$, so doubling the radiation dose decreases uncertainty by $1/2^{1/2}$, or 0.707. Doubling imaging time has the same effect, but this also has diminishing returns in terms of patient movement and the changing distribution of radioactivity.

The practical resolution of all the preceding questions is that most laboratories use a 64 × 64 computer matrix with 2– to 6–degree intervals (60 to 180 angular increments for 360–degree acquisition), and acquire data for 20 to 40 minutes. The total time and total number of counts are often kept constant, while such variables as dwell time and angular increment are varied. The amount of radionuclide injected is often at the upper limit of the activity range suggested in the radiopharmaceutical manufacturer's package insert. Specific details for particular organs are discussed in the chapter on clinical applications.

Gating

The newer SPECT systems permit acquisition of gated SPECT images. For the simplest of the gating methods, which used one ordinary-sized computer data file, the planar projection matrix was divided in half horizontally across the middle; end-systole was collected into one half and end-diastole into the other. When reconstruction was performed from the bottom to the top, each was reconstructed in its turn. For more than two images in the gated sequence, the computer must have a way to store the gated images at each angle and to access them for reconstruction. Of course, it takes more computer storage space and time for such processing, and the statistics of the images are poor unless longer times are used for acquisition.

Gating of heart and lung SPECT examinations will become more routine. It will provide both actual three-dimensional images of function and the opportunity truly to quantify volume of tissue or blood.

Patient-Following Orbit

The best resolution can be obtained from the Anger camera when the radioactivity is close to the collimator; a patient-contour-following orbit is a way to achieve this proximity. Newer SPECT systems have automatic patient-contour-following methods. A variety of mechanical solutions is possible for the single-headed system (Chapter 3), while a dual-headed system is limited to motion of the heads toward and away from the patient placed between them.

Patient-contour following does improve resolution, often measured as the contrast of a nonradioactive sphere in radioactive surroundings, approximating the imaging of a liver lesion (King et al. 1983; Croft, Teates, and Honeyman 1982) (Fig 5–7).

Patient-contour–following orbits in use today involve table motion, camera head motion, or both. In some cases the computer must adjust the position of the data in the matrix to maintain the rotational axis's central postition in the matrix, while in others this is not necessary, because the camera head follows a concentric-circles

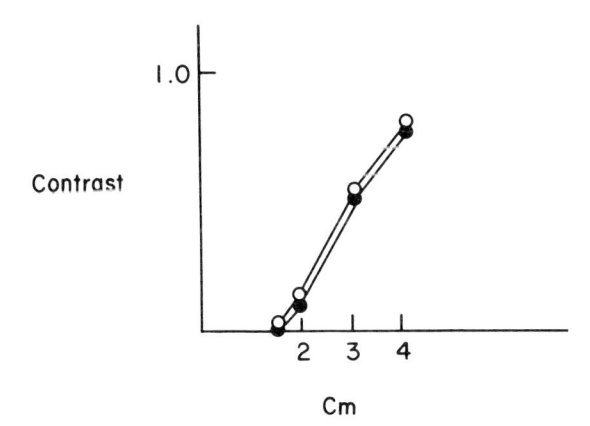

Fig 5–7.—The graph shows the improvement in contrast for spheres of graduated sizes for a contoured orbit around the Alderson organ-scanning phantom compared to a circular orbit (King et al. 1983).

orbit. Typically, the user "teaches" the system the patient contour before the start of image acquisition by moving the camera head or table to the positions of extremes of the patient ellipse. Since at very least patient movement contributes to poor resolution and at most it could cause the camera head to hit the patient, such motion should be prevented by attentive technologists. Some methods that move the table have the advantage of blurring out artifacts caused by camera nonuniformity, because a particular part of the patient is seen by different parts of the crystal. Imaging a series of point sources will permit a check of this system. It is important that the point sources be distributed around a volume to represent a patient.

A manual system, such as the one used in our laboratory (see Fig 3–20), requires well-trained technologists to operate it. The SPECT examination is begun with the camera close to the patient's anterior side. After determining that some change in path is required because the camera face is too close to or far away from the patient, the technologist stops the computer's acquisition of data, moves the camera head toward or away from the patient along a radius, reads the new angle on the gantry angle indicator, and repositions the patient couch to match the new angle. Camera acquisition is restarted. Point sources, placed on the patient so as to be in the camera's field of view but not to interfere with the image of the organ, allow us to tell when the patient bed has not been correctly positioned and, indeed, to use the computer to move the image of a mispositioned frame back into line. The rotating cine presentation is very helpful for picking up errors.

No matter what the contouring method, there should be a safe way to stop the camera when it applies too much pressure to the patient or to the imaging table. The stopping method should allow for restarting acquisition without the loss of any images, and with the loss of only one angular imaging period. The patient should be sufficiently well restrained so that having the camera graze him will not cause him to jump or move out of position.

Patient Positioning

The aim of positioning is to present the field of interest so the Anger camera can rotate around it in as tight an orbit as possible. When the patient is positioned optimally, the center of the organ being imaged is on the axis of rotation. The organ should not be out to the side because the center is the position with the least distortion. The organ must be visible to the Anger camera from all angles; if it is not, some of the data necessary for reconstruction will be missing and it will appear on the edge of the transaxial image. To prevent difficulties, a rapid manual or automated trial run is made to check the position of radioactivity in the field of view at all angles.

Acquisition of data for 180 degrees may allow the organ being imaged to be placed on the axis of rotation, off-centering the patient himself, for a semicircular path that hugs the patient.

Patients should be positioned as comfortably as possible on the usually narrow imaging table. Hospital gowns should be substituted for bulky or flowing clothing. Metal jewelry and buckles, braces, false teeth, and wigs should be removed for relevant portions of the body. Internal absorbers such as metal plates, joints, or pacemaker batteries should be noted, so the diagnostician does not have to guess what they are. The urinary bladder should be emptied, especially if it is a site of significant radioactivity. Radioactive catheters should be moved away from the body or positioned in the least distracting way. Thought should be given to the presence of any wires or tubes connected to the patient, so that they are not wound around the camera head or pulled out as the camera rotates; placing all such lines along the patient and taping them to him may prevent trouble during imaging. This process is reversed when moving the patient back onto his stretcher.

Arms should be placed over the head for trunk imaging. One normally thinks of supine imaging in nuclear medicine, but some laboratories have had success with the prone position for SPECT trunk imaging, because the arms may be removed from the field of view much more comfortably. Technologists should experiment to find positions that will make the patient comfortable; pillows, wedges, rolled sheets, and towels may be helpful. If the shoulders are the area of interest, consider what position will allow the greatest separation of the bones or will be the standard position giving the most information for comparison with other modalities. For imaging the legs, the feet should be positioned in a standard way, probably with toes pointed up and taped together. Confusion results when each patient is positioned differently; there is enough anatomic variation without adding other differences. Positioning straps should be used to restrain the patient lightly and remind him not to move. Bulky restraints will only interfere.

If the table is unstable and inclined to bob up and down in response to patient motion, a monopod may be fashioned for it that will not be in the camera orbit, but will help hold the table (Fig 5–8). This is more useful for imaging the human head (when the lever arm of

138   *Chapter 5*

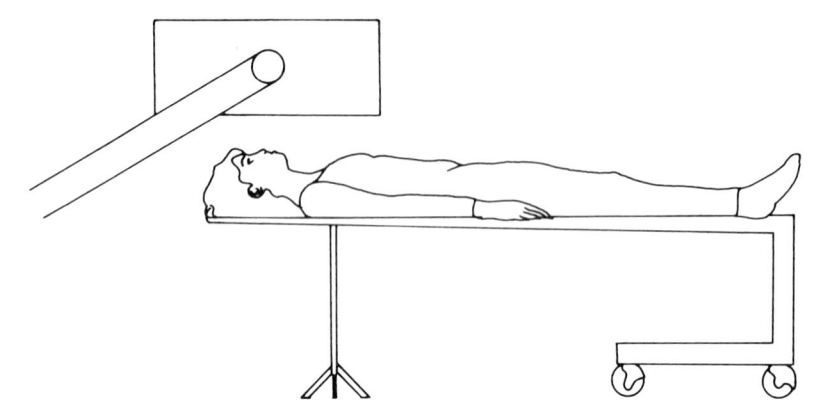

Fig 5–8.—A monopod supporting a cantilevered table for head imaging.

the table is the longest) or for tables that do not move to create the patient-contour orbit.

The camera and table should be secured against all possible undesirable motion before the examination begins. It is very annoying to realize that a procedure will have to be started over because the gantry is rotating around the pivot on the floor or because the table moves when the technologist brushes against it. The technologists must become thoroughly familiar with the gantry switches for the same reason: touching the wrong switch in the middle of the examination could necessitate beginning again.

A patient boundary for the attenuation correction may be selected before acquisition or may be calculated from the planar projection data, depending on the software. As was discussed in the chapter on theory (Chapter 2), attenuation corrections are often based on the assumption of uniform attenuation inside a simple geometric figure assumed as the body outline. This outline is either (1) an ellipse defined at the start of data acquisition by placing the point sources on the patient to inform the computer of the positions and lengths of the major and minor axes or (2) a simple geometric figure defined by the computer after examination of the planar images, using an edge-detection algorithm.

If sources are used to define the ellipse, they are placed first laterally, one on either side. If the patient is already radioactive, the sources must have enough activity to be visible in the presence of the radioactive organ. The computer algorithm that uses the data finds the centers of the sources' activity. The sources are also placed over and under the patient; the source underneath should be placed carefully so as to leave the patient correctly positioned for the examination. If it is attached to a string or holder, it can be retrieved without disturbing the positioning. The source should not be placed underneath the imaging table unless there is some correction made for the distance between the table and the patient's surface. The table has a significantly lower attenuation coefficient than the patient. One could resort to ultrasound, x-ray CT boundary detection, or transmission SPECT to determine the patient boundary, but these are not necessary to define an acceptable patient outline and would mean a much more complicated examination.

A pair or more of sources placed on the patient outside the plane of the organ (Friedman et al. 1984) acts as an aid for the technologist during acquisition and as a check and possible aid during reconstruction. Figure 5–9 shows sources on a patient during liver tomography. The sources should be radioactive enough to show while the patient is being imaged and during viewing of the planar images, but not so radioactive that they dominate the images. The creative use of marker sources can prevent identification errors. Much of the body is bilaterally symmetric; for these parts, a protocol that includes placing the marker closest to the head on the right side will help prevent

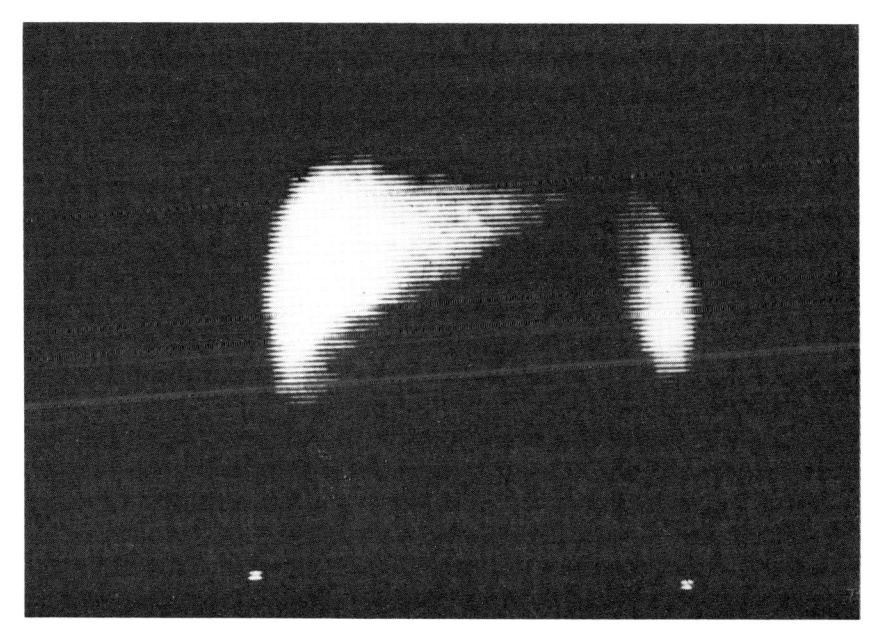

Fig 5–9.—Note the two sources on either side of the anterior image of a SPECT liver examination.

lateral misidentification, no matter what other changes from the usual imaging procedure have taken place. Marker sources can be used to bracket areas of interest or to locate structures in or on the patient (such as a radiation therapy portal or a surgical scar) that may not be obvious on the transaxial image. The sources can be aligned on the persistence oscilloscope, checked for alignment with a cine or sinogram presentation, and used as a guide to how far to raise or lower any misplaced images before reconstruction (but after any computer flood correction).

The marker sources may be used to check the position of the axis of rotation in the actual patient examination, or to judge whether patient motion or incorrect gantry and/or table motion has seriously compromised the examination. These problems are difficult to correct after the fact, unless there is specific software available allowing the realignment of the data (Fig 5–10 shows what would be necessary).

The collimator holes of the Anger camera and the axis of rotation must be perpendicular to each other at all times during acquisition (Fig 5–11). This relationship can be checked easily at only a few points during the acquisition, so it must be one of the given conditions of the mechanical connections in the equipment. The gantry should be leveled when it is installed, so that, barring a shift in the building, it will stay that way. A level gantry ensures that the axis of rotation is parallel to the earth's surface. If the head travels in a circular orbit, it can be set at the start, using a spirit level or some device for achieving the correct angle for an angulated collimator, and left that way during the whole acquisition. If the head travels in a

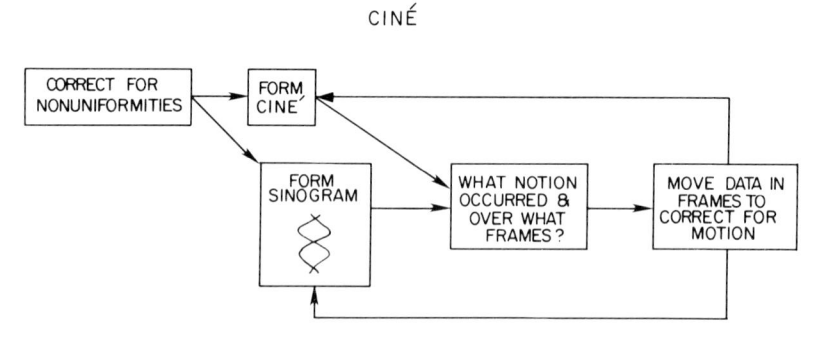

Fig 5–10.—Schematic diagram of what would be necessary if the patient moved during the examination: (I) determine movement: how far, in what direction and on what frames; (2) correct all the frames for camera nonuniformity, etc.; (3) move the patient frames back into place; (4) check cine and sinogram again.

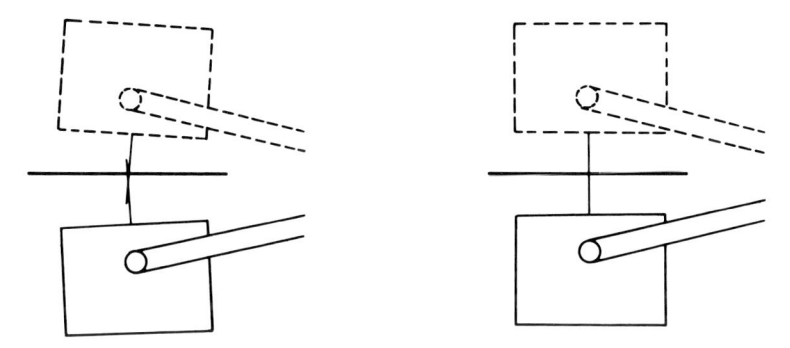

Fig 5–11.—The drawing on the right shows the camera head parallel to the axis of rotation, while the one on the left shows an angle. Note that on the left, the parallel collimator holes are not imaging the same slice all the way through the patient.

patient-contour orbit, there must be provision for maintaining the proper angle to the axis of rotation at all rotational angles. For any system in which the camera head is on a balance arm, the head, unless caused to remain level or correctly angled, will maintain its angular relationship to the gantry arm.

It has been remarked that although one can see the distortion that a tilted camera head introduces into phantom or point-source images, it is not possible to see such distortion on patient images. The only reply to this is that we must try to remove all the sources of distortion and error that we can, especially the simple mechanical sources of systematic errors, because the statistics of the imaging situation and the patient's involuntary motions will cause more than enough uncertainty in the results. Obviously, it is not necessary to go to fantastic lengths to eliminate the errors, but simple caution and the removal of mechanical problems visible to an observant eye cannot help but improve overall performance.

There are other considerations: some cameras and computers have a magnification mode, allowing magnification either of the center of the field or, often more usefully, any portion of the field, so that use may be made of more of the computer's matrix without increasing the processing time for the images. This mode has been used most often in planar cardiac imaging, since the heart is a small organ. It could be used for SPECT of small organs, such as the head, thyroid, and knees, always provided that the whole organ remains in the field of view of the camera at all angles. This should be tested before the examination is begun. If the computer's magnification mode is used, this test should be made also, but its performance may be complicated by not being able to see what the computer is acquiring.

PROCESSING

Processing turns the acquired data into diagnostic images and presents the physician with those images. The steps are diagrammed in Figure 5–12. The remainder of this chapter discusses the operation of each module and the effects of choices that are to be made by the operator or that have been made by the software authors.

Uniformity and Linearity Corrections

Corrections to uniformity, linearity, and center of rotation are performed before all other data processing because they presume the connection between the acquired data in the matrix and the camera face. After the computer has performed the corrections, the original data are replaced by the corrected data in all subsequent calculations. It is important that the corrections be appropriate because in some systems there is no second chance, since the original data are actually written over. An appropriate correction is one performed with the correction factors acquired under circumstances that match the SPECT acquisition circumstances as closely as necessary or possible.

When circular artifacts are seen in the transaxial images, the difficulty is with the correction routines. First, one locates the primary planar images and makes sure that file is secure against any changes or being written over. Then one can ascertain what corrections have already been made in the course of the acquisition and what their effect might be. If the wrong energy or collimator was used for acquisition, as soon as this is recognized, it may be able to be rectified by correction factors from a 30 million (M)-count image acquired by the

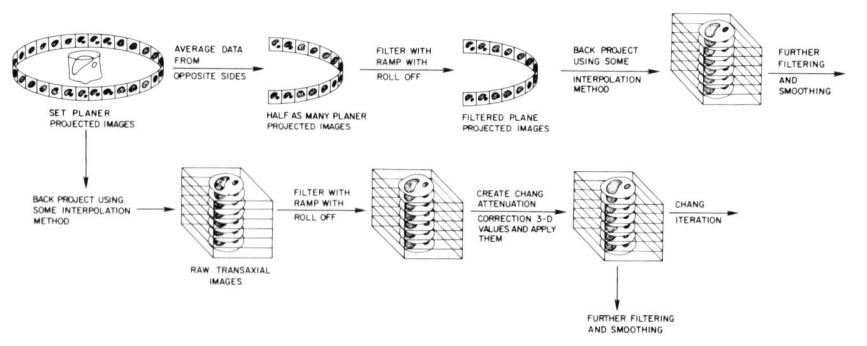

Fig 5–12.—The stages of processing SPECT information according to two common pathways. This diagram is similar to Figure 2–16.

computer under identical circumstances. The time might be put to better use imaging the patient again, however, though this is obviously much harder for the patient. If the correction has been for the wrong orientation or with a correction matrix for another energy or another time, starting the computer processing over with uncorrected patient data and the proper correction matrices should cure the problems, but only if the corrections are made by the computer and not the camera. When the camera makes the corrections, there is no solution for inappropriately applied corrections except to begin the examination over.

Patient-Contour Following

The patient-contour-following algorithm may involve having the SPECT images in different parts of the computer matrix at different acquisition angles. For reconstruction, the projection data must be put into the matrix so that the y levels are in line and so that the axis of rotation is in the center of the matrix on all the images. This could reasonably be expected to be an automatic process, which the operator would have only to initiate. If table motion to achieve a circular-elliptical orbit is part of the system, the uniformity corrections must be applied before the data are positioned in the matrix, so as to put the axis of rotation in the center of the matrix.

Creation and Use of the Cine Presentation

The cine presentation is created by storing the planar projection images in a play-back buffer. If marker sources placed on the patient are too radioactive their high counts will have to be overridden for a sensible cine presentation. This is because most computers automatically adjust the gray scale of each image to make the pixel with the highest count be the brightest pixel. If the pixel with the highest count is sometimes from a source placed on the patient and sometimes from the organ being imaged, the cine presentation of the organ will dim and brighten depending on whether or not the source is in the field of view. This is not helpful. The cine may be improved by adding another data point with a constant high count, higher than that in the source, to each image and then using the contrast enhancement functions to create an organ of suitable brightness and contrast. Such added counts should be placed well out of the field of view (for example, in one of the corners of the image).

Compensation for changes in maximum pixel counts and gray

level makes the cine much easier to look at. It should be adequately smoothed to remove disturbing flickering. Color does not contribute anything to the cine presentation and may make it impossible to appreciate the cine motion effect. The cine should be created and viewed at the start of processing to be sure the patient did not move and that the various corrections seem to be functioning properly. In addition, it is a very useful way to see the three-dimensionality of the organ; for those readers who have never seen a cine presentation of SPECT data, imagination can supply the essentials. Imagine a radioactive liver and spleen in a patient; now imagine these organs spinning in space as if suspended from a string. This is what the cine presentation looks like.

Creation and Use of the Sinogram Presentation

The cine presentation incorporates all the data of the examination, which may be distracting to the viewer trying to make a decision about patient motion. To simplify the information for the purpose of seeing whether the x and y positions of the patient activity distribution remained constant with respect to the axis of rotation, data from one particular point can be studied from all angles with a sinogram. A sinogram is created by abstracting the same line of data from all the planar projection images and creating a new image in which the x values are those of the planar image and the y values are determined by the angle (Fig 5–13). The image is called a "sinogram" because a particular point should follow a sine curve on such a presentation, if the data were acquired with a circular or concentric-circles orbit. Patient motion, any other discontinuities in data acquisition, or diffi-

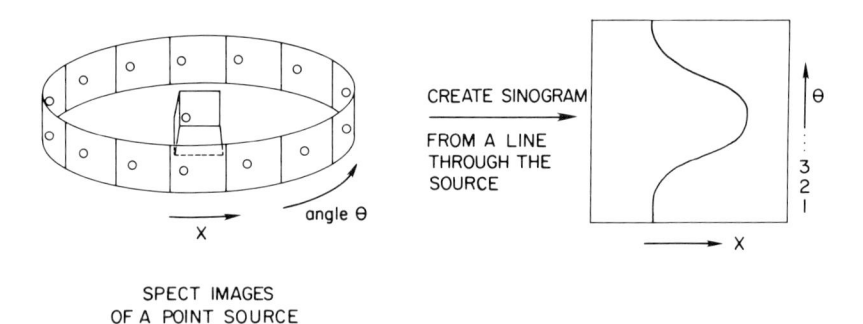

Fig 5–13.—A sinogram is made by selection of one line of data from each of the planar images making up the SPECT data and placing them in a matrix according to the angle at which they were acquired.

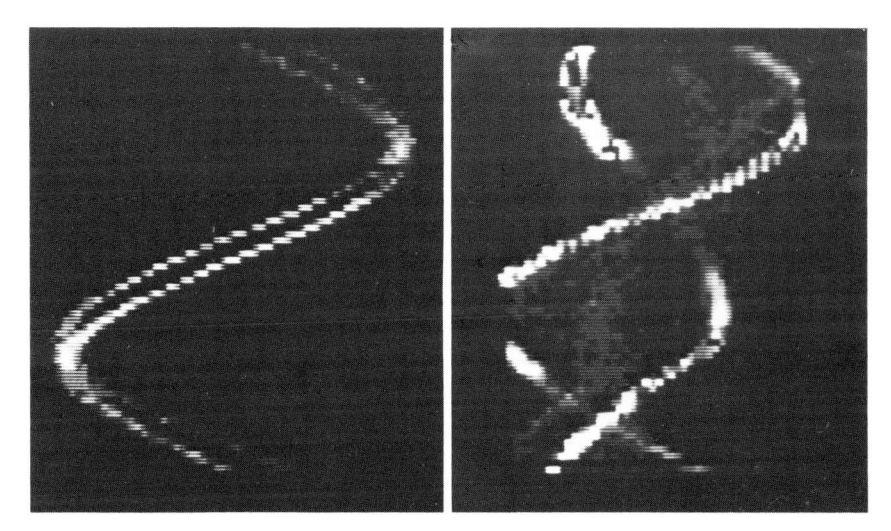

Fig 5–14.—The sinogram on the left is of a patient who did not move during the examination. That on the right shows a pattern of patient motion.

culties with computer matrix adjustments can be seen easily (Fig 5–14). If positioning sources were imaged during acquisition, a sinogram of them may be very useful. Lowering the upper end of the gray scale makes the whole sine wave visible.

Manual Realignment

Good technique should make the manual realignment of images unnecessary. In this imperfect world anything can happen, however, so computer programs that move data around in the matrix may save bad examinations or make mediocre ones better. Positioning sources on the patient that are imaged during the examination are markers for realignment. Since the sources will create multipixel Gaussian images, it is important to have a program to find the exact position of each source. If, in addition, a program to fit the sine wave in the sinogram is available, then it is possible to reposition planar images in both x and y dimensions.

Summing

In many commercially available processing routines, image data from opposite sides of the path are added together if there are 360 degrees' worth of data. This step would normally be part of the computer's

146 *Chapter 5*

automatic processing of SPECT data to create transaxial images. Since there are several possible ways to add the data together, it is good to know which is being used.

Chapter 2 discussed the most likely possibilities for ways to add opposing data together: arithmetic averaging and geometric averaging. Because the geometric mean better approximates an Anger camera with uniform response through a depth of tissue, it is most often used (see Fig 2–1). Figure 5–15 compares the full-width-at-half-maximum (FWHM) value for geometrically averaged data with that of the original data. Of course, the geometric averaging of information from opposite sides of the patient may actually cause a loss of resolution as the sharp information from the near side is mixed with the fuzzy information from the far side. This will happen even if opposite sides are not averaged together.

Filtering

The use of filter functions, either by convolution in real space (used by most commercial SPECT systems) or by multiplication in frequency space, was discussed in Chapter 2. The filters may be applied before or after back projection that creates the transaxial images. Planar projection data or the ensuing transaxial images are filtered to remove high-frequency statistical noise and the effect of the backprojection algorithm. Most commercially available SPECT software

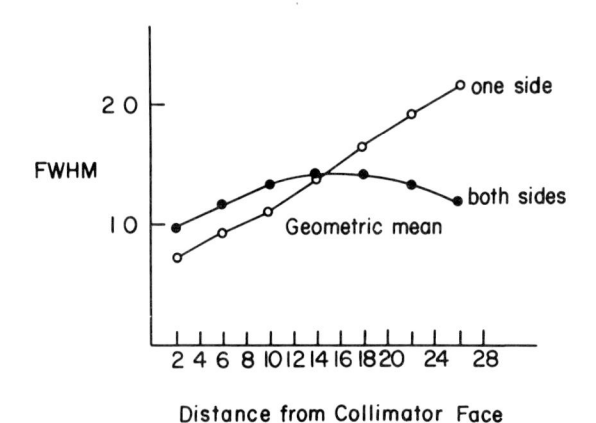

Fig 5–15.—A graph of the full width at half maximum (FWHM) for geometrically averaged data compared to the FWHM for data from one side, for a point source in a scattering medium. Note the degradation near the camera, but the improvement in the middle of the medium (Larsson 1980).

offers a variety of filter functions. In general, the choice of which to use depends on the statistical quality of the data; the more counts there are, the more the filter that is used may resemble the ramp filter and the higher the frequencies of which it can take account. Examinations that are count-poor benefit from smoothing filters. In every case the filters should not accentuate the noise or cause oscillations at edges.

It may not be too easy to discover what filters a particular SPECT system is using, since this comes under the heading of proprietary information, but it is important to have some feeling for what is happening in any particular system. If there is a series of filters, try them out on different kinds of images. If the filters are applied to the planar images before reconstruction, it will take patience to perform filter tests (Contino et al. 1984). Choose some unequivocal images for the tests. If the filters are to be applied to the transaxial images after reconstruction, it should be possible to create some very simple images, such as a point, a uniform circle covering part of the field, a flood image, and so on, and to see what the filters will do to them. One must be sure data are not oversmoothed so that they lose all definition or oversharpened so that extraneous detail is brought out. The filters should be tried on a range of patient data, from images with adequate counts to count-poor images. It is important not to take the vendor's word for the effects of the filters without trying them. The user must be the master of the system, not its slave.

Several issues in the area of filtering deserve discussion. One is the number of dimensions in which the filtering should be applied. The plane projection images are truly two-dimensional, so a filter that operates only in the x direction does not take into account contributions from other layers to the plane in question (King et al. 1984); if filtering is performed before back projection, the filter should be a two-dimensional matrix and not a one-dimensional line, but it should only incorporate the ramp-filter correction for the back-projection process in the x direction. If filtering is done after reconstruction, by convolution of the filter with the transaxial images, the same effect can be achieved by considering all the transaxial planes rather than each individual slice. Of course, this will be a three-dimensional filtering process (Fig 5–16).

Perhaps a more subtle question is whether to use a linear or nonlinear filter. They are different in that a linear filter operates on or is convoluted with all the data in the same way no matter what the value of a particular piece of data or its relationship to the neighboring points, whereas a nonlinear filter interacts with the data in some

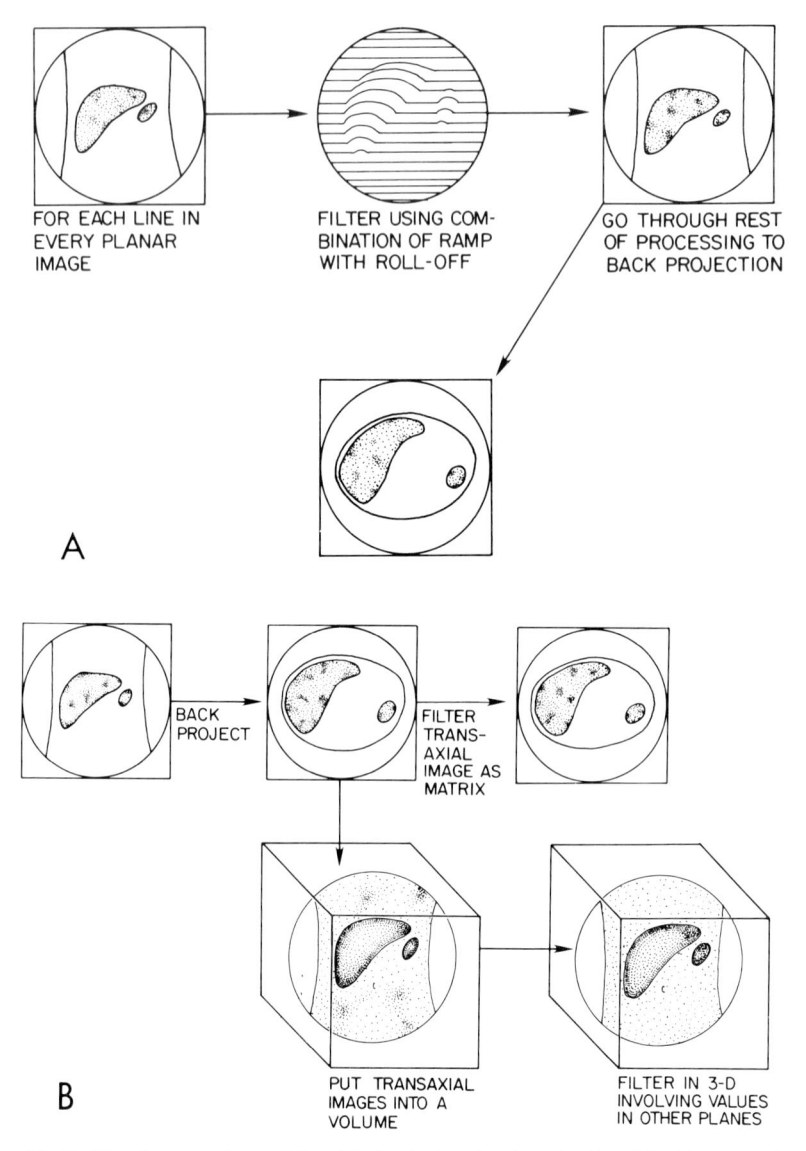

Fig 5–16.—A comparison of line filtering before back projection **(A)** with matrix filtering and volume filtering after back projection **(B)**.

way, such as by taking a derivative or only doing its operation if the value is greater than some threshold. Linear filters can be applied equally in Fourier or real space by transforming them and the data to which they are applied into the proper space. Nonlinear filters must stay in the space for which they were designed (usually real space) because their functional interaction does not transfer into the other space. A nonlinear filter can be designed to recognize and remove specific artifacts, to enhance features of certain shapes, or to perform any number of other specific functions (Raff, Nelson, and Ritenour 1984; Kircos et al. 1984). Streak artifacts of SPECT can be eliminated by nonlinear filtration. The user may have to decide on the threshold for such specific filtration and be sure that the images under consideration do not contain real information that might be eliminated by such a filter.

Attenuation and Scatter Corrections

Chapter 2 described a number of possibilities for attenuation correction. The first to be implemented on commercial systems (together with no attenuation correction at all) is based on a simplified set of assumptions. The patient is approximated by an ellipse of uniform attenuation, in which the radioactivity is uniformly distributed with an empiric attenuation coefficient of a bit less than the actual coefficient for that radionuclide in water. The coefficient is less than expected because scattered radiation adds counts back into the attenuated region; it would be overcorrecting to use the proper attenuation correction (Larsson 1980). This correction is applied before back projection.

The patient ellipse may be determined from measurements made of the patient width and given to the computer, from point source information acquired by the computer before the planar projection images, from the data themselves by considering the edge of the scattered image, from the reconstructed images by considering the edge of the figure in each slice, or from acquired Compton scattering images. If the ellipse is not formed from the planar projection data themselves, the corrected transaxial images should be checked to be sure the attenuation correction has been applied to the correct ellipse. If the patient and the ellipse are not in the same place, the attenuation correction routine will cut off part of the patient, ruining the images (Fig 5–17).

From this point, iteration to improve the closeness of the transaxial image's projections to the observed projection data would be the

150 *Chapter 5*

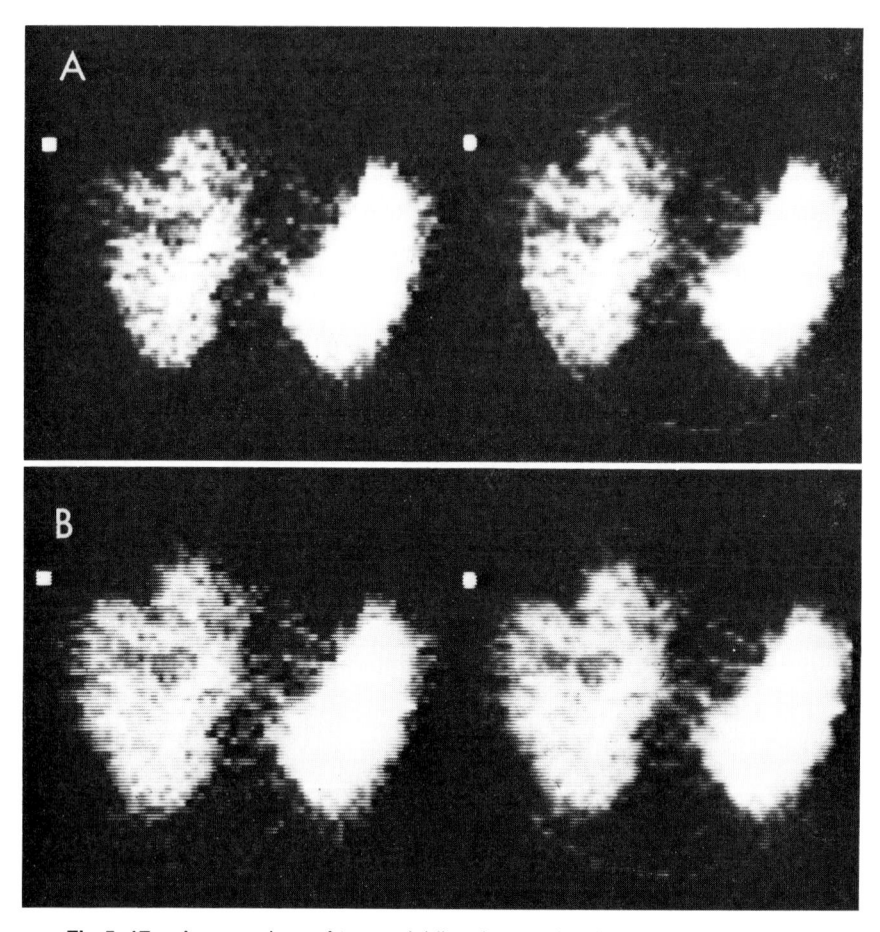

Fig 5–17.—A comparison of transaxial liver images in which the patient contour was displaced **(A)** and in which it was not **(B)**. The companion image in each case shows the contour that was used for the attenuation correction calculation. Liver activity outside the incorrect ellipse **(A)** is absent.

fastest way to improve on the estimated attenuation. Such an iteration might involve using projections at 90 degrees to the projection under consideration to improve the estimate of the position of the activity from a column of uniform activity to varying activities through the column.

The Chang (1978) attenuation correction also uses an assumed patient ellipse; it is an iterative correction applied after back projection (see Fig 2–8). Its essence is to consider the transaxial reconstruction pixel position in the attenuator and to correct for all the attenuation to which such a point would be subject. The attenuation correction is once again based on a uniform attenuator. The commercial software currently stops at this point. Chang provided for an iterative process of reprojection of the corrected transaxial images and correction by comparison to the original data. Each iteration is as time-consuming as the initial back projection and correction, so iterative procedures will not become an integral part of the software until the processors become faster.

It is possible to use data such as x-ray CT scans to give a detailed image of attenuation coefficients in the patient. Not only would such images increase radiation dose, examination time, and expense to the patient, but the images would have to be processed carefully to remove motion artifacts and be carefully aligned with the patient's cross-section to be sure that the attenuation coefficient data would be matched to the correct tissue. The care with which this would have to be done to avoid far worse artifacts makes the use of such additional scan methods seem unlikely in all but the most rarefied research settings. There are devices that would help in positioning and repositioning the patient in these situations (Conti, Deck, and Rottenberg 1982; Kearfott, Rottenberg, and Knowles 1984). Aligning the data and matching the sizes of the x-ray CT and SPECT images would be a considerable undertaking.

Attenuation correction is not possible in the usual way if only 180 degrees of data acquisition are used. Attenuation corrections based on uniform tissue cannot be made in the chest in any case, so the images are made without them in most systems in use.

Transmission SPECT images may be used to estimate attenuation in the patient or to provide data for other methods of attenuation correction (MacIntyre, personal communication, 1982). The images give a rough but adequate attenuation map that can be used to make the attenuation correction map for the Chang correction method.

Another method of making attenuation correction, which is more practical in some parts of the body than in others, is to assume an "attenuation reference man" model, perhaps with a series of scaled length variables, the values of which could be measured at the time of the examination or perhaps even supplied by the data themselves (Moore, Brunelle, and Kirsch 1982). The model would provide for the attenuation coefficients based on measurement from a large number of patients. This method has a great deal to be said for it in imaging the head, neck, and chest. Body outline and heart size could be ascertained from the images; standard heart, lung, and chest wall attenuation coefficients would be supplied. The attenuation calculation could even be made in the case of 180–degree data.

Thoughts about scatter correction (Chapter 2) have not been translated into commercial software as yet, except insofar as there are suggestions and instructions to use attenuation coefficients that are lower than the actual values for gamma rays of that energy in water, because scatter puts apparent counts back into an area from which attenuation has removed them. Scattering is very much a three-dimensional process, whereas attenuation is two-dimensional, so the corrections for scatter should be three-dimensional and involve all the data.

Back Projection and Interpolation

Back projection is the culmination of the whole mathematic process leading to transaxial slice images. Because discontinuous pixel data have been used all along the way and because the data must be back-projected into a square matrix, the pixels to be back-projected rarely hit their target pixels exactly. The contribution of more than one pixel of angular data to a particular pixel in the transaxial slice at a particular angle is accounted for by interpolation. Interpolation methods range from simply taking the closest pixel or nearest neighbor, called "nearest value" by Larsson (1980), to linear interpolation between the pixels in question, to interpolations involving larger numbers of pixels (see Fig 2–11 and 2–12). The nearest-neighbor interpolation is the fastest one to implement in the computer and is the equivalent of filtering the data with a rectangular filter, while linear interpolation means filtering with a triangular function (Larsson 1980). With a cutoff frequency for a 64 × 64 matrix of (1/0.6 cm), either method is a low-frequency bandpass filter, with relatively higher frequencies being passed by nearest-neighbor filtering.

More interpolation can be accomplished by considering the pixel as made up of a number of subpixels and subdividing the projection data as well. A set of projection matrices providing the geometric multiplication values for each point, based on the angle and positions of the projection subunits and subpixels, is large but need be calculated only once; it can be used with each successive slice (Fig 5–18). One might perhaps divide the pixels into 2^2, 3^2, or 4^2 subpixels, and the projection data into 2, 3, or 4 subunits. It is also possible to use linear (or higher-order) interpolation on the projection data according to the subunits (Fig 5–19). The number of operations for back projection increases by the multiplication factor applied to the projection

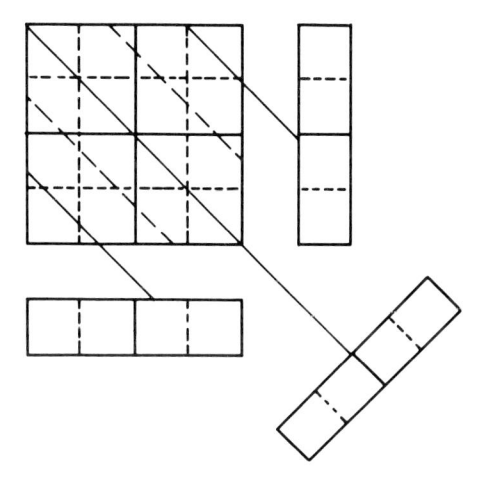

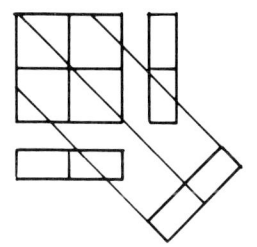

Fig 5–18.—A schematic drawing shows the pixel divided into subpixels and the transverse matrix subdivided to allow easy back projection of planar data into the transverse matrix.

pixel and the transaxial pixel. This is done to avoid losing hard-won resolution at this point by oversmoothing the results with too simple an interpolation.

The problem of resolution vs. sensitivity in nuclear medicine appears here, too. The coarseness of the angular sampling may not warrant fine interpolation; perhaps four subpixel and two plane projection subunits would be appropriate in most cases, leading to eight times as many operations for back projection. The results may be presented as they appear, that is interpolated, or added back together again to retain the matrix dimensions of the acquisition matrix. To

154 *Chapter 5*

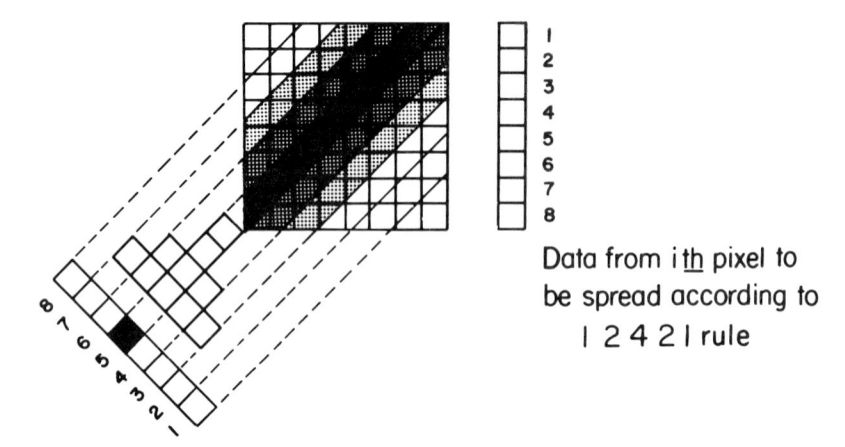

Fig 5–19.—Schematic representation of the use of higher-order interpolation during back projection.

Data from i<u>th</u> pixel to be spread according to 1 2 4 2 1 rule

interpolate more than this is to impute better statistical quality to the acquired data than they have.

The point was made earlier that information gathered on the opposite side from a source of activity has poor resolution by virtue of the distance from the collimator through a scattering medium. General Electric's Nowak back-projection algorithm (Nowak and Eisner

SQUARE BACK PROJECTION   NOWAK BACK PROJECTION

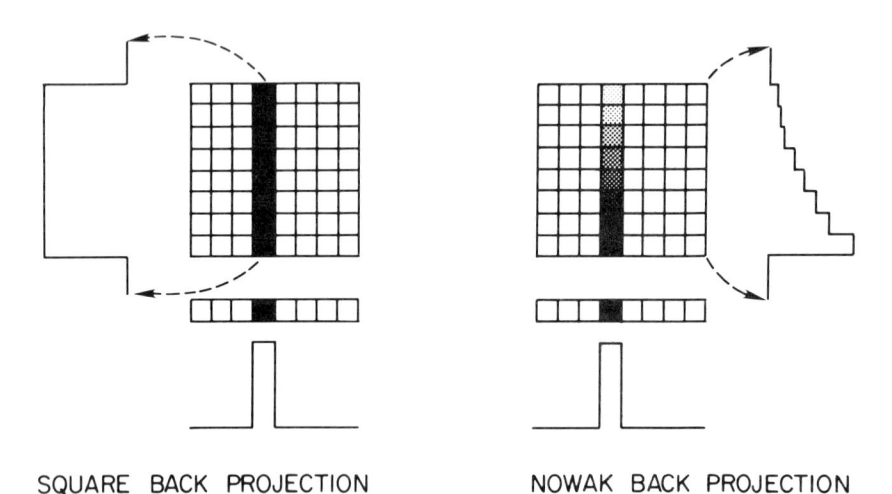

Fig 5–20.—Schematic illustration of the Nowak back-projection algorithm. The back-projected counts are weighted most heavily on the side of the planar projection rather than evenly.

1984) addresses this problem by weighting the projection data. Thus, instead of projecting a piece of information evenly across the transaxial matrix, more weight is given to pixels on the near side (Fig 5–20).

It was noted in Chapter 2 that many of the operations leading to the transaxial image could be performed in frequency space with a series of Fourier transformations. In practice, frequency-space manipulations are not done because, even with the use of so-called fast Fourier transform (FFT) algorithms, this approach leads to long computing times. As computers become faster and core memory becomes cheaper, some of these Fourier methods may become more possible and perhaps more popular. The two steps of Fourier and inverse Fourier transformation add noise to the resulting transaxial images because of the interpolations that must be made. Real space calculations do not have this problem.

VARIOUS OTHER VIEWS

The standard tomographic projection that results from using the available software is the transaxial slice. If other projections are desired, they are created from the stored transaxial data (Fig 5–21). The coronal and sagittal projections, which are orthogonal to the transaxial images, are the simplest to calculate. It should be remembered that since the transaxial images are computed first and may be two or more pixels thick, any slice that incorporates several transaxial slices will have to be interpolated to produce the same apparent resolution. Because the coronal and sagittal sections are derived from the transaxial sections, it is wise to go back to the transaxial sections for any decision-making or numeric calculations.

Various views are useful for various organs. For the head, one could produce reverse Townes views to match x-ray-transmission CT of the head more closely; one might want to look at coronal views of the liver or view the sagittal planes of a set of gallium images. One might wish an oblique view to slice a bone lengthwise. In the heart in particular, as is further discussed in Chapter 8, there is a need to fix on a standard projection and develop an automatic or semiautomatic way to achieve it. We have become accustomed to looking at and thinking about thallium-201 planar imaging in a particular way; SPECT may be able to make the conceptualization easier by standardizing all heart imaging.

156 *Chapter 5*

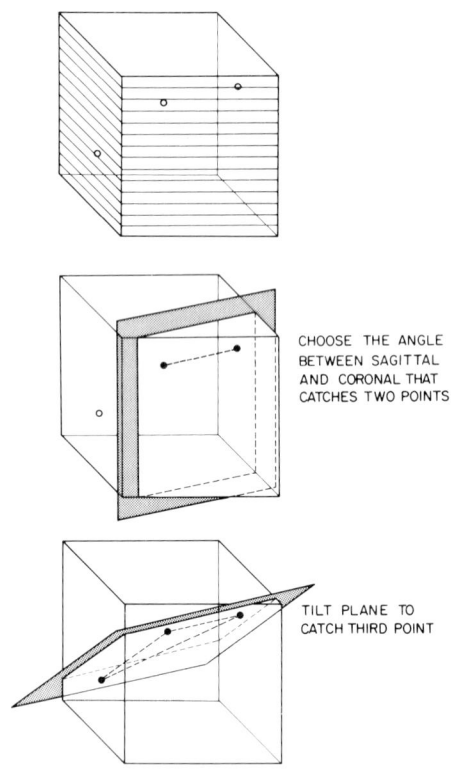

Fig 5–21.—Schematic illustration of the process for making oblique slices from transaxial projections. Note the process for achieving an oblique projection containing the three point sources.

SMOOTHING AND CONTRAST ENHANCEMENT

Prior to creating hard copy for viewing, more computer processing may be desirable. The usual aim is to clean up the images, eliminating noise and extraneous detail. Most nuclear medicine computer systems and indeed most SPECT systems have a set of smoothing filters available. No more smoothing or contrast enhancement should be used than is necessary because images become muddy and clouded when they are oversmoothed. Just as one might wish to view rectilinear scanner images with a diffusing lens or at some distance to make their details run together, or use contrast enhancement to bring out certain details, these techniques can enhance the appreciation of the information in SPECT images. Similarly, however, the user's ability to view the images without the aid of such devices comes with experience. Just as the rule in rectilinear brain scanning was that there should be evidence of background counts in the hemispheres, contrast enhancement of any clinical image should not be used to the extent that all background is removed. Correct contrast is needed to be sure that all the details are visible and that defects are not created where none exist. Experience will lead to techniques for assessing each kind of clinical image.

Besides the obvious method of contrast enhancement, which involves moving the lower threshhold up to black out the lower-count pixels of the image, there are much more subtle methods. For example, the relationship of the gray scale to the image can be examined (Pizer 1981), and a scale that fits the image better than a linear scale can be used. At least the following two issues should be considered in this connection: (1) differences in count rate that are not statistically significant should not be emphasized, and (2) one of the most useful images comes from having the same number of pixels at each gray level. Naturally, the ordinarily presumed linear relationship between the gray level and the number of counts in a pixel is disturbed by this kind of processing. X-ray CT uses the windowing approach very successfully to achieve contrast enhancement over the range of attenuation coefficients. Digital angiography is employing the same techniques to produce more comprehensible images.

Display

Without getting into the thorny area of what kind of oscilloscope and what matrix size to use to display and photograph nuclear medicine images, with special reference to SPECT, several display concepts should be examined. The object of display and hard copy devices is to make the information available to the diagnostician. To the extent that the film makes them portable, the images are available anywhere. To the extent that the images really exist in digital form in their file on the computer disk, to be considered with the aid of the computer, the computer presentation should be brought to the physician in the form of a display terminal that can be used at the time and in the place where other diagnostic nuclear medicine images are read. We are slowly becoming aware that the computer should fit comfortably into the diagnostic setting. Only the combination of the computer and the diagnostician can get the most value out of the information.

The next best thing to actual access to the computer file at a display terminal may well be videotapes taken from the computer display. The videotape images must be made according to an established protocol that allows for no special manipulations or decisions unless the technologists are versatile and very well trained. Obviously, videotape provides an inexpensive, portable medium that does not tie up the computer or require the physician to learn how it works, but it does not provide the versatility of the computer. Contrast enhancement, smoothing, new views, and reprocessing are not options with the use of videotape.

The usual way to display SPECT and other CT data is as a series of images proceeding in stepwise fashion from one extreme of the organ to the other, either on film or on a CRT screen. Keyes (1981, 1983) reviewed the display problem. The images are photographed on film using a formatter that generally allows for six or nine images on one sheet of film. The formatter may be an integral part of the camera or computer, or it may be added separately. The system must be tuned to prevent the images from having too much contrast. (Photography represents yet another filtering process.) It is illuminating to create a gray-scale image of a number of bars; 16 gray levels are enough to show the effects. One can photograph the gray scale image and see how many of the gray levels are actually visible on the film (Fig 5–22). This experiment gives an idea of the range of the film and the part of the intensity scale that is actually being portrayed. One must do everything possible to make the visible intensity range as long as possible and to make it fit the range of the organ being imaged. A protocol should be developed for the photography, so that a uniform series of images can be produced. With reference to computer processing, it may be necessary to use one technique of smoothing and contrast enhancement for viewing the images on the screen, and quite another for photography in order to achieve hard copy that seems to look like the screen. One should not be satisfied until a satisfactory image can be made reproducibly.

Three-dimensional data are difficult to appreciate in a series of two-dimensional images. Especially difficult are internal details and connections between details seen in neighboring images. A number of techniques have been advanced to make three-dimensional viewing possible. The simplest of these is cine presentation of the projection data, which appears to make the radioactivity distribution rotate in space on the screen. This effect can only be achieved in black-and-white or shades of gray or another color; the rainbow color table is too distracting. The basis of the cine technique is that the human

Data Acquisition and Processing **159**

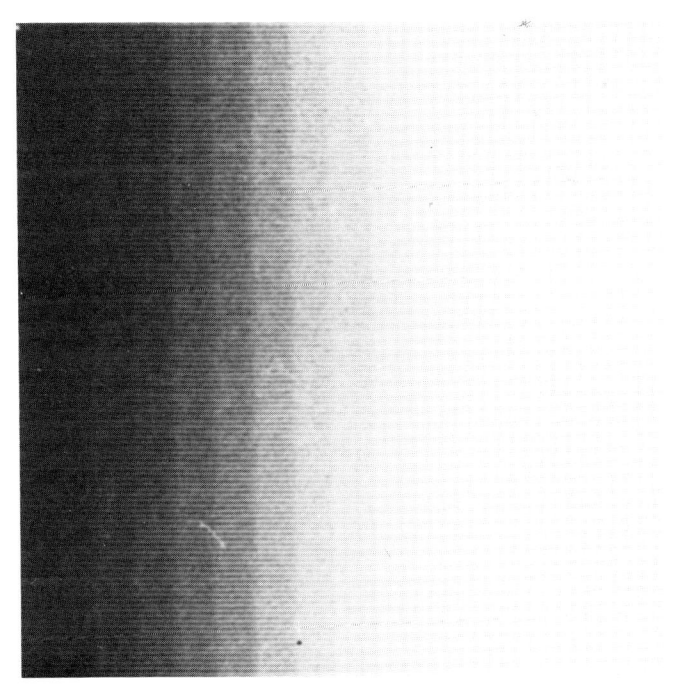

Fig 5–22.—A typical formatter image of a set of gray bars of even-intensity steps. As many bars as possible should be visible.

brain assumes that the activity fading out is actually going behind the organ as the images are shown in rapid sequence. Many details on the exterior of the organ, or details that are quite radioactive, can be appreciated in the cine presentation, but of course, it really does not make deep "cold" lesions appear much more obvious than they do on planar projection images. Video presentation for cine is very acceptable. Hard copy devices that show the same sort of cine images have been developed; they may be based on the creation of a loop of 35–mm images. Other devices have been created to project a three-dimensional image into space (Bradley-Moore and Woloshuk 1980) for viewing without the use of a computer.

The reconstructed images can be viewed in cine too, but this may not be so helpful because cine will only show a series of plane images without a focus. The diagnostician does not seem to be zooming up the axis of rotation, for example, because the planes of data already gone through do not fall away on the sides. It is surely possible to use some computer game techniques to make three-dimensional images.

Three-dimensional images have only begun to be available. The Mayo Clinic three-dimensional CT scanner (Behrenbeck et al. 1983) was accompanied by software that allowed data to be viewed in many novel ways, including the selection of a plane along which to split the image to see the inside. A prospectus has been presented (Batnitsky et al. 1982) describing three-dimensional computer reconstructions of brain lesions from x-ray CT images. The paper is complete with clinical examples, including several in which the radiation therapy isodose surfaces are visible in the images. The program allows for de-emphasis of the skull in the images, so that the brain, ventricles, and lesions might be seen more easily. Figure 5-23 is a SPECT image from this system. Such a system has been developed specifically for use with SPECT (Minato et al. 1983).

Gated SPECT presents the necessity adding a fourth dimension, time, to the display. The cine presentation of a rotating beating heart is a real possibility. Naturally, the appreciation of such examinations in two-dimensional presentation on film would be extremely difficult, so access to the information on a CRT screen with image-manipulation capability should be rapid. The area of four-dimensional imaging may represent another area of technology where techniques developed for nuclear medicine images may be very useful for x-ray imaging in the future.

Quantification

Quantification was mentioned in a general way in the discussion of theory, but must be treated more thoroughly here, and with respect to various organs, because it is really a practical topic. Quantification is not wholly theoretical because if the instruments had sufficient sensitivity for really good statistics and resolution for fine-grained images, and if, as well, the problems of attenuation correction and scattering were solved, there would be little problem with it. This is not a world of fully solved problems, so partial practical solutions are used until better ones come along.

The first aspect of quantification is measuring the volume of some radioactive region using SPECT. This can be done either by

---

Fig 5–23.—Three-dimensional image of a brain tumor. **A** is a transaxial slice through the tumor and **B** is the three-dimensional image of the head created from SPECT slices. (Courtesy of D. F. Preston, University of Kansas.)

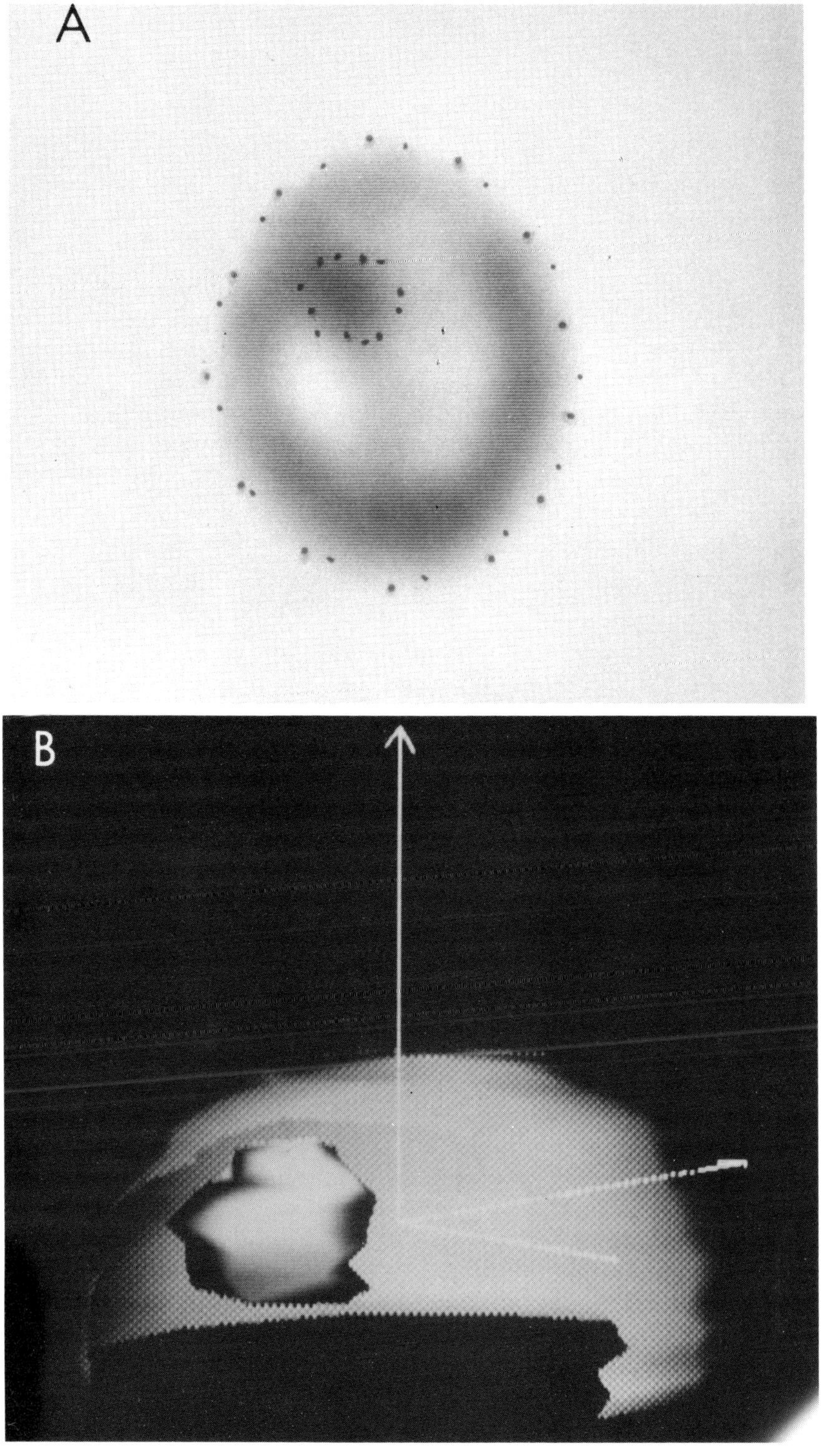
A
B

counting the number of voxels that contain the organ or by measuring the number of counts that are seen when the volume is filled with a well-mixed radioactive fluid. Let us consider the first of these, which is more appropriate to SPECT.

The hard decisions about measuring organ volume by counting the voxels are those concerning the location of the edge of the organ. Edge detection was discussed in connection with the attenuation correction, but it is more critical for volume measurements. The threshold method depends on the relationship of the counts to a local or global maximum. The second-derivative algorithm is based on the shape of the curve of activity vs. position; the edge is located at the point where the second derivative is zero, which is the point of steepest descent of the data. Threshold-based edge detection is much easier, but the proper threshold must be selected. An edge-detection method for volume measurement must be verified. Tauxe and others (1982) and Tauxe and Todd-Pokropek (1983) attempted to verify volume measurement using a set of phantoms; their conclusion was that a threshold of 46% of the maximum activity in a volume of interest for volumes above 1 liter and 45% for volumes less than 1 liter would allow them to estimate the volumes correctly. Soderborg and coworkers (1983) analyzed the problem and found it to be more complex, but were in fact using a threshold of 45% for volume calculations. In the meantime, the original authors (Tauxe and Todd-Pokropek 1983) repeated the measurements on another SPECT system and found that a threshold of 36% was required for accurate volume measurements. The difference between the systems presumably was in the reconstruction software, although perhaps it was in the filter, which was not specified. They also noted experiments with more complex edge-detection methods that did not seem to work well with clinical data, because the contrast of the organs under their consideration—the kidneys—differed. Volume measurements should be based on the transaxial section data directly, with appropriate account taken of the fact that the transaxial section may be several pixels thick so that some interpolation between slices may be appropriate. One cannot rely on the algorithms that interpolate between transaxial images to create smooth coronal or sagittal sections that are good for volume determination, especially of small structures. Because of the potential clinical importance of volume measurements, many more experiments will be carried out in this area.

The second aspect of quantification is measuring the quantity of radioactivity in a particular portion of the organ being imaged. This area has created a stir because of the many questions surrounding its precision and accuracy. The value measured may actually be the reason for the imaging examination, or it may be used to provide a value for an enclosed volume of radioactivity such as might be contained in the heart. The results of processing are important, because the quantification of SPECT is so often expected to create a map of the distribution of radioactivity, voxel by voxel, rather than to result in the sum total for a volume of interest in which the relationship of the individual voxels to each other is not of any quantitative utility. In addition, noise in the final image that results from noise in the planar projection data may mean the difference between useful results and trash.

As noted previously, a great deal of the problem with quantification lies with the difficulties of attenuation and scatter correction; another part lies with the resolution of the Anger camera and its modulation transfer function. The camera does not permit the resolution of high-frequency changes. This means the boundaries between areas become smoothed and the cutoff point for the counts is not obvious. Some three-dimensional techniques for recognizing and using regions of interest have been developed (Huesman 1984; Schlusselberg, Lewis, and Simon 1984).

An investigation was conducted into various quantitative properties of a dual-head SPECT system (Jaszczak, Coleman, and Whitehead 1981) with a phantom under experimental, not clinical, conditions. The results point to some of the problem areas for quantification (Chapter 2). It proved to be possible to make an estimate of the activity in 2– to 6–cm-diameter spheres provided one already knew their volume and had some information about the resolution of the system. The imaging situation of patient activity distributions is not so ideal; it must be modeled carefully. It is not clear to what extent one might be able to use the following algorithm: (1) image a phantom with a series of volumes of the proper kind to find the threshold to use; (2) use that threshold with patient data to find the organ volume; (3) knowing the organ volume and other properties of the instrument, such as point-source response, find the activity contained in the volume. In high-contrast situations, this could well be possible. When the contrast is lower, it would seem to be more difficult because the computer algorithm might not be able to recognize the volume by thresholding.

Practical advice about quantification is not to use any method clinically until it has been tried experimentally on the same SPECT system (hardware and software) with the acquisition and reconstruction values used for patients. It even makes sense to test the proposed method with a range of count densities from the high-count situation to that of a suboptimal patient image. Volume calculations can be expected to be most successful for high-count–high-contrast images.

Other problems are those of all three-dimensional quantification. Partial voluming comes from the presence of a gradient of activity within a voxel, so that the activity seen is a combination of high activity in part of the slice with low activity in the rest. The thicker the slices are, the greater the problem will be. In addition, artifacts of motion and of reconstruction affect the activities seen in a particular area. Motion artifacts are usually radial streaks, while reconstruction artifacts may be streaks or ringing at the locations of great contrast, or bridges between radioactive areas. Any variation from the expected attenuation, such as may be caused by the patient's arms at his sides or extra absorber in the patient or in the imaging table, will affect count density and quantification.

IMAGE STORAGE, NETWORKING, PACS, AND SPECT

The final step of the SPECT process to be considered is archiving the data. Many laboratories elect to save film hard copies of the patient information and nothing more. In the course of ordinary clinical work this may well be sufficient. If it becomes necessary to compare the patient with himself at some other time or to make new measurements on old data, however, there must also be some way to store the planar projection data or the transaxial images. Stored planar projection images must be uniformity corrected or the relevant flood image must be stored too.

Nuclear medical digital data have been stored on magnetic media: tape (either reels or cassettes) or large disks. Floppy disks take too much file room space. Preparation for the all-digital radiology department has included extensive study of the requirements for digital networking, storage, and recall. It would be sufficient for nuclear medicine to tie into such a system so that images might be stored and recalled, probably not through a display station of the radiology system, but back into the active areas of the nuclear medicine computer. We should look forward to compressing the data to $1/10$ to $1/5$ of its size, which will help a great deal with storage problems. Processed SPECT images in their turn might well be available to the radiology network for comparison with x-ray CT and ultrasound images in relevant places. At this point we can see the practicality of such a system, but only prototypes have been created and none of the major interfacing or storage difficulties has been solved. It is expected that the economics of such an all-digital department will be favorable because it will avoid the high cost of the silver content in film. There is nothing about SPECT that makes analog or film imaging necessary.

BIBLIOGRAPHY

Batnitsky, S., et al. Three-dimensional computer reconstructions of brain lesions from surface contours provided by computed tomography: a prospectus. *Neurosurgery* 11:73–84, 1982.

Behrenbeck, T., et al. Some imaging characteristics of the dynamic spatial reconstructor x-ray scanner system. In *NATO Advanced Study Institute on Diagnostic Imaging in Medicine*, ed. R. C. Reba, D. J. Goodenough, and H. F. Davidson. The Hague: Martinus Nijhoff, 1983, pp. 254–271.

Bradley-Moore, P. R., and Woloshuk, E. A. Stroboscopic analyzing monitor: an optical instrument for creating a "transparent solid" three dimensional display. In *Single Photon Emission Computed Tomography and Other Selected Computer Topics*. New York: Society of Nuclear Medicine, 1980, pp. 159–167.

Chang, L.-T. A method for attenuation correction in radionuclide computed tomography. *IEEE Trans. Nucl. Sci.* 25:638–643, 1978.

Coleman, R. E., et al. Collimation for I-123 imaging with SPECT. In *Emission Computed Tomography: Current Trends*, ed. P. D. Esser. New York: Society of Nuclear Medicine, 1983, pp. 123–133.

Conti, J.; Deck, M. D. F.; and Rottenberg, D. A. An inexpensive video patient repositioning system for use with transmission and emission computed tomographs. *J. Comput. Assist. Tomogr.* 6:417–421, 1982.

Contino, J., et al. Performance index: a method for quantitative evaluation of filters used in clinical SPECT (abstract). *J. Nucl. Med.* 24:P88, 1984.

Croft, B. Y.; Teates, C. D.; and Honeyman, J. C. Single-photon emission computed tomography of the liver. In *Digital Imaging: Clinical Advances in Nuclear Medicine*, ed. P. D. Esser. New York: Society of Nuclear Medicine, 1982, pp. 271–282.

Floch, J.; Alazraki, N.; and Wooten, W. SPECT and planar image detection of hot lesions in a chest phantom using Ga-67 and Tc-99m (abstract). *J. Nucl. Med.* 24:P51, 1984.

Friedman, J., et al. Motion detection and correction in Tl-201 SPECT imaging: a simple, practical method (abstract). *J. Nucl. Med.* 24:P70, 1984.

Huesman, R. H. A new fast algorithm for the evaluation of regions of interest and statistical uncertainty in computed tomography (abstract). *J. Nucl. Med.* 24:P89, 1984.

Jaszczak, R. L.; Chang, L.-T.; and Murphy, P. H. Single photon emission computed tomography using multi-slice fan beam collimators. *IEEE Trans. Nucl. Sci.* 26:610–618, 1979.

Jaszczak, R. L.; Coleman, R. E.; and Whitehead, F. R. Physical factors affecting quantitative measurements using camera-based single photon emission computed tomography (SPECT). *IEEE Trans. Nucl. Sci.* 28:69–80, 1981.

Kearfott, K. J.; Rottenberg, D. A.; and Knowles, R. J. R. A new headholder for PET, CT, and NMR imaging. *J. Comput. Assist. Tomogr.* 8:1217–1220, 1984.

Keyes, J. W., Jr. Display of three-dimensional tomographic images. In *Functional Mapping of Organ Systems and Other Computer Topics*, ed. P. D. Esser. New York: Society of Nuclear Medicine, 1981, pp. 219–226.

Keyes, J. W., Jr. Image motion and depth perception: a key to improved three-dimensional display. In *Nuclear Medicine and Biology Advances*, Proceedings of the Third World Congress of Nuclear Medicine and Biology. London: Pergamon, 1983, pp. 2169–2172.

King, M. A., et al. Preliminary characterization of the properties of a new rotating SPECT imaging system. In *Emission Computed Tomography: Current Trends*, ed. P. D. Esser. New York: Society of Nuclear Medicine, 1983, pp. 91–104.

King, M. A., et al. Two-dimensional filtering of SPECT images using the Metz and Wiener filters. *J. Nucl. Med.* 25:1234–1240, 1984.

Kircos, L. T., et al. Comparison of planar images and SPECT with Bayesean preprocessing for the demonstration of facial anatomy and craniomandibular disorders (abstract). *J. Nucl. Med.* 25:P71, 1984.

LaFontaine, R., et al. ROC demonstrated improvement in lesion detectability using asymmetric photopeak windows (abstract). *J. Nucl. Med.* 25:P104, 1984.

LaFontaine, R.; Graham, L. S.; and Stein, M. A. Effects of asymmetric photopeak windows on flood field uniformity and spatial resolution for scintillation cameras (abstract). *J. Nucl. Med.* 25:P22, 1984.

Larsson, S. A. Gamma camera emission tomography. *Acta Radiol.* (Suppl.) 363:1–75, 1980.

Minato, K., et al. Three-dimensional display of single photon ECT imaging. In *Nuclear Medicine and Biology Advances*, Proceedings of the Third World Congress of Nuclear Medicine and Biology. London: Pergamon, 1983, pp. 3651–3654.

Moore, S. C.; Brunelle, J. A.; and Kirsch, C.-M. Quantitative multi-detector emission computerized tomography using iterative attenuation compensation. *J. Nucl. Med.* 23:706–714, 1982.

Mueller, S., et al. SPECT imaging with the long bore collimator: loss in sensitivity vs improved contrast resolution (abstract). *J. Nucl. Med.* 25:P106, 1984.

Nowak, D. J., and Eisner, R. L. Distance weighting for improved tomographic reconstructions (abstract). *J. Nucl. Med.* 25:P54–55, 1984.

Pizer, S. M. Intensity mappings for the display of medical images. In *Functional Mapping of Organ Systems and Other Computer Topics*, ed. P. D. Esser. New York: Society of Nuclear Medicine, 1981, pp. 205–217.

Polak, J. F.; English, R. J.; and Holman, B. L. Performance of collimators used for tomographic imaging of I-123 contaminated with I-124. *J. Nucl. Med.* 24:1064–1069, 1983.

Raff, U.; Nelson, T. R.; and Ritenour, E. R. Improvement of SPECT imaging for myocardial perfusion studies using a medial filter preprocessing technique (abstract). *J. Nucl. Med.* 25:P14, 1984.

Saw, C. B., et al. SPECT imaging (140–364 keV): influence of photon scattering and penetration on backprojected noise within tomographic plane (abstract). *J. Nucl. Med.* 25:P90, 1984.

Schlusselberg, D. S.; Lewis, M. H.; and Simon, T. R. Computer-aided analysis of three-dimensional radiopharmaceutical distributions in serial ECT acquisions (abstract). *J. Nucl. Med.* 25:P90–91, 1984.

Soderborg, B., et al. Re: determination of organ volume by single photon emission tomography (letter). *J. Nucl. Med.* 24:1197, 1983.

Tauxe, W. N., et al. Determination of organ volume by single-photon emission tomography. *J. Nucl. Med.* 23:984–987, 1982.

Tauxe, W. N., and Todd-Pokropek, A. E. Reply to re: determination of organ volume by single photon emission tomography (letter). *J. Nucl. Med.* 24:1198–1199, 1983.

Tsui, B. M. W., et al. The design and clinical utilities of a fan beam collimator for a SPECT system (abstract). *J. Nucl. Med.* 25:P5, 1984.

6

Whys and Wherefores of SPECT

As Keyes (1982) pointed out, the place of SPECT in the panoply of clinical nuclear medical modalities is uncertain. He and others examined its economics and utility and concluded that 15% to 20% of patients might benefit from the procedure and that it costs 15% to 20% more than planar imaging. Thus, allowing for a margin of error, the cost seems justified, especially in view of the fact that the buyer has gained a camera, not lost an imaging room. The instrument is generally useful for all of the procedures that Anger cameras perform and has the advantage that it can often be positioned more easily than other cameras.

REASONS FOR USING SPECT

Because SPECT acquires information from a full circle around the patient, it makes available an image that does not have to be viewed from the perspective of a particular angle, with some details being hidden. At last, clinicians can see behind an organ. Because the background can be separated from the target, the contrast of the images is improved over that available in planar projection images. Anatomic localization and details of lesions are improved (Kuhl, Edwards, and Ricci 1973).

Keyes (1982) wished to make extremely clear that even if receiver operating characteristic (ROC) analyses of the value of SPECT did not show it to be any improvement over planar imaging, this would not mean that it has no benefits. He believed that SPECT can be helpful not only in the full three-dimensional depiction of lesions in the head and liver, but that it should be used in all examinations of complex structures. There are problems, of course, if the activity distribution changes too rapidly for adequate SPECT acquisition. When optimized by special collimators for SPECT, the sensitivity of the camera is not so much worse than the probe-based instruments, while it has the advantage of collecting all of its slices at once.

Over and over again in the nuclear medicine literature there are examinations of the benefits of a particular advance, with attempts to measure these benefits with ROC or some other analysis. While there is no doubt as to the utility of ROC analysis, there are also benefits that cannot be measured, particularly not in the institutions that are doing the measuring. It is not possible for an investigator in a research setting to measure the benefit of a technique for the average practitioner of nuclear medicine. The effect of many of the advances has been to raise the overall standards of nuclear medicine being practiced, although there may be no rise for the institutions that are already at the top. One of the hidden benefits of the recent advances is to increase the confidence of practitioners in the diagnoses made in their laboratories. Used with a good Anger camera with good quality control, SPECT gives them confidence in their diagnoses by providing three-dimensional images. These are of greatest value to the experienced reader who also has access to images from complementary modalities.

PROBLEMS WITH SPECT

It is relevant in this discussion of the advantages and shortcomings of SPECT to separate the difficulties that are intrinsic to the technique from those that could be altered by better engineering. Breakthroughs must be sought to solve the intrinsic problems, while pressure can be put on manufacturers, engineers, and programmers to do something about engineering and software drawbacks.

The intrinsic problems have to do with the nature of emission imaging. A source of unknown strength and distribution lies in a body of unknown attenuation and scattering capacity. In addition, the source is of such strength that its counts must be described using Poisson statistics, in the range where the statistical uncertainties form an unsatisfactorily large fraction of the counts. The mathematic formulation of SPECT reconstruction seems to make the uncertainties worse than they are in planar imaging.

Count-rate limitations can be addressed in several ways: the detector-collimator system could be improved so that it would record a larger percentage of the emanations from the source; the collimators alone could be made more sensitive; the effects of Poisson noise could be countered more effectively in the mathematic production of images. A set of images containing several million counts in a volume of 1,000 cc should yield reasonable uncertainty if great attention is paid to using algorithms for noisy data (Oppenheim, 1981; Herman and Lent 1976). Great things are done with noisy data in the space program and for national defense; the same kinds of efforts might pay off in medicine. Sensitivity can be addressed by altering the shape, size, or composition of the detector or of its collimation. Current work in this area is on the use of multicrystal detector systems for the head and the addition of one or two more Anger cameras for the body.

Photon attenuation and Compton scatter will always be with us, but may well be tamed by systematic study of their effects and proper tuning of the camera energy window. Current wisdom suggests a narrow, centered window (Croft, Teates, and Honeyman 1982), but careful research might find that wide or off-centered windows (King et al. 1983) actually yield better images with the proper acquisition and processing. Both attenuation and Compton scattering may profitably be addressed mathematically in the course of the reconstruction. The practical approaches to attenuation correction in various parts of the body are instructive (Larsson 1980; Chang 1978) and with more computer power, better things may be able to be done in the future. Compton scattering has also been treated by Egbert and May (1980), who emphasize the use of sensible time-saving computer methods, as do Axelsson, Msaki, and Israelsson (1984) and Jaszczak and coauthors (1984). The use of models to gain some mastery over the problems of processing will be repaid handsomely if quantitative imaging becomes necessary and useful.

Improvements in Anger camera resolution have not been great recently. SPECT resolution depends on camera resolution and, with spatial uncertainties just as with statistical uncertainties, the combination of a large number of images mathematically seems to make the uncertainty in the results worse, just as can be expected from statistical theory. In addition to the uncertainties introduced by the camera, patient motion itself contributes its own.

The current perplexities regarding shape and size of the Anger camera head and patient-contour–following rotation paths must be addressed by engineering experts, as must camera nonuniformity and nonlinearity. Each camera system is only as strong as its weakest part. There should be enough attention to engineering details so that the cameras, under real-life conditions, are stable within normal variations of temperature, electrical current, and technical competence; the gantries and patient couches should not wobble or creep. The computer programs should fulfill all of the vendor's promises. Then attention can be given to the hard issues.

There will always be patients who are larger than the field of view of the camera or instrument being used. The user must make the decision about the suitability of a SPECT examination for such a patient, given that the whole organ under consideration must be in the field of view during the whole examination if the reconstruction is to be performed properly. Such large persons also strain the capabilities of the imaging table, and thus questions should be raised about safety during the procedure.

For some, the necessity of giving serious attention to quality control for a SPECT system will be a drawback. It may be late for them to "get religion" and join the congregation of those of us who feel seriously about the indispensability of such testing, but there is no time like the present. The small percentage of the workday that quality control occupies will more than pay off in terms of instrument performance and examination quality.

GENERAL CLINICAL APPLICATION OF SPECIAL SPECT PROPERTIES

Keyes (1982) believed that SPECT quantification is possible and that it can be useful not only to measure activity as a function of position, but also to measure volume.

Quantification of a volume can be useful many different ways. A lesion may be compared as to its size and shape at two different times. The size of an organ such as the kidney may be of use in deciding on the prognosis after transplantation. SPECT may provide some of the many values in comparisons of renal function. The actual volume of ventilated or perfused lung would be much more accurate in helping to make lobectomy decisions than is the current method of quantification of planar images. Cardiac stroke volume and ejection fraction could be measured using the actual volume of the chambers, rather than volumes inferred from activities that are subject to all the problems of attenuation uncorrected for in planar techniques.

Quantification of activities can be used for the following purposes: to create a graph of activity as a function of time for a particular area, to compare activities across an organ such as the brain for differentiating normal from abnormal areas, and to quantify the amount of activity in an organ at a particular time, as in the thyroid. However, SPECT will not prove very useful in producing activity-vs.-time curves unless and until the examination can be done more quickly. In comparing activities within an organ, SPECT must be used carefully, because, in spite of the fact that it improves contrast, it still does not reproduce the activity distribution accurately. It would seem that SPECT would excel in quantifying the amount of activity in an extended organ, since background considerations are eliminated. However, since quantification is bound up with resolution, attenuation, and scattering, both in the volume and in the plane of the slice, some unscrambling of the relationships by filtering may well yield images whose activity distributions match those of the object being imaged. Here, as throughout the discussion of quantification, it should be remembered that when images are said not to be quantitative, this does not mean that "hot" is "cold" and "cold" is "hot."

RESEARCH OF THE FUTURE

More research is needed into ways to correct for attenuation and scattering so that the results may be truly quantitative. It would be good to achieve this without resorting to x-ray CT imaging or other methods that extend the time, cost, or radiation dose of the examination. Mathematic filtering may provide answers.

There will be explorations into the dynamic use of SPECT; the more flexible instruments will be essential to this research. There is a great deal of interest in multicrystal SPECT, especially for cerebral blood flow work. The multicrystal systems have the advantage of speed and sensitivity in a limited area.

Research is necessary in areas that will allow the full exploitation of the power of SPECT in diagnostic imaging. Radiopharmaceutical research to find technetium-99m–labeled cerebral blood-flow agents and cardiac perfusion agents would cause a flowering of SPECT and nuclear medicine in general. Antibody imaging excites the imagination, but, at present, the contrast is so poor that even SPECT cannot help it, unless a dual-nuclide technique with subtraction of images is used.

CONNECTION WITH TCT, NMR, AND ULTRASOUND

Clearly, SPECT is in the mainstream of modern medical imaging together with x-ray CT, digital radiography, ultrasound, and nuclear magnetic resonance (NMR or MRI [magnetic resonance imaging]). Used creatively, it can allow the further exploration of functional imaging in areas where anatomic differences do not shed any light on the disease state. It is a companion to the other techniques, especially x-ray CT and NMR, and gives images that can be compared directly with those from both of these modalities.

CHOOSING AND PURCHASING A SPECT SYSTEM

Needless to say, shopping for a SPECT instrument carries all of the hazards of shopping for a camera and computer system, plus a few more. The camera must be the very best; the computer must perform all the usual nuclear medicine computer operations and have up-to-date SPECT acquisition and processing software. It must be capable of doing the examinations and be easy to operate, both for SPECT and for conventional imaging. Potential users must become knowledgeable about the SPECT technique even if they have never really participated in it. If the buyers have no familiarity with the various functions of nuclear medicine computers, they should become acquainted with the capabilities of the nearest x-ray CT scanner for an idea of the range of capabilities that should be available.

Obviously, gaining experience with the technique in a setting similar to that for which it is being purchased is advisable. One way of doing this is to visit a site and see if actual participation in the process is possible; technologist and physician might go together to learn more than either could alone. If direct participation in a patient examination is not possible, the visitor should ask to serve as a subject with a few sources placed on him and then take an active part in reconstructing the images. This is the time to ask questions about the various steps and make a list of both questions and answers. It is a good idea to talk to users of different systems and become familiar with the appearance of the images. Good counselors will not tell a shopper which instrument to buy, but will provide relevant questions, helpful information, and anecdotes. The availability of a good vendor service organization is also important. For example, the camera may need more than the usual amount of work to maintain its uniformity, and uniformity is vital to SPECT.

The following are factors that must be considered when purchasing a SPECT system: patient-contour–following orbit; Anger camera head shape; Anger camera engineering, such as stability, uniformity, and linearity; computer power; sensitivity; how the system will be used; and vendor(s) with a real interest in SPECT. After considering how the system has been used elsewhere, each new user must picture how the system will be employed in the setting of his laboratory. Of course, the buyer is looking for a vendor or vendors who will remain interested in SPECT and continue to improve the software for data acquisition and processing.

Modifications of an orbit that allow closer following of patient contour for better resolution are being made from several directions; however, some cannot be applied in all situations, such as two-headed SPECT systems. The manual method requires careful attention from technologists and cannot be practiced with all the versions of commercial acquisition software. The automatic methods must be carefully thought out to avoid injuring the patient or achieving useless orbits that are no better than the circular ones they replace.

Anger camera shape is critical to a close approach to the body, since any camera head with too thick a "rind" does not permit satisfactory proximity to the human head. Solutions to this problem include the flat-sided camera, a smaller camera head with thinner edges, and the angulated collimator.

The internal engineering of the camera head is important to stability, uniformity, and linearity. It is difficult for a particular camera to surmount flaws in design that do not permit stable operation. A potential user should ask to see quality control test data from a real camera of the type under consideration. These can only be obtained from a user of the system; the salesperson will not have it.

Computer power and storage capacity are important for gated and dynamic studies of the future and for the rapid performance of reconstruction. It may not seem important to be able to reconstruct quickly in some circumstances and laboratories, but the buyer should determine whether or not it might be desirable to call back raw data from a previous examination or series of examinations for review. If so, consider the frustration of a reconstruction time of perhaps ten minutes for each of these examinations, or of being able to load only one or two examinations and their reconstructions at a time on a disk for review. The would-be user should select a storage device that is commensurate with the amount of data to be stored; one must be especially careful not to choose a medium that will not allow storage of the largest dynamic studies, unless there is no desire to keep these. If possible, one should see the computer in action and see what it can do under normal operating conditions, such as simultaneous acquisition and processing. What happens if a gated study is being acquired simultaneously with SPECT processing? What other processing is allowed? Can anything else be done while a SPECT study is being processed? Does the full use of the computer slow down the processing? See what the effect of doubling the number of acquisition angles or quadrupling the matrix size is on processing speed. How easy is the computer to use? Does the number of options seem limited at the current time, and what are the plans for more software capability? It is foolhardy to buy promises for the future unless one is in some position to fulfill them oneself if the vendor does not.

The buyer should be wary of all combinations of camera, computer, and software because each has its own problems. A camera purchased separately from the software may not be capable of rotating in the way the software wants it to. Software purchased for a computer may not in fact connect the particular camera and computer, or may require quite a bit of extra hardware in order to perform satisfactorily. Even a system purchased from one vendor may not actually have the software and hardware flexibility available on some of the systems purchased from separate vendors.

The issue of sensitivity is important, especially in the face of the low amounts of radioactivity administered or appearing in certain structures to be imaged. Sensitivity is being enhanced by the addition of another (or perhaps two more) camera head to the system so that data may be acquired two or three times faster. Since these multiple cameras do not have exactly the same properties, they must be very carefully aligned and tuned together for their images to be anywhere near as good as those of one camera. The computer may be called upon to make the final balancing of the cameras, just as it corrects uniformity. In many instances, new collimators may help sensitivity and resolution; the fan-beam collimator improves sensitivity and resolution in the head, for example.

General advice is to look for sturdy hardware with a very good Anger camera attached, that will image all parts of the body well. One should buy an up-to-date computer. The software will be rough at first, but will improve with age (provided the vendor remains in the market). There is no cure for bad or mediocre hardware, but software can be changed. A Dun & Bradstreet report can be very useful for predicting the financial future of the company and for a look at its prospects.

BIBLIOGRAPHY

Axelsson, B.; Msaki, P.; and Israelsson, A. Subtraction of Compton-scattered photons in single-photon emission computerized tomography. *J. Nucl. Med.* 25:490–494, 1984.

Chang, L.-T. A method for attenuation correction in radionuclide computed tomography. *IEEE Trans. Nucl. Sci.* 25:638–643, 1978.

Croft, B. Y.; Teates, C. D.; and Honeyman, J. C. Single-photon emission computed tomography of the liver. In *Digital Imaging: Clinical Advances in Nuclear Medicine*, ed. P. D. Esser. New York: Society of Nuclear Medicine, 1982, pp. 271– 282.

Egbert, S. D., and May, R. S. An integral-transport method for Compton-scatter correction in emission computed tomography. *IEEE Trans. Nucl. Sci.* 27:543–548, 1980.

Herman, G. T., and Lent, A. Iterative reconstruction algorithms. *Comput. Biol. Med.* 6:273–294, 1976.

Jaszczak, R. J., et al. Improved SPECT quantification using compensation for scattered photons. *J. Nucl. Med.* 25:893–900, 1984.

Keyes, J. W., Jr. Perspectives on tomography. *J. Nucl. Med.* 23:633–640, 1982.

King, M. A., et al. Preliminary characterization of the properties of a new rotating SPECT imaging system. In *Emission Computed Tomography: Current Trends*, ed. P. D. Esser. New York: Society of Nuclear Medicine, 1983, pp. 91–104.

Kuhl, D. E.; Edwards, R. Q.; and Ricci, A. R. Transverse section scanner at the University of Pennsylvania. In *Tomographic Imaging in Nuclear Medicine*, ed. G. S. Freedman. New York: Society of Nuclear Medicine, 1973, pp. 19–26.

Larsson, S. A. Gamma camera emission tomography. *Acta Radiol.* (Suppl.) 363:1–75, 1980.

Oppenheim, B. E. An overview of the technological problems in rotating camera SPECT systems. Presented at the Single-Photon Emission Computed Tomography Symposium, Durham, North Carolina, May, 1981.

7

Quality Assurance: Acceptance Testing and Quality Control

Quality assurance is the philosophy and general approach taken to assure that the product, in this case medical images, is up to the standards that have been set for it. Quality control encompasses the specific procedures necessary to achieve quality assurance. In addition, when performed regularly, these procedures permit an easy relationship with, and mastery of, the instrument in question.

Mastery implies interest in, knowledge about, and a regard for the proper function of the instrument. Each piece of equipment seems to have a personality, and part of its behavior includes a willingness to perform correctly for certain people and not for others. It can also go awry physically, just as humans do, and require diagnosis and treatment. The speed with which its ailments are attended to will depend on someone's having rapport with both the instrument and the repairman. Although mastery does not require becoming a slave to a machine and its needs, a SPECT system should not be treated so casually that the images become too bad to be ignored. There is a middle ground, consonant with available time and energy, and with the intended clinical use of the instrument. Mastery allows the most efficient use as well as intuitive troubleshooting when something is wrong.

A broad discussion of quality assurance should cover all the parts of a nuclear medicine examination, including the people as well as the equipment.

HUMAN FACTORS

The human participants are those being examined—the patients, those performing the examinations—the technologists, and those making diagnoses—the physicians. Because SPECT involves a considerable investment of time, money, and energy, it is worthwhile for all the participants to be prepared. Patients require screening, perhaps some specific preparation, and instruction about the conduct of the examination. Technologists must be carefully trained, with refresher courses and tests as time goes along; the equipment does not go untested, so neither should the persons who operate it. Physicians also require special training; they cannot assume that because they understand all about planar imaging, SPECT is known territory.

The patient variables are the least controllable. Attempts can be made to be sure that patients are able to tolerate the supine or prone position, and are noncombative or even cooperative. A host of examination-specific attributes, such as whether or not they are fasting or hydrated, must be ascertained. The referring physician's eagerness to have a test performed for a particular patient often overrides certain apparent contraindications. This being the case, the technologists must be yet better prepared.

Technologist training should first be in basic nuclear medicine technology for an understanding of the field and its practical aspects. This knowledge must be extended, because SPECT is more technically complicated than ordinary static imaging and even more than some of the more complex dynamic examinations, perhaps not in data acquisition, but in processing. The joy of this is that with proper care in positioning and selection of acquisition variables, and use of a well-tuned and quality-assured instrument, good data can be collected by a reasonably alert, well-trained technologist. In the processing steps, SPECT requires a level of experience that leads to real understanding and discernment. Not every technologist will be able or will care to come to this point.

Physicians also start with basic nuclear medicine. A bit of background in x-ray body CT or ultrasound will be of added benefit because the transaxial plane is a new angle for looking at the human body and experience is needed to gain familiarity with the projection. Beyond the unfamiliar anatomic projections, there is a large number of variables to become familiar with, because the practitioner should know the effect of a particular acquisition or processing choice on the resulting images. Thus SPECT will be a badly used technique without the interest of its users in maintaining quality from start to finish. Since the physicians are ultimately responsible for everything in the nuclear medicine laboratory, they must take the lead in insisting on adequate and continuing training for themselves and their technologists, as well as quality assurance, maintenance, and timely upgrades for the SPECT instrument.

Lest my physicist colleagues feel left out of the discussion, I must state that they have not been included because I feel it is possible to do good SPECT examinations and achieve adequate quality assurance without a physicist on the premises. It is the physicist's place to bind together all the ideas of this chapter and to use them in everyday practice and teaching.

THE SYSTEM

The whole practice of quality assurance is a field in itself, much more developed in x-ray imaging than in nuclear medicine (Gray et al. 1983). Without the possibility of employing a flying squadron of quality-control experts (which might be appropriate in a large institution with several active SPECT units), it is possible to keep on top of the variables of a SPECT system with a reasonable time budget and at reasonable intervals. Following the lead of the book just mentioned, sample forms for quality control procedures for SPECT should be developed. The reasons for the tests and the test interpretation are discussed in the remainder of this chapter.

At the very heart of quality assurance is the principle of comparison of the instrument's present and past performances. Acceptance testing involves testing some of the variables once and for all, and others for the first time to begin the comparisons. For satisfactory comparisons, data must be acquired and recorded in a standard fashion. Data acquisition and processing should be operator independent. Systems involving several parts must have all their components and interfaces checked and put through their paces. The computer can be a very useful adjunct to quality control testing in addition to being one of the components to be tested.

Comparison of past and present performance is a way to observe stability in the instrument and in the whole system. The time (or space) frame for such testing may vary according to the needs of the instrument and the operators. Stability is important to routine operation. Having a measure of the speed with which a certain value is varying enables the user to know when to collect a new set of correction factors or when to have the instrument retuned. If a value seems to depend on a rapidly varying environmental property such as room temperature or electrical noise, one can try to correct both the instrument's dependence and the environmental difficulty. An Anger camera should not be a huge thermometer, and the temperature in a nuclear medicine laboratory should not fluctuate by more than several degrees, even on a hot summer day.

Comparison can only be made if records are kept, so record keeping is important to quality assurance. One should be thoughtful, however, before starting yet another notebook or pile of films, or filling yet another computer file. The user should try to consider which information is of long-lasting value (because it gives a standard to live up to or is one clue to a trend) and which is of evanescent value (necessary for the day's information but of no importance in several days or weeks).

It would be well to get two ideas out into the open. The first, as has already been stated, is that there should be routine quality control testing for a SPECT system. It will come in the form of special tests and of critical examination of patient images. The special tests should take only one-half hour per day or less, unless a problem is suspected, and generate perhaps one piece of film, one piece of paper, and a small computer file or addition to a computer file. The second important idea is that quality assurance must involve making use of the information that is gathered during testing. If the information is not going to be used, it should not be bothered with, and neither should SPECT, because it will prove unrewarding. In addition, any person using the images, whether a newly trained technologist or an experienced physician, should maintain a critical eye and not be afraid to speak up. Poor, nondiagnostic images from out-of-tune equipment represent wasted time and radiation dose to all concerned.

One school of thought would have us design quality-control phantoms so that the results could be read directly off the images, as when a photomultiplier (PM) tube is very obviously much more or less sensitive, or when one quadrant of a bar phantom is or is not visible. The other school would have us quantify observations to give numeric descriptions of the instrument's performance. Both of these views have validity, with the former obviously taxing the phantom designer more than the instrument tester or the computer programmer. Since reliance on computer processing for the presentation of the data has become almost complete in the case of SPECT, however, it seems that the numeric outlook must at least supplement the qualitative one. Thus one must use the computer and special software in testing. As the numeric measurements are adopted, they should be standardized, perhaps using the National Electrical Manufacturers' Association (NEMA) (1980; Muehllehner, Wake, and Sano 1981) recommendations as a guide, so that users and manufacturers are all talking about the same properties of the instrument. Special attempts must be made to keep the tests sensible and comprehensible so that their obviousness is unmistakable.

The SPECT instrument must be tested as a static device and as a tomographic device, so as to separate the factors and simplify troubleshooting. In addition, since the whole instrument combines camera and computer through an interface, all of the parts must be tested, separately and together. Thus acceptance and quality control testing could be fairly time consuming. This discussion is a recommendation for neither the minimum amount of testing that one can get away with nor an exhaustive quantity that leaves no time for clinical work or for the other duties of the technologist, physician, and physicist.

Decisions about how often to perform a particular test are made with reference to several standards: How rapidly can a particular property of the instrument change? How much does a measurable change matter? What is the testing interval mandated by regulation or other written standards? Since each system is an individual, it is impossible to set testing intervals for them all. Local practice should be in response to the behavior of a particular instrument. The acceptance testing period should give users familiarity with the instrument's characteristics and allow the repair of the most objectionable dysfunctions. Beyond this, adhering to a testing schedule is important, but so is the intuition born of experience. When a particular error is suspected, a procedure designed to examine that property should be performed whether or not it is time for the test. System failures do not come on schedule.

CAMERA QUALITY CONTROL

This chapter is organized according to the following general outline of quality control of the Anger camera, the computer and interface, and the SPECT system: what to test, general methods, what and how to image, what to record, what to do with the information, interpretation, and comments. These sections aim to be methodical rather than exciting and to lead to a quiet pride in the performance of good routine examinations; the opposite of this is the exciting and disheartening practice of examinations in which poor equipment and procedures cause, at best, nondiagnostic examinations and, at worst, the false-negative and false-positive results that SPECT is supposed to help prevent.

The Anger camera will not function properly unless all of its components are working. Thus correctly peaked and set energy window, sensitivity, uniformity, linearity, resolution, and any effects of uniformity and other corrections must all be tested, although perhaps not all with the same frequency. The sensitivity and uniformity of the Anger camera are basic to SPECT because all the systematic nonuniformity errors multiply in the production of transaxial slice images. Thus tests, techniques, and standards suitable for plane projection work are not adequate for SPECT.

Not only is energy peaking the variable to begin with in working with an Anger camera, or any other thallium-activated sodium iodide [NaI(Tl)] detector system, it is the rock on which the operation of the system is founded. For the Anger camera, the best count rate is found around the photopeak, and the most uniform and linear images are produced there. Off-peak operation is now being used more in SPECT, with computer corrections, than ever before, but it must remain suspect until proved to be an acceptable mode of operation for a particular camera.

The visual tests of camera uniformity performed on 3 million (M)-count images do not go far enough. One can devise numeric tests to discover something about the statistics of the counts forming the image and the degree of uniformity, but a visual test of certain computer-formed images is very much to the point. These may be fairly elaborate images of mean ± 1 standard deviation (SD) or images of the difference between two relevant test images. The routine given below may be substituted for the analog quality control procedure used daily for most Anger cameras, since it goes beyond the analog procedure.

The NEMA standard method for uniformity testing was predicated on local nonuniformities causing artifacts that might be perceived as lesions. The method does not consider that the large nonuniformities that can show up as ring artifacts on transaxial images would be a problem (Fig 7–1), so it is not directed at discovering these. The bias toward the detection of small nonuniformities makes reliance on the NEMA format as the sole arbiter of uniformity unwise, although the camera should meet this standard too. This is especially important if quantitative imaging of any kind is being attempted, because thresholds have to be based on some high count.

Linearity goes right along with uniformity and is closely con-

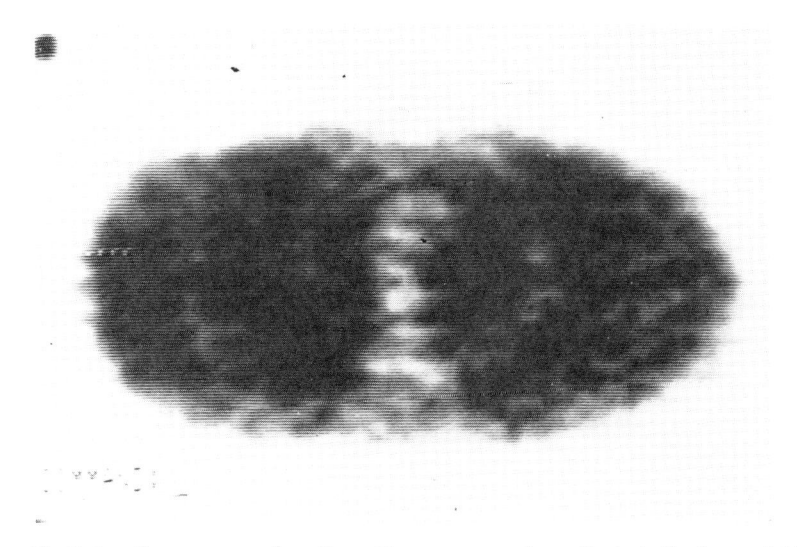

Fig 7-1.—Camera nonuniformities will appear as a ring artifacts in the transaxial image. Any nonuniformity visible to the naked eye on an analog image will cause a ring in the transaxial image.

nected to the energy window setting. Pincushion and barrel distortions are common in the modern, light-guideless cameras unless they are carefully corrected. Linearity is obviously important, especially since nonlinearity may be the real cause of nonuniformity. Camera manufacturers have realized this and have begun providing automatic microprocessor-based circuits that get at the roots of energy instability, nonlinearity, and nonuniformity (Chapter 3). In an older camera, it is possible to correct nonlinearity using a grid phantom in much the same way as nonuniformity is corrected (Brookeman et al. 1972; Spector et al. 1972) except that it is more difficult and time consuming. Because of the trouble involved, no one makes this correction if the camera is not designed to do it automatically. It is obvious that nonlinearity should have an adverse effect on SPECT images, but the need to resort to elaborate and time-consuming methods to eliminate nonuniformity is not obvious. Mercifully, new camera designs are making the question moot.

Resolution and sensitivity are derivative properties of the system that are observed after the other tests are made and the instrument is ready to operate. Resolution is of interest not only on the surface of the collimator but at depth in a scattering medium. As such, it is a useful property to measure in a planar fashion, but much more interesting to measure in the three dimensions as a property of the whole SPECT system. Therefore, much more is made of resolution later in this chapter.

The processes of determining and storing, in some way, a uniformity correction and of deciding whether that correction is adequate are different. The correction itself should involve 30 M or more counts, while its adequacy might be tested with one-tenth that many. Of course, if the correction is found to be inadequate, a new correction must be stored.

The general method for Anger camera quality control tests is to have the camera image a known object under a standard and recorded set of conditions and to look at the image and at other recorded variables, such as counts in a unit of time per millicurie in the test object. The SPECT quality control protocols generally add acquisition of the image by computer, the use of more counts than are required for pure analog imaging, volume comparisons, and some computer programs to test the data and make numeric comparisons. In no case should the computer calculations be substituted for the pattern recognition capability of the human eye and brain. Since the quality control for the camera involves the computer and vice versa, the process of testing and tuning sounds somewhat circular. If the computer is used to test the camera and the computer is not working, then how can one be sure of anything? Luckily, some rather basic tests of each part will allow the system to be set to start the spiral of testing and tuning.

The influences of room temperature changes, line voltage instability, presence of moving or intermittent sources of gamma or x-radiation, and magnetic flux can cause intermittent difficulties with camera stability. According to the camera's situation, each of these difficulties must be sought, experimented with, and solved. Testing a suspect system at different hours of the day or "surprise" testing just after a clinical study may reveal problems not seen in the routine testing times of early morning or after-hours.

Energy Peaking and Window Setting

Research has shown that correct centering and stability of the energy window are central to finding uniformity and linearity acceptable. Therefore, quality control of the camera usually starts with attention to the energy window and recording the energy spectrum and window every day. This may be done with the collimator in place with a solid or liquid source, or without the collimator, using a point source.

Most Anger cameras are equipped to allow the user to examine the spectrum of the PM tubes on the crystal as a whole array. A few allow the user to look at spectra from individual tubes, but this is not an everyday event. Tubes are tuned by service people, often very laboriously. When an older camera is tuned, count rates for individual tubes are maximized, then a bit of judicious detuning is added to prevent a hot center or a hot edge or a particularly hot tube. This detuning to achieve as much basic uniformity as possible is at the root of problems encountered when operating with the energy window deliberately offset from the peak, because tube response there will not match the way it does on-peak.

The energy window should be examined and set using an extended flood source (to be discussed in more detail) and enough activity to be certain of the position of the peak in the window. A source like that used for subsequent uniformity testing should be used, so that systems for which the certainty of position of the window in the peak depends on the count rate will have adequate counts to determine the peak position. Systems that show a spectrum should be using an adequate count rate in the display so that the user is not forced to deal with inadequate statistics. Poor statistics will be evidenced by a changed appearance in the spectrum from one spectrum image to the next. If this seems to be the case, one can combine the highest count rate on the count-rate meter with a spectrum display that seems to be peaked. A well-peaked instrument gives the highest count rate together with a satisfactory spectrum.

A standard offset window can be determined by the simultaneous occurrence of a particular spectrum (guaranteeing the offset to the correct side of the peak) with a particular fraction of the maximum counts in the centered window. The protocol thus requires centering the window before offsetting it (LaFontaine, Graham, and Stein 1984). Obviously, statistics must be adequate for reproducibility in such cases, implying the need for 10,000 to 20,000 counts per second across the whole camera face, so that decreases of 5% to 15% could be measured well.

It should be understood that an Anger camera must be peaked at least once every working day as the first action before using it. It may be repeaked or checked during the day; some laboratories have insisted on spectrum or gray-wedge and uniformity images before every patient examination. The camera should be peaked with a source, not the patient, because the patient incorporates too much scattering medium. Each and every radionuclide should be checked; often this means the camera is tested and set in the morning with technetium-

99m and then repeaked when other nuclides are used during the day. Preset pushbutton settings allow the preservation of values determined for a particular nuclide. The technetium-99m spectrum, the voltage value to produce it, and the window width are recorded and filed with other quality control data for that camera for that day. If the computer allows storage of spectra, it would be useful to have them for comparison, although such data cannot be used to rescue any examinations, but only to prevent future difficulties and chart past performance. Because individual tubes are not tested, it is difficult to appreciate all but the broadest shifts in energy spectrum.

When several radionuclides are used together, the system must be observed very carefully. Spilldown is usually a linear phenomenon in which scattered counts and counts from lower-energy peaks of the higher-energy nuclide appear in the lower-energy nuclide's window, in proportion to the number in the higher-energy window. Spillup in NaI(Tl)-PM tube detector systems is usually a nonlinear phenomenon, depending not only on the number of counts in the lower-energy window but on the total count rate. Thus a proper test for spilldown and spillup requires the use of sources of several activities, all presumably within the count-rate range in use. There is no point in studying the system in count-rate ranges in which it will not be used.

The energy variable is so basic to the operation of the system that variations in energy spectrum of individual PM tubes are the cause of nearly all variations in uniformity and linearity beyond the fixed one caused by the geometric arrangement of the tubes on the crystal. Because the individual tubes are so numerous and difficult to isolate for testing, uniformity is the property that is observed, but it should always be remembered that an energy-related problem is probably the basis for a difficulty.

Sensitivity and Uniformity

The point was made earlier that while energy differences and shifts are at the heart of changes in the Anger camera as a detector of radiation, uniformity is what is measured to detect these changes, because it gives us the whole picture all at once. We really are interested in how the camera behaves as a unit, and it should be tested that way.

The uniformity phantom is not used merely to test to see how uniform the image is, as in the good old days, but it teaches the camera or the computer a pattern that can be applied as a correction factor to the clinical images. The modern camera, when uncorrected, is quite nonuniform in its response, so it must have the correction factors not only for SPECT but for all operations.

Quality Assurance

There are two ways to measure uniformity: intrinsically, with a point source with the collimator off and a lead ring to cover the outer row of PM tubes; or extrinsically, with a large flood source of some kind and the collimator on. The following discussion covers the use and advantages and disadvantages of each, as well as their utility under certain circumstances. Feeling runs high about the proper way to create a uniformity image, and there is no general consensus. Because the arguments for and against the particular methods are familiar, they are presented in outline as follows so direct comparisons can be made among points.

Point source:

1. Easy to make with any nuclide
2. Small amount of activity and radiation exposure
3. Collimator off, lead ring in:
   a. Cumbersome, crystal unprotected
   b. Hard to get the source far enough away
   c. Cannot be rotated
   d. Potential backscatter; room background problems
   e. Does not integrate collimator into system
4. Guarantees uniformity of counts themselves
5. Can not easily be incorporated into scatter medium measurement
6. Can be used with lead bars, hole phantoms, other patterns
7. Easy to shield source against scatter from its holder

Sheet source:

1. Not all nuclides can handily be incorporated
2. Large amounts of activity and radiation exposure
3. Collimator on:
   a. Normal operating mode, crystal protected
   b. Sheet source sits on collimator
   c. Can be rotated, if source hangs on
   d. No backscatter problems; background controlled
   e. Tests the collimator as part of the system
4A. Solid sheet source—cobalt-57:
   a. Uniformity problems
   b. No filling problems
   c. Only cobalt-57 available
   d. Must be replaced every 6 months or tolerate lowered count rates
4B. Liquid sheet source:
   a. Can be well mixed
   b. Filling problems, bulges, etc.
   c. Can be filled with several nuclides
   d. Can be used for long time

4A. Solid sheet source—cobalt-57: (cont.)	4B. Liquid sheet source: (cont.)
e. No mess if dropped	e. Messy if it breaks

5. Can incorporate scattering medium between source and collimator
6. Can be used with lead bars, hole phantoms, other patterns
7. Some scatter accepted with use of sheet source

The issues raised in the outline are important, but the discerning reader can soon see that there is no one correct solution to the problems (Rogers et al. 1982). It suggests some possibilities for standard operating procedures. First, routine uniformity checking and correction-image formation can be performed with a point source or a properly filled sheet source in the technetium-99m energy range, provided that the user is satisfied that his collimator is not a source of error. The solid cobalt-57 sheet sources are very convenient, but not uniform enough. If elaborate measures (Oppenheim and Appledorn 1985) are used to find an image of the cobalt-57 sheet source separately from camera nonuniformities, the source must subsequently be positioned exactly in the same way in the computer matrix and, of course, a new image must be measured whenever a new source is purchased.

A point source, used with the lead shielding ring, should be of such an activity that it does not stress the count-rate capabilities of the camera, including not only the counts in the window, but those excluded, since the PM tubes must still be detecting the radiation whether it ultimately falls within the window or not. The point source should be hung, if possible, about 7 camera field-of-view diameters away from the crystal face, symmetrically, so that there is no close scattering medium to confuse the issue. Other sources of ionizing radiation may also confuse the camera; these may be in the laboratory upstairs, the dribble of activity on the floor from yesterday, the x-ray CT unit across the hall, the radioactive patients in the hall, or the radiopharmacy. A camera with the collimator off is a very, very sensitive instrument with a wide angle of acceptance. In one laboratory, the point source is put on the floor and a lead apron is draped around the camera head to shield it from the radiopharmacy area. The lower-energy nuclides such as thallium-201 will be even more difficult than technetium-99m, because lead x-rays from shielding higher-energy gamma rays enter the thallium-201 window. A distance of 7 camera field-of-view diameters is suggested to cause the gamma-ray flux at the center and edge of the field of view to differ by less than 0.5%. At five times the field-of-view diameter, the error is about 1%, which may be acceptable if an adequate number of counts is collected, because the point source does put out a perfectly uniform flux in all directions if it has been properly constructed and used. If the point source is encased in a lead shield with a hole in it, some thicknesses of copper shielding over the source and the lead shield are recommended to avoid the lead x-rays and other scattered radiation (R. Adams, personal communication, 1984).

The point source method may have to be used under all circumstances for a camera that must "learn" the separate energy peaks and uniformity correction images for each radionuclide that will be used with it.

A liquid sheet source has its own peculiarities, but has the added advantage for the SPECT system that the uniformity-correction image can be collected with the correct collimator on the camera. This is important because collimators can cause enough differences in uniformity to degrade SPECT reconstructed images (Farrell, Cradduck, and Chamberlain 1984). In addition, the liquid sheet source can be attached to the camera face, so uniformity images at all angles can be compared. The problem with the liquid sheet source lies in the deformability of the plastic from which it is constructed. No matter how uniform the void inside the empty source may be, when it is filled with water it changes shape in many positions. When the source is opened to receive a new charge of technetium-99m it is usually stood on its edge and bulges, with the result that more liquid could be poured into it than it should hold. After it is closed, this extra liquid will cause a hot center. A fair amount of pressure on the open source exerted while putting the screws back into the holes will force it back to the correct size; too much pressure will cause a cold center. If the source is attached to the collimator and rotated with the camera, it will bulge on the lower side. These difficult handling procedures increase the user's radiation dose. Inventive minds need to institute a search for liquid sheet source designs that incorporate ease of filling, portability, and dimensional stability in all positions. Even great thicknesses of plastic have not proved rigid enough. Other workers have fallen afoul of chemical reactions that corrode metals in the presence of saline. The source should be fitted with clamps that allow it to be fixed to the collimator so that it can be used at various angles of rotation without requiring a person or some jury-rigged apparatus to hold it. It should be light enough for the SPECT system to rotate it, together with the camera head and collimator.

Since nuclides other than technetium-99m are not usually used with a liquid sheet source in most laboratories, energy peaking and

190 Chapter 7

uniformity correction images for other nuclides must use point sources. The collimators used for the other energy ranges should be checked with the technetium-99m sheet source initially and at intervals such as yearly, or after they have received wounds in the laboratory battles, to be sure they are not introducing nonuniformities.

It is suggested that the following combination of sources be used for creating and checking uniformity images: technetium-99m in a liquid sheet source for the major check every day, point sources in the intrinsic mode for other nuclides, and a large solid source, if there is one available, for rotation, because it does not deform (English, Polak, and Holman 1984).

There are also some camera-specific questions to be asked: Does the camera require a new uniformity correction at every new energy? For on-peak operation? For off-peak operation? Is the correction good for all window widths? What is the optimum width at which to collect the correction image? Is the correction collected in multiple windows for multiple-peak operation (as for gallium-67)? Is it applied to multiple peaks if collected at one peak setting? Is there provision for corrections to all windows under true multiple-window operation, in which there is a separate image for each window? What provision is there for correction of spilldown and spillup? Obviously, routine operation with technetium-99m with a peak-centered window does not require answers to these questions. Other modes of operation do, however, so they warrant thoughtful testing of the actual instrument to be used.

For a stable camera, the following protocol is recommended: Using a liquid flood uniformity source, one collects 30 M counts in a computer image, with the same matrix dimensions as will be used for clinical work, at count rates that are not excessive for the camera. Thirty million counts was chosen, because in a 64×64 matrix, there are 10,000 (10 K) counts per pixel, or an acceptable statistical sample. The 30 M-count image is used to correct succeeding clinical images, if necessary. It is also used to check the quality of 3 M-count images taken on succeeding days, also corrected with the 30 M-count image. The corrected 3 M-count images are viewed on the computer monitor and archived on film with contrast enhancement thresholds of 50% to 60% on the lower side. Such enhanced images should have a salt-and-pepper random appearance, rather than any suggestions of structure. If structure can be seen, it indicates drift in the camera uniformity pattern and a new 30 M-count image should be collected and the process repeated. Obviously, this is an exercise in futility for an unstable camera. In the newer cameras, PM tube spectra and sensitivities may be continuously corrected by a microcomputer.

If circuits in the camera, exclusive of the computer, collect and apply the uniformity correction, as in the older GE 400T camera, the camera may not be using a satisfactory algorithm or adequate statistics in its processing, so that the uniformity will not be good enough for SPECT. The same, of course, may be true for some automatic computer-collection protocols, so the user should be sure that he knows what the computer is doing when it is collecting and creating a uniformity correction image.

In adapting this procedure for use in a particular setting, adjustments of the numbers of counts acquired and the matrix size are made to fit the usual SPECT imaging situation of the laboratory. For acquiring a uniformity correction image, one uses the same matrix size and two to three times as many counts as the total number in the SPECT study.

At no time during the testing or use of a SPECT system should the camera's maximum permissible count rate be exceeded. The loss of counts due to dead time produces distortion and is unacceptable in any circumstance. For the ordinary large-field camera, 20,000 to 50,000 counts per second depending on the camera is a sensible upper limit, meaning that 30 M counts will take ten to 25 minutes to acquire.

The users should be aware of the maximum count-rate capabilities of the instrument, and also that some digital systems now have correction circuits that attempt to provide replacement counts for those lost to dead time. Such corrections should be used carefully, because significant dead-time losses usually mean that the energy spectrum has lost its usual peaked quality and that the full width at half maximum (FWHM) has greatly broadened. In a sense, the excess counts are leaking out of the window at higher and lower energies. If this is a differential effect across the field of view of the camera because the source distribution has high and low count-rate areas, then parts of the image are affected and others are not. The dilemma of nuclear medical imaging is that, just as count rates that would yield good statistics for images acquired in short time intervals are approached, the NaI(Tl)-crystal-PM tube system is unable to handle them. Because the circumstances of testing for the maximum count-rate characteristics of the system (the collimator off and a point source) can represent a shock to the camera's system, it is not recommended that this test be performed often, or that a "naked" crystal be flooded with large amounts of activity, no matter what the source. The camera should be treated as a delicate instrument, physically and electronically.

The same 30 M-count image can be used for correction until it is no longer a true image for the camera, or it can be replaced at regular intervals, such as weekly, according to a schedule.

The 30 M-count image should itself be examined visually and with computer enhancement for any untoward detail. In many cameras, the PM tubes will be visible. This is acceptable though not desirable, but very active or very inactive areas should be viewed with suspicion as signs of future trouble. With a little practice one can learn the expected image, rather like the face of a friend. Computer processing and contrast enhancement of the daily images bring out detail and make the mathematic comparisons useful.

In testing the adequacy of the 3 M-count daily test images, numeric measures of camera uniformity should be used. These should be made with reference to the number of counts in the images. To say that a system has a uniformity of 5% without an associated count density per pixel is meaningless, since uniformity is a statistical property and depends on the number of counts under consideration. In addition, a percentage measurement is not so useful as one that compares nonuniformity with the statistical uncertainty of the image, which can be expressed by the standard deviation. To practice such a comparison, the average number of counts per pixel in some selected field, either the central field of view or the useful field of view, is calculated. Then NEMA (1980; Raff, Spitzer, and Hendee 1984) differential and integral nonuniformity (or another measure if so desired) are calculated and expressed as a number of standard deviations. In a 64 × 64 matrix, with a camera circle of radius equal to 32 pixels, 3,056 (or 95%) of the 3,217 pixels that constitute the circle should have values inside ± 2 SD. The number of pixels that lie outside the range of ± 2 SD can be calculated and compared to the ideal. An image may be formed of a corrected uniformity test image, with the thresholds placed to eliminate all areas where counts are outside ± 2 SD. The image is important because it shows whether any troubles are concentrated in some way that might cause a reconstruction artifact or whether the nonuniformities seem random. The human eye and brain can make this determination easily.

Planar sensitivity is usually measured in connection with uniformity. A record is kept of the amount of activity used in the standard procedure for collecting and checking the uniformity image, and the times of calibration and use. At the time of uniformity imaging, the count rate is recorded and the count rate per activity unit is calculated and recorded. Obviously, standard procedures must be used or the number is meaningless.

Several problems can be diagnosed through quality control procedures. When the uniformity image changes in part of the image, the difficulty may be that one of the PM tubes is loose; this has been the most common problem. Tubes are generally round or hexagonal. Round tubes slide easily onto the grease and can be installed easily with no air bubbles between the quartz front window and the crystal, but they can slide out of line and be pushed off the crystal by lever-type action of the plate and springs that hold the tubes on the plug end. Hexagonal tubes are harder to install correctly, because there is only one way to put them in and they cannot be twisted back and forth in the grease to remove air bubbles. Since there is only one way that they fit together, they stay in place better and conform to the back plate.

Once the PM tube-to-crystal coupling has been eliminated as a reason for nonuniformity, the crystal and electronics must be examined for problems. Crystals become damaged and can turn yellow from the action of air and water on the sodium iodide, but this is rare. The electronics of the camera head may be faulty; each tube has its own energy-tuning circuit. Small changes in energy peaking will cause large changes in the image, so the energy peak and window must be carefully adjusted. Each manufacturer approaches the camera head differently, so users must work with service personnel to learn the characteristics and idiosyncrasies of their systems. The service-person should demonstrate what the out-of-tune condition looks like so that it can be recognized.

Linearity

Linearity is a measure of how closely the camera is able to image a straight line as a straight line. Linearity is important because the SPECT system integrates signals from a slice all the way through the patient. Variations in linearity affect the resolution in the x and z directions in the transaxial image and the actual thickness of the slice in the y direction. Poor linearity will cause a general loss of resolution in three-dimensional work.

Some of the newer camera systems learn a linearity correction, but in other cases the user is only observing the linearity, which is a derivative property of the energy window setting and the physical design of the crystal-PM tube connection. The NEMA method for observing linearity is satisfactory, but other bar phantoms can be used with equal success.

If the camera is to learn a correction, the manufacturer's instructions should be followed for storing the correction. Linearity testing can then proceed by standard methods. In this case, the user should ascertain what the statistical quality of the information collected is and with what resolution the linearity correction is being made, lest it actually contribute error rather than correct it.

In the NEMA method, a special linearity and resolution lead bar phantom with 1–mm slits 30 mm apart is used intrinsically with a point source behind it. Counts are collected in a 64 × 64 or 128 × 128 matrix, with at least 1,000 counts in the high-count pixel. The operator uses a special computer program to find the position of the slits of the phantom along the direction parallel to the slit, which reflects the linearity. Functional images to reflect the degree of linearity could be made. Analog images should be made of the data as well. The absolute and differential linearity are calculated after the test is performed with the slits parallel to both the x and y axes. It is possible to tune some cameras to eliminate most linearity defects, while others will always show wavy lines.

There are many other ways to test linearity. One can use orthogonal hole phantoms, parallel-line equal-spacing (PLES) phantoms, the Hine-Duley bar phantom or some other linear pattern, or even sources made with radioactive tubing in straight rows. If the pattern runs only one way, it must be turned and used in both the x and y directions, since the x and y linearity circuits may work separately. One may do this test intrinsically, as in the NEMA method, or extrinsically with the collimator on and a sheet source behind the lead pattern. If the camera is tested with the collimator on, one must beware of moire effects or interference between the collimator holes and the holes or spaces in the phantom plate. Moire effects can also occur between the computer matrix and the other elements.

Depending on the final use to which the information is to be put, it may be stored only as an analog image or it may be acquired and analyzed by computer. The testing bears a great resemblance to resolution testing, but the critical points to look for are different.

Linearity testing, whether carried out by the intrinsic NEMA method or other ways, should be performed once a week or more often, depending on the utility of the results and the stability of the instrument. The results should be marked and filed for reference and used for later comparison.

The NEMA linearity tests include a test of the ability of the camera to sense the same position at different energies. Any serious difference in the intrinsic position of a multiple-peaked source, such as gallium-67, at different energies should call into question the adequacy of the energy window settings or the built-in correction routines, which could well be mispositioning the source. Deviations should be adjusted before trying multiple-peak imaging, because there would be a degradation in resolution when the images did not register properly, since the axis of rotation would be in different locations in the matrix for different nuclides.

Resolution

Resolution is a measurement made to test the system's ability to separate one structure from another spatially. Because there are so many kinds of structures to be separated, many tests of resolution have been proposed and are relevant, although perhaps only in a limited setting. Resolution is a derivative measurement; for SPECT, it may be derived as much from the software as from the hardware. This discussion of Anger camera resolution mentions the standard methods of measurement; later resolution is discussed in the SPECT setting.

The NEMA standards approach the question of resolution in several ways. First, intrinsic resolution, with the collimator off and a point source flooding the resolution and uniformity bar pattern just mentioned, tests for full width at half maximum (FWHM) and full width at tenth maximum (FWTM) of the 1–mm slits of the same phantom as is used for linearity measurements. Beyond this, the same profiles can be used as line-spread functions for the calculation of an intrinisic modulation-transfer function (MTF) for the camera. To test the camera with the collimator on, the range of patterns discussed for linearity testing above has been used, along with alternating wedges of different-sized bars. If the resolution is meant to be read qualitatively from images of these phantoms, there should be a section of the bars that the camera can barely resolve, so that one can see when the camera loses a bit of resolution and the bars can no longer be seen. Point and line sources can be used to obtain point- and line-spread functions from which an MTF for the system can be calculated. Further steps in resolution measurement require imaging in the presence of a scattering medium of varying depth. In some laboratories, this might mean a bar phantom separated from the collimator face by thicknesses of plastic, while in others it means a container of water surrounding a point or line source for a series of measurements with an increasing depth of water between the source and the collimator.

Any and all of these tests are relevant for SPECT, but a great deal of time can be used performing them. Only the simple testing at the collimator face need be done on a weekly basis, performed with the linearity testing; information recorded and saved should consist of at least an image and perhaps the results of computer processing. The most sophisticated processing could include functional images of FWHM and FWTM over the camera face, to display variation graphically, so that poorer areas of the detector could be seen.

There will clearly be a variation of resolution with collimators, since they are optimized for various purposes. In addition, because resolution is affected by the number of scintillations generated in the crystal by gamma-ray interaction, there is a variation of resolution with gamma-ray energy using the same collimator. This property is of special interest when images made with different nuclides are being compared, because the structures have softer edges with the lower-energy nuclides.

COMPUTER AND INTERFACE QUALITY CONTROL

By virtue of using the planar images in mathematic calculations to produce the transaxial image, SPECT puts stringent requirements on the camera-computer connections. Although the general idea is still to be sure that what the camera sees is what the computer records, there is more subtlety for SPECT. Exactness in position and distance must be part of the relationship of the data acquired by the computer to the activity distribution seen by the camera. The x and y axes of the camera must be lined up with the x and y axes of the computer matrix. The axis of the gantry's rotation comes at the center of the matrix. Proper alignment means that the process of back projection will combine data from a particular volume element in the patient, imaged at all angles, into a voxel in the transaxial image. Misalignment will degrade the resolution of the system. The distance between one pixel and the next in both the x and y directions must be the same and it must be known so that the computer can perform attenuation corrections.

Both the camera and computer have timing capabilities. They are used to time frame lengths and deliberate pauses after movement and before data acquisition in SPECT. The computer also finds the heartbeat frequency in gated studies. On occasion, the timing capability of either the camera or the computer can be in error. What seems to be causing the problems, such as a computer timing board or chip, should be discovered so that it can be fixed.

Analog-to-digital converters (ADCs) are the final interface between analog camera data and the computer. If the camera emits digital signals, the ADC of the computer will be unnecessary. The ADCs are responsible for turning the analog x and y position signals into digital information and must be tested to be sure that the positions are correct and that all the pulses they are presented with are recorded by the computer.

For SPECT, the camera gantry's rotation is controlled by the computer, which tells it when to rotate and how far around to go. Incorrect angular stepping will cause data from an inappropriate angle to be acquired, making nonsense of the reconstructed images.

Gating is one of the other functions the computer handles for the camera-computer system. The computer senses the heart rate from the electrocardiograph (ECG) attached to patient leads; it divides the cardiac cycle into a specified number of segments for data acquisition. Multiple-gated SPECT, in which images are acquired for a series of cardiac segments at each of the angular increments of the SPECT acquisition, represents the ultimate in camera-computer cooperation for data acquisition. Obviously, multiple-gated acquisition must be as efficient as the rest of the system.

The general method for testing the interface between the camera and the computer and the acquisition process is to have the camera image a known object, with computer acquisition, and see if the digital images and variables match the analog images and variables, where the variables include numbers of counts, distances, and acquisition times. The disconcerting part of testing and analyzing the results is that the camera and computer's automatic processing may make it difficult to be sure what the camera is really imaging or what the raw information being passed to the computer is like. It should be, but is not always, possible to bypass the corrections so that a simple one-to-one correspondence should exist between the input and the output.

Center of Rotation—X-Axis Offset and Straightness

The x and y axes of the camera must correspond to the x and y axes of the computer matrix, with no rotation. The correct alignment is mechanical: the PM tubes must be placed on the crystal so that the y axis of the camera will be straight up and down in the computer matrix. There should be positive positioning devices inside the camera shielding to assure the stability of the correspondence. The center-of-rotation test described below, if performed at various positions along the y axis, will evaluate this relationship. If the camera image never seems correctly positioned in the matrix, the axes should be checked.

Two special calibrations of the ADCs are required for SPECT. The first of these is to assure that the axis of rotation falls in the center of the computer matrix, for the correct calculation of back-projected images (Fig 7–2). This means that if the lower left-hand corner of the computer matrix is $x = 1$, $y = 1$, the axis of rotation should fall in $x = 32.5$ in a 64×64 matrix, or $x = 64.5$ in a 128×128 matrix. If it does not, the transaxial reconstruction of a point source will be a little open circle, giving an idea of the degradation of resolution in SPECT images that this problem causes.

The correct x-axis offset (called center of rotation) may be tested manually, automatically, or semiautomatically by the computer software. A manual check involves imaging a point source from above and below and recording the data with the computer. One finds the position of the point in each of the two views; since the image of a point source will not be a single pixel, one must determine where the source actually is by using a Gaussian or bell-shaped curve fit, mathematically, graphically, or by eye. The average pixel position of the point is found by dividing the pixel distance between the points in the two matrices by 2 and adding the value of the lower pixel position. The result should be 32.5 (for a 64×64 matrix, if $x = 1$ is the first pixel) $\pm$ 0.25 pixels. The relationship should be tested in different parts of the camera image. If the axis of rotation does not fall at the correct location, one may use the point sources as a guide to resetting the ADCs or fill a scalp-vein catheter with radioactivity (or use another line source) and tape it to the exact middle of the collimator face. The desired pixel position is marked on the relevant oscilloscope screen with a marker, and the ADCs are adjusted until the image of the line source lies on the marked line. Then one rechecks the center of rotation with the point source method. Obviously, a more sophisticated apparatus would hold a line source straight and could be used to test the axis alignment as well as the offset; such a line source may well be in use already for extrinsic resolution measurements.

The test should be performed as often as the instability of the system warrants, after ADC service or PM tube regreasing, or once a week when resolution and linearity checks are made. Experience with most systems suggests that this variable is stable over a period of months.

Quality Assurance 199

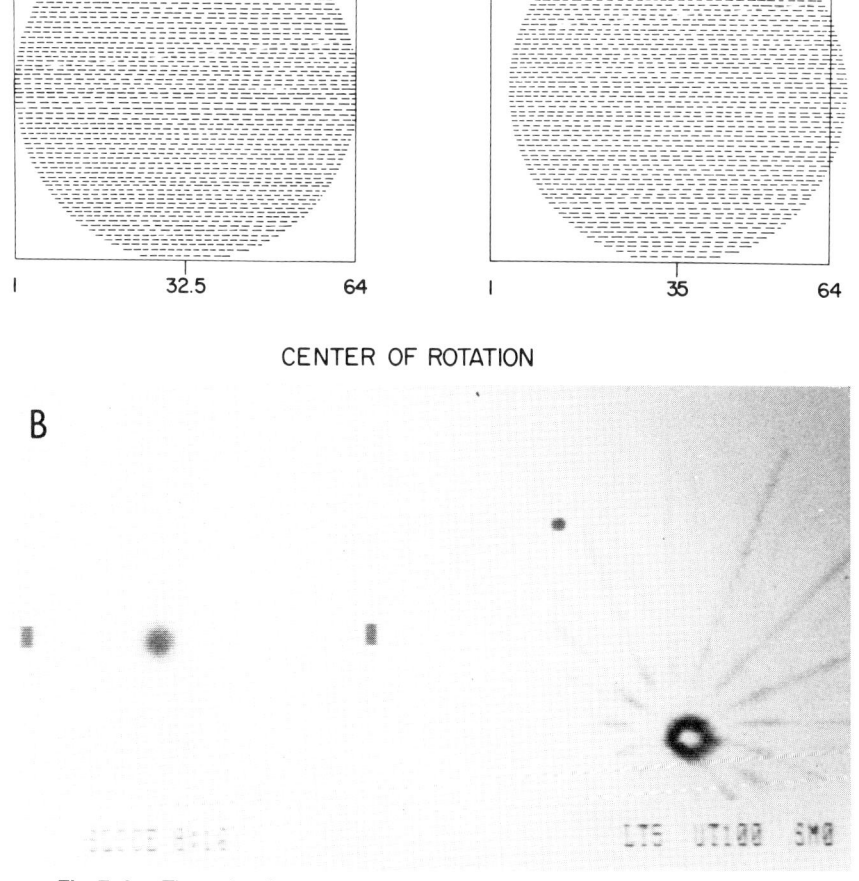

Fig 7–2.—The axis of rotation should fall in the center of the computer matrix as shown in **A left,** not off to one side as is shown on the **right.** In **B** a point source imaged with the axis of rotation in pixel column x = 35 of a 64 × 64 matrix gives a transaxial image as shown on the right.

Whenever the axis of rotation is found not to be in the center of the matrix, it should be repositioned. Some SPECT system software permits setting the axis of rotation in the correct location, which can also be described as setting the correct x axis offset, with software. The program accepts data from a point or line source and automatically puts the y axis in the middle of the computer matrix. Even though the computer is doing the correction, it is well to find out the magnitude of the correction, because the field is narrowed by twice the number of pixels by which the system is out of manual alignment. For other systems, manual offset settings are the only ones possible; the operator must manually do this with a tiny screwdriver. In either case, the system should be checked to be sure that the x-axis offset is correct.

X and Y Axis Distance Calibration

The SPECT attenuation correction program needs a correspondence between the size of a pixel and distance in the real world in order to apply the attenuation coefficient, expressed as a fraction of counts attenuated per millimeter, across a distance of the thickness of a patient, expressed as a number of pixels across the computer matrix.

This calibration is normally made when the computer software is installed and is typically about 6 mm (= 40 cm/64) to the pixel for a 64 × 64 matrix with a large-field camera. The best way to make this measurement is to image two point sources that can be accurately positioned a known distance apart. See how many pixels apart they are (again performing a Gaussian fit to the pixel data). The distance in millimeters is divided by the number of pixels for the result, and this is supplied to the SPECT software. Gross changes in the camera image-matrix correspondence affect this relationship. One should find out what the SPECT program does if the camera's zoom or blow-up mode is elected; it may correct for this or it may not.

Beyond the necessity of having the correct distance calibration, it is good Anger camera-computer practice to be sure that the image which the camera field makes in the computer matrix is round and that it fills the matrix. This guarantees correspondence of distances in all directions and maintains the distance calibration. A monthly test of these properties can be combined with the linearity and resolution checks.

Timing of Camera and Computer

It is important that both the camera circuits and the computer know how to keep time and how to stop acquiring an image when a preset time has elapsed. This should be true for all the various modes of operation. Many things can go awry with the timing control mechanisms, so it is not possible to conceive of tests that will catch all the errors. The ones that can interfere with routine operation should be tested for.

One checks both the camera and the computer with a good watch or stopwatch and against each other. Each instrument is set to collect information for one minute and both are started together. One must watch very carefully to see if a difference can be discerned in the times at which they stop. They are tested in all common modes of operation that depend on time. This need not be done more than once a year or when trouble is suspected.

Cameras' timing circuits depend on digital thumbwheels for their settings. The control mechanism for ending acquisition is digital and may be based on binary numbers in actual operation. If one of the digits no longer can register both binary values, certain time settings may not cause acquisition to stop at the preset value. Such an error seems like a random one until it is examined closely.

When the internal clock that the computer relies on for timing data acquisition goes awry, the times the computer thinks are correct do not match real time. Since each computer may have two or three internal clocks, it may be possible to use one to check another.

ADCs as Data-Transfer Devices

The ADCs translate analog x and y position pulses of the camera into digital information for the computer; the so-called z signal from the camera identifies pulses within the energy window. Testing ADCs is a matter of testing the information acquired by the camera and by the computer to see if it looks the same and to see if the numbers are the same, always provided no correction factors have been applied to one set of information that have not been applied to the other.

During daily uniformity and sensitivity testing, the images acquired by the computer and the camera should always be compared as to their visual and their numeric content. If the two instruments are set to acquire a preset number of counts, one must determine whether the numbers of counts acquired are in fact the same to within some satisfactory statistical accuracy and whether the acquisition times are the same. The information found by each should be written down and the images stored.

The hardware components being tested are cabling, ADCs, and computer buffers. The most likely to fail is the cabling, with ADCs next in line. Cable failures may result in the acquisition of a single line, horizontal (y cable failure) or vertical (x cable failure). When the z cable fails, nothing comes through because the z signal triggers the positioning of the data. Cable failures may also result in strange dropouts, causing high counts in the 1,1 position. Note that the computer matrix has its origin in a corner, while the camera matrix has its

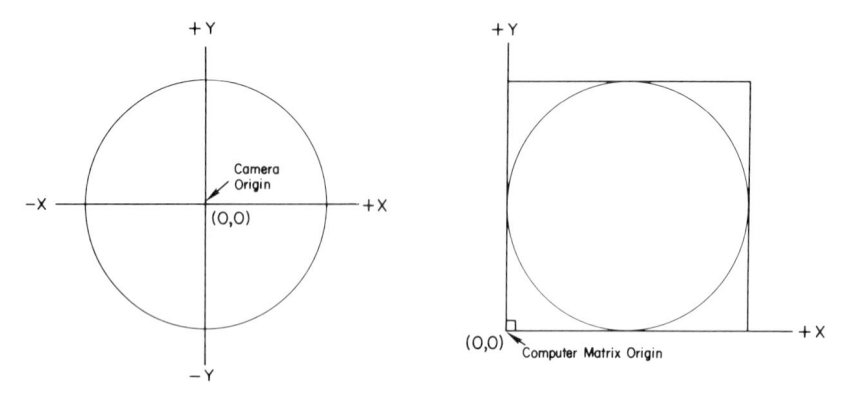

Fig 7–3.—The camera x and y axes cross in the middle of the camera field at x = 0, y = 0. The computer matrix origin is in the lower left hand corner and may be called x = 1, y = 1.

origin in the center (Fig 7–3), so there is a shifting of origin between one instrument and the other, for which the interface is responsible. When the ADCs themselves fail, they can no longer correctly position signals and must be replaced.

If subtle differences exist between the analog and digital images, the effect of changing the camera's position switches should be explored. Does the difference seem to follow the switches or does it seem to depend on the computer's matrix position? Is the difference really in the acquired numeric data or does it just appear on the oscilloscope screen? Screen-only errors are most often associated with the display hardware. Can a trained individual reproduce the problem, or does it only seem to happen to novices?

Computer-to-Camera Interface for Gantry Control

Information is passed in both directions between a SPECT camera and the computer. The computer signals the camera to move and to stop. Step-and-shoot and continuous operations differ, but in both cases the starting, stopping, and timing must be according to the operator's instructions. In discontinuous operation, the camera should start on command, advance the correct angular distance, pause for the correct amount of time before starting data acquisition, acquire for the correct time period, and then advance. In continuous operation, the gantry must rotate at an even speed and it should go the correct angular distance around, not stopping short or overshooting the end. The computer may or may not know at what angle the camera is positioned, but it must be able to count time or distance from the beginning.

To discover if the angular steps are the correct size, one should use markings provided by the manufacturer, or a template created for the purpose, to check the angles. The template should fit on the gantry in a way that some prominent piece of the rotating part points at it; the template should be marked to show the places where the gantry should stop. This motion is tested quarterly and the information recorded. During routine clinical operation, it should be noticed if the instrument does not finish at the point at which it started in 360-degree operation.

To discover if the dwell time in discontinuous operation is correct and the same around the circle, or to discover if the rotational speed of continuous operation is constant, one can image a constant source attached to the camera head as it rotates. Point sources will do; so will the uniformity sheet source, if it is equipped with clamps to fix it to the collimator. The acquired data are collected with the computer. If room background is not a problem, the total counts in the images are compared as a function of angle. There should be no variation that cannot be accounted for by statistical uncertainty or decay of the source. This test should be performed quarterly and when suspicions about gantry motion arise, and the results recorded.

If the camera stops when it is not supposed to, it may be that the signal is not large enough or that extraneous electrical noise is interfering. Some laboratories have found that electrical noise from the photoprocessor was responsible. Careful attention to cable shielding and termination in both directions will prevent difficulties.

Gating

If the instrument is used for gated acquisition, it should be tested in the gated mode as well. Gated acquisition is a highly technical procedure. The system must be able to recognize the ECG signals and use them to synchronize the gating of a set of frames.

When the system fails to recognize the ECG signals, it is often because the cables have failed. While testing to see if contact has been re-established, any regular signal will suffice: ECG signals from a technologist, an electronic device to emit regular pulses, or even rhythmically tapping the leads together. To see if the timing is correct, an electronic device that emits regular pulses is much better than either of the other two maneuvers. There are commercial devices for testing ECG instruments that can be used to test the gating instruments.

Testing gated acquisition itself can be as simple as imaging a uniformity sheet source while using an electronic pulse and observing whether the counts are identical in all the intervals. It is recommended that this be done periodically, especially when acquisition software is changed, to be sure the system works as it is supposed to. Quarterly testing is recommended, to be performed at the same time as the test for SPECT timing. If gated SPECT is being used, a three-dimensional heart phantom should be imaged and reconstructed to see if the images accurately represent the volumes.

There have been a number of observations of delay time difficulties in the ECG monitors used for multiple gated acquisition; these difficulties become most acute at high heart rates (Powers et al. 1982).

SPECT SOFTWARE QUALITY CONTROL AND SOFTWARE FOR QUALITY CONTROL

Beyond acceptance testing of software, discussed in a later section of this chapter, and the continuing educational process for all the users about its proper use and capabilities, there is very little need to test the software itself. If some sort of difficulty develops in the system—e.g., a particular mode of acquisition becomes impossible—it would be rare that the software would have developed such an error, so the hardware should be examined until the error is found.

Because there are increasingly more points at which a value or piece of information supplied by the user is employed in a number of programs, it is possible that the user misunderstands what information is required and therefore has supplied it incorrectly. Examples might be incorrectly performed x-axis offset data acquisition, incorrect attenuation correction values, incorrect millimeter-per-pixel distance, application of correction factors from incorrect uniformity-correction matrices, or the use of the wrong activity or distance units. Rereading the documentation and/or experimentation will often provide an answer.

The software may in its turn be made more useful in the search for such errors by supplying, when asked, various information. The computer should store, and be willing to share, values of the attenuation correction, millimeters-per-pixel distance, acquisition date of the uniformity-correction matrix, identity of the filter used, and other variables used in the calculation. To the extent that the best transaxial images will be those for which the variables of the calculations have been tailored to the radionuclide, radiopharmaceutical, patient organ and configuration, collimator, information density, and acquisition values, it will be necessary to see that the best set of variables has been used and to be able to compare images in which small adjustments have been made.

A discussion of software for quality control is almost entirely speculative because, although programming exists for some of the functions, it is not put together in a package to be applied to Anger camera or SPECT images. The progress of software development has been interesting. It has been pointed out that while chemists, for example, have at their immediate disposal all of the knowledge and tricks of the trade of their colleagues and their scientific ancestors, the programmer must learn a great deal of his craft from the absolute beginning. This is like reinventing the wheel, and takes a great deal of time and energy that could be put to advancing knowledge. As SPECT matures, we might expect to see a body of quality-control software develop much as the acquisition and processing software of nuclear medicine has.

There already exist programs for testing and setting the x-axis offset. These programs should not only perform this function but should give some indication of the magnitude of the correction that has been applied. It is possible to imagine two ways to perform this correction and to decide which is preferred. In one method, the computer finds where the center of the camera image falls in the matrix and creates an additive correction factor to be applied to all incoming x pulses to move them over so that the y axis will be in the middle of the matrix; this correction is only active when SPECT acquisition is occurring. This is not a preferred method, because the uniformity correction factors to be applied by the computer will be formed from an image that did not have the benefit of a software x-axis offset, so each correction will be offset just a bit from the area it is meant to correct. Also, the field of view is diminished by twice the width of the pixels that fall outside the matrix before the correction, because they represent overflow and cannot be brought into the matrix. In the second and preferred method, a special program in the computer finds where the position of the center of the camera image falls in the matrix and permanently corrects the x-axis offset of the x-ADCs, so that all incoming data will be correctly positioned, whether for SPECT or not. In addition, the x and y gain should be under the same kind of software control. Most of the older systems have no control over the first, and less desirable, correction.

To test to see which correction a system has, one should inquire about adjustment of x and y gain and offset. With the system out of adjustment, one acquires a planar image of a uniformity sheet source to fill the whole camera field of view. Then the x-axis offset-adjusting program is run and another planar image is acquired of the uniformity sheet source. If the image has clearly moved in the matrix, the software corrects all the data the computer is acquiring; if it has not, the x-axis offset program should not be used. Rather, the offset should be adjusted by screwdriver, at least until it is very close to correct.

Planar sensitivity and uniformity programs should be easy to incorporate into SPECT software. Once they are, perhaps information may be stored and used in the computer instead of being recorded on film and by hand. Future comparison would be much easier in the computer than with sheets of film. It has been suggested herein that different images and images of the average count ± 2 SD would enable the user to find and follow difficulties much more easily than he can with analog images, which may suffer from formatter intensity variations.

At the heart of measuring linearity and resolution and of finding the x-axis offset is the exact measurement of position of a maximum or minimum count in the computer's matrix. In some cases, only a modulation transfer function is required, while in others the position of a point source must be fixed in two dimensions. This calculation can also be used by the software, which finds the position of sources on the patient used to inform the computer of the patient's shape for attenuation correction calculation. Once the position of the minimum or maximum is known, MTF, FWHM, FWTM, and a host of other uses can be made of the information.

The computer programs available for the formation of functional images should be strengthened and made more readily available to the average user. A particular application of such programs would be to provide functional images of FWHM and FWTM, as well as linearity, in any specified plane for which there were data available. The NEMA calculations of differential and integral measures of camera performance should be part of the package.

SPECT QUALITY CONTROL

The preceding sections of this chapter have been adding complexity to the quality control protocols for a simple Anger camera making analog images. That process continues now in the discussion of quality control methods for the SPECT system, especially because a system that produces three-dimensional images must be tested in three dimensions (Greer, Jaszczak, and Coleman 1982; Greer, Coleman, and Jaszczak 1983; Greer et al. 1985; Harkness et al. 1983). Also, the methods for testing a SPECT system require a leap of faith—the SPECT software has to be assumed to be able to create transaxial images from a set of planar images. Once this correspondence has been tested, routine quality control procedures can be based on it.

The SPECT system properties that should be tested are the mechanical motion and its safeguards, sensitivity, uniformity, resolution, volume threshold measurement, and patient-contour positioning for attenuation correction. Variation of the image with rotational angle should be tested periodically to be sure no problems have appeared since the acceptance testing. The formatter or device for making hard copy images should also be tested as part of the SPECT system and as one of the ordinary nuclear medicine instruments.

The general method for testing a SPECT system follows the guidelines above: the camera images a known test object, and the computer and the operator together record the instrument parameters and make measurements on the transaxial images.

Mechanical Motion

The mechanical motion of the gantry and its response to instructions from the computer were discussed in the previous section, but necessary tests of the gantry and its computer interface were not exhausted. The various mechanical motions of the camera gantry and/or patient imaging table should be tested to see that they ensure a coherent set of images. If rotation path shape is set by the technologists, there should be periodic checks of their acuity. It is also necessary to test any built-in safety devices that prevent the instrument from crushing the patient or sweeping him off the table.

The most modern SPECT systems have automatic means of minimizing the collimator-to-patient distance. This is done by moving either the camera head or the patient couch. No matter what motion is used, there are safety devices to prevent injury to the patient. In some, gears slip, while in others the system locks and refuses to move until the contact condition is changed. The safety mechanisms should be tested every day by running the camera slowly into an immovable object to be sure it will stop. Each laboratory, or at least each vendor, should consider the most likely set of circumstances in which a patient might be in the way of the motion of the system;

these circumstances should be simulated in the test procedure. In most cases, two technologists should participate, one as the test object and the other to stop the system. The best designs for gantries are probably those that allow a slipping motion in case an obstruction is met; at worst, these slip when they are not supposed to, as when carrying a heavy collimator or the uniform sheet source, and must be tested as described in a previous section to be sure that they complete the full rotation around the circle. For Anger-camera SPECT, it is really not possible to design a gantry that will never touch a patient; a large circle of rotation means the collimator face is much too far from the patient. A design such as that of an x-ray CT unit is not of much use for a SPECT instrument.

The simplest test of the whole mechanical system is to place a few adequately sized point sources on a human being and acquire a set of SPECT images of them, using all of the mechanical capabilities of the instrument. A technologist may be the test object or a patient may be used in the course of an examination if the sources will not interfere. One must make sure the sources will potentially be in the field of view at all angles, although they may appear to be hidden by the body. The reason for using a human being instead of one of the cylindrical phantoms that are discussed below is that the instrument can only truly be tested with an object with all the complexity of the human anatomy. A perfectly cylindrical object is not much of a test, especially if fairly elaborate table and/or gantry motion is involved.

Data analysis consists of a close examination of a sinogram of each of the sources and a cine of the images. This is performed as often as necessary for the technologists to be capable of producing good images, when there is trouble suspected, or at six-month intervals.

Another facet of the mechanical operation that should be checked periodically is the level position of the camera head during rotation (or the position at some other specified angle, as with the angulated collimator). The camera head should have a spirit level on it that can be read at various positions. It should be checked that a camera head which is set to be level at the start of the rotation remains so during the whole circuit. This test should be done monthly and reported along with the other monthly tests.

For completeness, the test for the mechanical rotational motion is mentioned again. Variations in rotational speed or timing of the pauses for data acquisition can be detected by rotating the camera with the uniformity sheet source attached. It should be noted during data acquisition whether the gantry is in the correct position at the correct time and whether it does actually go 360 degrees around when instructed to, or by how much it deviates. The data are analyzed to see if the same number of counts is collected at each angle. Data acquired in this test can be further used as described below for testing the performance of the camera with respect to uniformity as a function of angle.

Sensitivity, Uniformity, Linearity, Resolution, Attenuation Correction, Volume Calibration, and Energy Effects

There is no doubt that instrument performance imposes some special constraints on the quality of the examinations performed with SPECT. The instrument should therefore be tested in the three-dimensional mode to see what the performance of the instrument is and to learn to recognize the effect of instrument performance on the images. In going from two to three dimensions, a leap is made from the possibility of a reasonable number of quality control tests to an unreasonable number, unless order is imposed on the testing process. The basic idea is to have a camera that performs well in two dimensions and to know what that performance is. Then a limited number of tests in three dimensions should serve to define the boundaries of the system's capabilities. It is of little use to perform a sophisticated and sensitive test on a SPECT system whose camera cannot perform well on the planar tests, because the camera will not improve when it is rotated, nor can it contribute anything but distracting errors to the reconstructed images.

Sensitivity, uniformity, linearity, resolution, attenuation correction values, and volume quantification are properties of the system to be measured at depth in a scattering medium to approximate the circumstances of the SPECT examination. From quality control tests, the user can get an idea of the performance of the system in the clinical setting. To permit the smallest number of time-consuming tests, phantoms have been devised to incorporate the testing of several of these variables at once. The camera should be performing in the same fashion over its whole active area, so that tests performed with one part of its surface will produce results that are representative of the performance of any part of the camera face.

The attenuation correction is based on the assumption of an elliptic (or other simple) shape for the patient contour. If the calculation is made by the software, based on information it gleans from the clinical data, the assumed shape should be correct unless the contrast between the source and the background is too great. Such might be the case with I-131 sodium iodide in the thyroid of a hyperthyroid patient 24 hours after administration. The computer algorithm might not have enough points to find the neck outline. It is wise to test this possibility with a "hot" source in a scattering medium.

Before embarking on collection of data from a three-dimensional phantom, it is wise to be sure that the camera performance does not vary with rotational angle. This can be detected by rotating the camera with the uniformity flood source attached, as described above for testing the mechanical rotational motion. Three million counts acquired at each of 16 or 20 angles around 360 degrees should suffice to show gravity or magnetic field dependency. The images are compared by subtracting them from a standard image as described in the section on acceptance testing.

A three-dimensional phantom is needed for sensitivity, uniformity, resolution, and volume threshold testing. There are currently two commercially available SPECT phantoms (Fig 7–4). Each features a watertight cylinder into which test objects may be firmly fixed. The phantom must be large enough to simulate the patient imaging situation, but small enough to carry around when it is full of water.

Because it is desired to image the cylindrical phantom as few times as possible, all of the test objects must be packed together and each used in as many ways as possible. Each of the sections of the phantom is described separately, but the tests will be performed on data acquired all in one rotation.

The question of how often three-dimensional testing of the system should be performed is paramount. It would seem if the system is operating routinely well, that these tests might be performed monthly. Assembling the phantom and filling it with activity will become routine after a few trials; imaging should take less time than a patient examination because the postioning time should be less. Data processing time may well be more than that for a patient examination because of the execution of special programs that perform the numeric calculations, but one might expect that less than two hours total should be required once the procedures become routine. Of course, laboratories in which research is being performed on system performance or production of new software or hardware will require more frequent and more elaborate testing.

For sensitivity and uniformity measurements, the best test is a section of phantom with no test objects in it. The phantom should have one section, at least 2 cm wide, that is devoid of objects. The section must be this wide to avoid the effects of partial voluming from neighboring sections. For sensitivity and uniformity measure-

Quality Assurance **211**

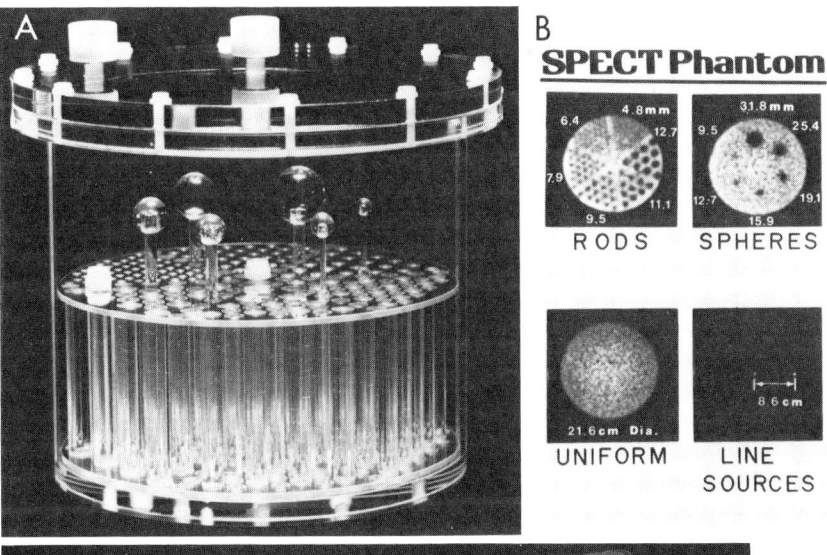

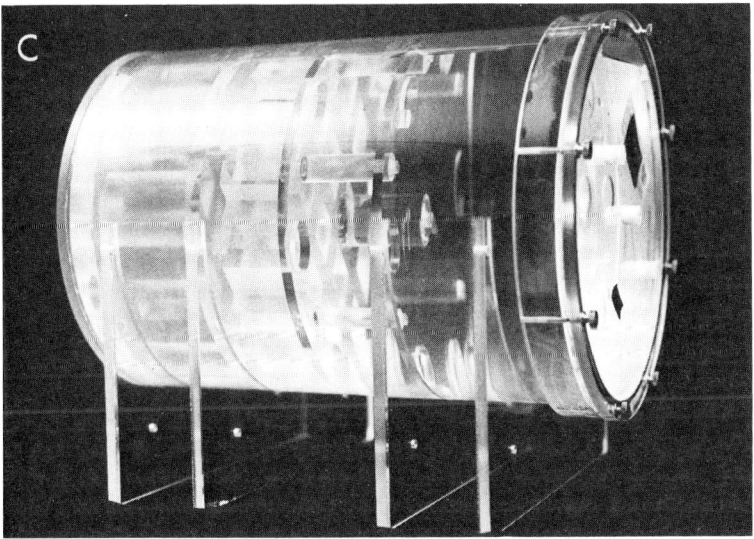

Fig 7–4.—Two commercially available cylindrical SPECT phantoms. Note the variety of inserts. **A** shows Data Spectrum's Model 5000 Deluxe SPECT Phantom, with **B** showing images of this phantom. (Courtesy of Data Spectrum Corp., Chapel Hill, N.C.) **C** shows another phantom by R.A. Carlson and J.T. Colvin.

ment, the cylinder is filled with a technetium-99m solution of known specific activity and is mixed thoroughly. It may be helpful to know the total volume of the cylinder, so that the specific activity in microcuries (μCi) or kilobecquerels (KBq) per milliliter may be found after technetium-99m is added to this volume and mixed. The cylinder is imaged, with counts collected at a rate consonant with camera dead time and on the high side of patient study counts. One must not collect too many counts, or special uniformity checks of the stationary camera will have to be performed just to assure the information in this test. Then one reconstructs to form the transaxial images, using the appropriate attenuation correction. This can be done without attenuation correction to ascertain the proper attenuation coefficient for the system. The images are examined for uniformity using the computer's thresholding and uniformity analysis programs. One should have standards for the uniformity and statistical uncertainty as a function of count density. One cannot expect the kind of uniformity that is expected in planar imaging. The images are recorded. If the center is more radioactive than the rest, the attenuation correction was overdone. The reconstruction should be repeated with a lower value for the attenuation coefficient.

If the calculation of the ellipse for the attenuation correction is made from point source data supplied to the system at acquisition time, one should be sure that the data are used correctly in the calculation or that the ellipse and the object are matched. If the software calculates its own ellipse from scatter or from separate Compton scatter images, the ellipse must be correct for the whole phantom. The computer should put the ellipse it is using in the calculation some place where the user can find it. The accuracy of the ellipse is tested by superimposing it on a transaxial image of the cylindrical phantom. A film of this image should be part of the results of the quality control imaging of the cylinder phantom.

Next one calculates the sensitivity, expressing it as cps-ml per μCi or cps-ml per KBq, which means that the pixel size in centimeters is used in the calculation. The thickness of the transaxial voxel must be included in the calculation. A typical SPECT camera system has a sensitivity of 200 to 400 cps-ml per μCi or 5 to 10 cps-ml per KBq. One need not feel apologetic about this sensitivity, but remember that the system is capable of acquiring 15 to 20 slices of data at once, each with this sensitivity.

Several benchmarks of resolution can be incorporated into the cylindrical phantom, but one must be thoughtful about how to use them in the setting of quality control testing with the smallest amount of time expended. Caution must be exercised to be sure that the inserts do not cause moire effects with the collimator or the computer matrix or even with the SPECT reconstruction software.

A qualitative measurement of resolution may be gathered in the course of measuring the volume calibration, using a series of plastic spheres that includes one at or below the resolution threshold. After reconstruction, transaxial images of the spheres are filmed. The contrast of the spheres as a function of diameter may be calculated. The volume quantification software should be used to calculate sphere volume; the correct threshold value used with this software should give the best estimate of the volumes. It is appropriate to test the volume threshold in the range of the usual clinical applications, since it may be slightly volume dependent. The threshold is dependent on the count densities, filters, and other acquisition and processing factors, so these should be matched to the clinical situation and noted as part of the information. Absolute quantification of the activity in a volume requires special phantoms, designed for the specific circumstance under which patients are to be imaged (Macey et al. 1984).

For resolution and linearity testing, one section of the phantom can be devoted to a set of linear test objects. One phantom design provides an insert that looks like ice cubes. Linearity can be measured along the lines. The blocks are large enough so that the shoulder on the side of the block can be used to compare the square shape of the block with the actual shape presented in the image. The MTF provides the best comparison of these two spread functions. One should save images of the results of these tests.

If more time is available for resolution testing, hot line sources, made with micropipets designed for measuring hematocrit, are placed at several points in the SPECT phantom and surrounded by nonradioactive water. They are imaged and the transaxial images reconstructed. The line spread functions and modulation transfer functions are found for each. All the conditions of acquisition and reconstruction, including all filtering, must be noted. The micropipets may be used for resolution measurements in the presence of the uniform background, but account must be taken of the background.

Most of the use of Anger cameras to date has been with energy windows centered around the photopeak of the radionuclide in use. SPECT may well be increasingly done with a window offset to the high-energy side of the peak. Because such a setting has a distinct effect on the uniformity of the camera, it is well to carry through testing of its effects into three dimensions. After it has been ascertained that such operation is satisfactory and it is used for clinical imaging, all testing should be carried out with the window offset normally used in clinical imaging.

In designing phantoms it is well to keep in mind the conditions of patient imaging. If a SPECT system is used largely for a specific examination, it is well to test the system specially for performance under similar circumstances. At times, even good-sized animals, such as dogs, may be inadequate to simulate human beings. One must be careful during testing, especially in situations of camera or test object movement, to separate all the various effects. For example, one would like to be able to separate internal from external effects on the inner workings of the camera head and distinguish these influences from gantry movement or source movement.

The Alderson liver phantom, surrounded by scattering medium, can be easily used with SPECT, although the rectangular plastic box must be rethought to approximate the human contour more closely and one must be sure the whole assembly can be put on its side. This phantom has the advantage of not having a series of regular defects or sources to interact with the mathematics or the collimator, but it has the disadvantage that repeated images must be made to determine mathematic characteristics of the system.

Formatter and Other Hard Copy Devices

Since many images are ultimately presented for diagnosis as hard copies made from computer images, they must contain all the diagnostic information that the computer makes available. The wrong set of variables for a formatter can render invisible all the detail that was present after computer processing.

A series of quality assurance tests is recommended for the display devices in use in the nuclear medicine laboratory. For the analog camera, intensity, sharpness, and dot size and shape must be examined on the primary hard copy device every day, and artifacts that develop must be fixed. The computer's hard copy device must be similarly tested. It also has certain image manipulation controls for its oscilloscope, such as contrast, brightness, and exposure time, which may drift with time. A gray scale is a good control image for a formatter. As part of the weekly tests in a laboratory, an image of the gray scale should be made. The image should be examined to determine how many of the levels can be seen, and the instrument adjusted to meet the standard for the laboratory. If different kinds of images are produced, there may need to be a number of different settings, just as there are for the hard copy devices attached directly to the Anger camera. Specific test images may be used, or a specific part of the gray scale may be required for the result to be satisfactory for use with a particular examination.

SPECIFIC KINDS OF PROBLEMS: THEIR DIAGNOSIS AND CURE

Artifacts to Look for on Patient Examinations

Far more patient examinations than quality control procedures should be performed on the SPECT system. Therefore it makes sense to use patient examinations for continuing quality control. Depending on the situation, film images of some of the tests, such as a sinogram, a uniformity-correction image, or patient-contour outline, should actually be required as part of the patient's record for a SPECT examination.

Patient motion during data acquisition causes artifacts in the SPECT images. The technologists must carefully immobilize the patient without using apparatus that might interfere with the examination and must instruct the patient and watch him during the procedure. Imaging marker sources on the patient and their subsequent presentation on a sinogram or cine allows the operator to see if there was a motion problem. Sinograms of a line of data through the organ of interest are very helpful too (Fig 5–14).

The cine and sinogram should be examined for traces of patient motion, incorrect patient couch movement during the examination, and downright mispositioning in which the organ of interest does not lie in the camera's field of view at all angles. The sinogram may be photographed as a permanent record of the quality of the examination. It can even be helpful in moving misplaced images to the correct position. Point sources placed on the patient may be especially helpful as markers, but it is essential that they be firmly attached and not move around with the patient's clothes.

The cine should be examined for other details. If a shadow shows across the image at a particular angle, it must be identified. Shadow artifacts may be caused by arms and by metal absorbers in the patient couch, or in or on the patient (Fig 7–5). The usual attenuation corrections will not correct for these artifacts, so there will be a shadow across the image too. A very "hot" injection site can be a serious problem in reconstruction; programs can be developed to remove this sort of artifact.

It is possible to see only the grossest kind of angularly dependent

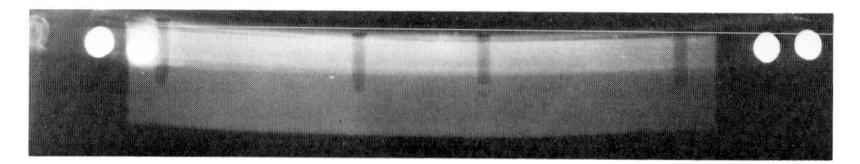

Fig 7-5.—This portable x-ray image shows that the end of the SPECT table is made of denser material than the rest of the table. It also shows the snaps in the table cover. This part of the table should not come between the camera and the patient.

difficulties on the cine images, such as a PM tube that is poorly coupled to the crystal, but these problems should be looked for.

Next the transaxial images should be examined. Does their sharpness correspond to the sharpness of the planar projection images? The reconstruction process cannot work miracles and does give a noisier image, but the two sets of images should belong to the same family statistically. The filter used in the reconstruction must be appropriate to the count density of the examination. The films should be examined to be sure an adequate number of gray levels is visible and that diagnostic detail is not lost from either end of the scale.

Are there rings or arcs around the center of the image? Is a bull's-eye visible (see Fig 7-1)? The ring artifact is caused by nonuniformity; arcs are caused by nonuniformities that are angularly dependent. Were the images uniformity-corrected before reconstruction, either by the camera or by the computer? Was an inappropriate uniformity correction applied, as for the wrong nuclide or another time? Arc artifacts, showing angular dependency, can be tested for by rotating a uniformity sheet source as described above.

Does the transaxial image show the patient lying on his back in the so-called obstetric position? Or is he on his stomach? Are right and left correctly marked by the computer? The images may be rolled over if the patient was put feet-first into a normally head-first imaging system. The camera position switches can wreak havoc with a SPECT acquisition, even making impossible a reconstruction without a rotation of each frame of data. The SPECT software may enable mirroring and rotating the images so they can be photographed in the standard form. Photography should be in a standard form so there will be no questions when the films are reviewed at a later time (Fig 7-6).

Does the resolution of the system seem to be seriously compromised? Could there be problems (1) with the angle of the camera head to the axis of rotation during acquisition (or correct angle in one of the angled collimator imaging situations), (2) with the center of rota-

Quality Assurance **217**

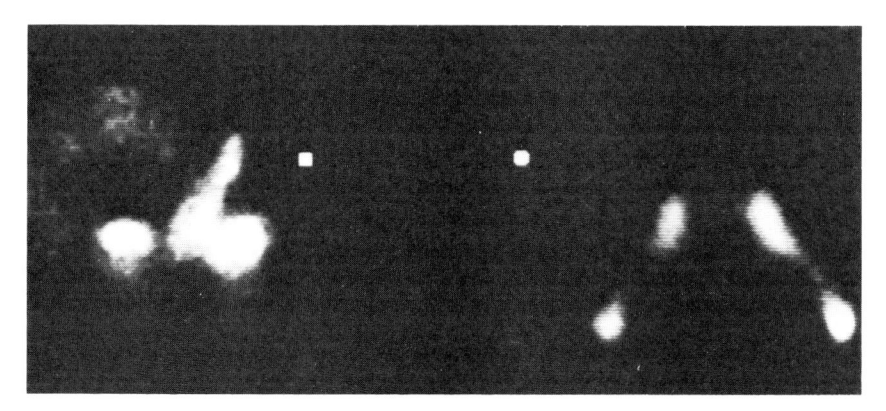

Fig 7–6.—Clinical image of pelvis 3 hours after the administration of 20 mCi of technetium-99m medronate (MDP). On the left is the anterior view of the patient. On the right is one of the reconstructed transaxial images, just as it came from the computer after SPECT processing, with the patient's right marked by the bright square on the left side of the image. Notice that the transaxial image is upside down and that the right marker does not mark the right-hand side of the patient, because the patient was imaged with his feet pointing into the gantry circle. The GE 400T camera console switches were used to create an upright planar image, but the SPECT images were all upside down and mirrored.

tion, or (3) with larger path diameter than necessary? Was an unaccustomed filter or interpolation method used in the reconstruction? Any of these could cause resolution problems; the cine and sinogram may give clues only to some of them. The image of a point source is really a center-of-rotation check, so one must reconstruct the point source part of the image if there are questions about the center of rotation. Examination of the cine may show when the collimator was close to the patient surface and when it was not; when detail seems to be in good focus, the collimator was closer to the patient. The incorrectly angled camera head may show detail that is acceptable in the center of the image but worsens toward the edges.

One artifact is caused by patient motion between the time of creating an ellipse for attenuation correction and starting the rotation. In this case, the ellipse will not be in the right place, so part of the patient, and perhaps the organ of interest, will be cut off by the edge of the ellipse before reconstruction. A zero-order remedy is to reconstruct without attenuation correction. A first-order solution is to change the ellipse parameter values to match the observed position of the patient; usually there is sufficient background scatter to allow estimation of the patient outline. If attenuation correction is made, it may be helpful as a quality control measure to photograph the patient contour superimposed over a transaxial slice to be sure that they match (Fig 5–17).

If the attenuation correction is performed using the wrong value, the image may have a "hot" or "cold" center. If there is no clue to what value was used, one should try reconstructing again, first using no attenuation correction and then trying the supposedly correct value again. A set of cylindrical phantom images may be stored for testing difficulties in case the system does not seem to perform correctly. It is possible that the patient actually has a relatively more or less radioactive center.

INSTALLATION AND ACCEPTANCE TESTING

Most practitioners of nuclear medicine are excited at the arrival of a new piece of equipment. The natural impulse, like a child at a birthday, is to open the package and start to play with the contents immediately. Later, again like the child, the new users may become disenchanted with the toy on learning some of its faults. Famous physicists and engineers connected with the field have been telling us for years to be more circumspect in the start-up of new pieces of equipment; we have been urged repeatedly to perform the acceptance tests and get to know the equipment before imaging the first patient. Will we ever learn?

A good, thorough round of acceptance tests will make the users confident of their prowess and knowledgeable about the capabilities and shortcomings of the equipment. There is no substitute for experience for both technologists and physicians.

Acceptance and initial testing of a SPECT system should settle some questions forever (and may raise some specters for the future, too). Initial testing in the laboratory gives values that can be compared with the manufacturer's preshipment values to establish a norm or a starting point for the instrument.

Mechanical Set-Up

The mechanical set-up of the instrument will probably be done only once, so it should be done correctly. Glue and permanent cement are used to install the gantry and, for some instruments, the patient imaging table. Once the installation has been made, the gantry can be moved only with difficulty.

Installation of the camera should include careful gantry leveling so that the rotation ring is perpendicular to the earth's surface. The patient couch should be perpendicular to the rotation ring and should be positioned so that the camera can pass the couch, if at all possible, because it makes some kinds of tests and camera head manipulation much easier. There should be markers on the gantry to correspond to angles of rotation so that the rotational angular increment can be checked easily. Marks should indicate when the gantry and the patient couch are lined up perpendicularly, since the couch may roll on a track while the camera head may possibly rotate around on a pivot on the floor. A scale should show the angle the gantry arms make with the rotating ring; there should be a spirit level on the head.

In a well-designed system, the gantry arms that hold the camera head should be rigid and not droop, either when the camera is pointing down (0 degrees) or up (180 degrees) or when it is placed at 90 or 270 degrees. If the camera head will pass the patient couch, the couch is used as a fixed point. The gantry arm and camera head are leveled at 0 degrees; a point is marked at the height of the axis of rotation, on the camera head, and by the height of the patient couch. Then the camera is rotated around to 180 degrees; the mark should be at the same height. If it is lower, the gantry arms are bending. The same maneuver is performed for the camera head on its side, comparing 90 and 270 degrees. Flexible gantry arms indicate a permanent instability in the system and may lead to failure of the arms through metal fatigue. The flexing of the arms causes the head to move in an orbit that does not correspond to the back-projection calculation; an orbit caused by flexing gantry arms does not have the center of rotation in the center of the matrix at all angles, while the circular orbit, even if of different radii, does. In addition, the drooping head may mean that the camera head is not parallel to the axis of rotation at all angles, which causes further loss of resolution and distortion in the images.

If the camera head will not pass the patient couch, some very careful measurements should be performed. One should watch the spirit level as the head is rotated (provided the angle of the head to the gantry arm is fixed), since the bending arms will cause the head to go out of level between 0 and 180 degrees. The sides are harder to test.

The patient couch must be aligned parallel to the axis of rotation and aimed straight into the center of the circle of rotation. This facilitates the camera head's clearing the sides of the couch during the course of rotation, although it is not otherwise necessary in the operation of most systems. It also assures that the patient will be in the same position in the matrix if the couch is moved to compensate for camera head movements.

Usual Anger Camera Tests

When the mechanical installation is complete and the cables connect all the parts together, it is time to test the camera as a camera. Since some of these tests require the use of the computer, the computer must be tested to be sure that it operates as a standard nuclear medicine computer.

Because the NEMA standards (1980) were not developed with SPECT systems in mind, NEMA tests are not the ultimate for SPECT camera performance. They should be made, however, and the camera should be seen to perform very well. A test for larger-scale difficulties and patterns should be used to augment the NEMA differential and integral uniformity tests that seek to avoid misidentification of small lesions.

The quality control tests described on page 181 can be used for the camera and will help the user acquire a feeling for the capability of the camera. The initial tests will form the basis for future testing of the system, so they should be thoroughly performed, even if some will be found to be superfluous later.

Camera-Computer Interface Tests

Once the Anger camera and the mechanical parts of the system are shown to be intact, the system is rotated under automatic control. One should go through the whole gamut of quality control tests described on page 196, checking out the camera-computer interface and the gantry motion. All the advertised motions are tested under operator and computer command. All the safety features are tested. One must make sure that the SPECT acquisition and camera motion can be stopped on command. Then one tests to see if the examination can be resumed at that point or if it must it be started over. This depends on the software and is a factor that must be known.

The camera has now been put through its paces and is seen to be properly connected to the computer. The next set of tests is to be sure that it can keep its integrity while rotating.

Angular Dependence of Images

Now comes the most troublesome set of tests, which is also very important. They are aimed at showing whether or not there is some angular dependence in the images the system acquires. The question of the influence of gravitational and magnetic fields on the PM tubes should be approached when the camera is installed and then need not be considered again unless the camera is moved, its motors or brakes are serviced, extensive electrical work is done in the area, or a nuclear magnetic resonance (NMR) unit is moved in next door. Since the difficulty came to light several years ago (Williams et al. 1981), recently produced cameras should be protected against most magnetic field problems.

Magnetic field and gravitational effects may be hard to separate, but it is worth trying. Gravity will not change significantly with time or instrument placement, but the magnetic fields may be altered and could become a renewed problem at a later date.

All of the positional effects on the rotating camera must be tested for at the same time and the contributions of various problems to the difficulties observed must be sorted out. The test consists of rotating the specially designed, nondeformable, flood-uniformity phantom discussed earlier. The phantom may be carried on its own gantry or attached to the camera head, but it must itself be insensitive to positional changes. Several images (16 should be enough) are acquired around the circle using the camera's own drive motors, not manual operation, if possible. Three million counts per image are acquired and stored on the computer. The count rates used must be in the same range as those used for flood uniformity work. The images are corrected in the usual way with the 30 M-count image. One image is selected as the standard (usually that acquired in the same position as the 30 M-count image) and subtracted from the other images. The contrast is enhanced and the results are evaluated: What sort of detail is visible? Does some specter suddenly arise in several of the images? Has the camera cable come between the source and the collimator face (this will not happen if they are clamped together)? Does one now notice that the camera goes "clunk" at one or more positions as it rotates? The obvious problems are corrected and a second set of images is made, accounting for the problems with explanations based on gravity for as long as possible.

The force of gravity is felt by the contents of the camera head and may have some untoward effects. Examples of gravitational effects on camera head are (1) the whole head contents may be able to shift from side to side, crystal and all; (2) the PM tubes may be floating free on the surface of the crystal, able to slide as a group from one side to the other, or to come uncoupled from the crystal; (3) the dynodes in a PM tube may be loose and move around as the tube changes position; or (4) temperature gradient changes within the camera head may cause shifts in PM tube behavior and energy peaking. Each of these problems will give a separate symptom.

The movement of the head contents is usually perfectly obvious—a noise or significant vibration, rather like a loose collimator, can be heard and/or felt as the camera head rotates. Positioning spacers may be required inside the camera head or the whole assembly may need to be tightened.

If the PM tubes are free to slide on the crystal or light-guide face, the result may be anything from one tube obviously coming uncoupled and all the rest seeming to need frequent recoupling, to the PM tube coming completely out of position vis-a-vis the light guide or mask. The movement may have peculiar relaxation properties—the return to a "normal" image when the camera head is put back in the starting position. The PM tubes may need to be recoupled.

Gravitational problems inside PM tubes are the bêtes noires of physicists doing scattering measurements, who test their PM tubes at all angles to put them through their paces before beginning any experiments. Dynodes are little pieces of copper clipped into an insulator in the PM tube and may be unstable. Dynode movement will show up as a shift in the energy spectrum of the tube at the angle in question. If there is any suspicion of dynode movement, the tube should be replaced. Shaking the suspected tube gently may produce a rattle.

Changes in temperature gradient caused by changes in the camera head position may affect one tube or all the tubes; a single sensitive tube may be seen to have a problem and be removed. If all the tubes behave the same way, the problem should be studied as carefully as possible, so that some means of correction, such as a fan or a layer of insulation, may be found. Johnson and co-workers (1983) detail some of these phenomena and their effects on the images.

Magnetic field effects may be caused by the influence of any stray magnetic field, even the earth's in extreme cases. Common sources are the brakes or motor associated with gantry movement, large high-current–carrying wires nearby, NMR units, or other large pieces of equipment. The dynodes contain copper that is diamagnetic and the head is mostly diamagnetic lead; these metals should not themselves be sources of magnetic field effects that could be expected to have hysteresis or "memory." Iron in the camera head or in the moving part of the sytem could well be a problem. The effect of a magnetic field is to bend the path of the electrons between one dynode and the next in a PM tube, moving the tube off its tuned energy setting. Because of a potential problem that has been observed (Williams et al. 1981), a special alloy, mu metal, to shield the PM tubes (the sensitive part of the system) from magnetic fields has been incorporated in various ways (for example, placing sleeves of mu metal around each tube, wrapping each tube in mu metal, and/or inserting a band of mu metal inside the camera shield). It is to be hoped that the shields do not interfere with the placement of the tubes on the crystal or with the ability of the silicone grease to attach the tubes securely to the crystal or light guide; retrofitted devices often cause such problems.

When the only explanation of a problem is the magnetic field gradient in the area around the camera, test this effect. It may emanate from the gantry motor and brake assembly. A compass can be used to see if measurable fields are involved. Also, a stronger magnetic source can cause the same or more exaggerated effects. What kinds of electrical and magnetic devices are in the area, and can they be turned off for a test or shielded for the long run? The camera manufacturers' answer to magnetic influences has been to incorporate mu metal shielding. Are the shields in place?

Since the effect of a magnetic field is to bend the electrons as they stream from one dynode to the next, a varying field means variation in energy spectrum of the affected tubes. Thus it would be desirable to test the energy spectrum of any suspect tubes at the angles at which differences are noted. If only one or two tubes seem affected, the dynodes may be moving in the gravitational field or they may be specially sensitive to magnetic effects; these tubes should be replaced. If the whole image changes, all the tubes are feeling a force. The test for energy spectrum shift is best done with the collimator on (making it difficult in those cameras where the tube locations are certain only with the collimator off) because (1) it is hard to rotate most cameras with the collimator off and (2) as the naked camera faces different directions, it will be looking at a wide variety of backgrounds, which may well overpower the point source used for testing. Camera service people usually face a naked crystal toward the floor or ceiling to avoid such problems. Cameras are very sensitive to spots of technetium-99m spattered on the floor, to the radiopharmaceutical area, to radioactive patients outside the room, and to x-ray units in the vicinity. All of these influences are disconcerting during a test and may contribute to incorrect conclusions, so one must come up with a way to look at individual tube energy spectra with the collimator on.

Software Installation and Testing

Installing software is sometimes a simple process and sometimes not. It may depend on the kind of computer, the various options that are to be implemented, and complications in the options. Usually the user will have to bear the responsibility for installing new software after the initial installation, which will be performed by an applications specialist from the vendor. How does the user, who may not be very knowledgeable about computers (and may not want to become very knowledgeable, either), approach the installation process so that the applications person need not be called back every time a software update is sent? The secret is for everyone to keep exquisitely detailed notes of everything that is happening. No one can assume that it will be possible to remember anything six months or two years hence. The printer should be used to echo all operations; all the pieces of paper it produces should be saved and labeled with the date and time so that one can reconstruct the order of events. The verbally oriented user may want to dictate all the steps being taken and have the notes transcribed to accompany the printer-generated record. Someone should be designated to be in charge of the archives.

Another helpful hint is that the users should read the documentation carefully. The old adage, "When all else fails, read the instructions," is never more true than with computer operation. Experienced users are far more likely to ignore the documentation because it contains so much material that they already know. It is very helpful if the manufacturer makes the effort to highlight changes or include a description of them for such persons.

All programs should be preserved in a back-up copy from which the software could be completely regenerated if need be. The master disk that comes from the vendor should never be put into routine use, but should be used in the computer only long enough to make a copy of the programs with which all operations can be performed. When software updates are distributed, the same should be done with them. They will often come with instructions for implementation as well as programs that will put them into place. One must keep copies of everything and file them neatly so they can be referred to. When major changes in software occur, they are documented as to date, nature, and their effect on the images if relevant. This will make it possible to tell whether information retrieved from the patient files was processed by an old or new method and how it might compare with an examination just performed. The farther nuclear medicine gets from simple Anger camera images, the more necessary this will be.

If there are questions about the software, it helps to write them down. Then one can try to find answers in the documentation or by consulting the manufacturers. Another idea is to try experiments to see whether the answer is really right there.

A set of protocols for the computer can be compiled just as for the rest of the nuclear medicine examinations. For example, the acquisition and processing protocol is kept with the rest of the examination protocol; a second copy is kept with the computer for ready reference by the operators. In addition, a hard copy is kept of command sets or program listings that are required. If all the magnetic media should be destroyed, it should still be possible to re-create the system between new software from the manufacturer and the local listings. Without these listings and magnetic back-up, which is usually available, it is necessary to begin all over again to re-create the local system.

It is not so easy to make the programs that are written locally as neat and tidy as those that come from the manufacturer, but it should be tried. A scheme should be developed into which all the local programs will fit, so that there need not be a new program written every time some small change in procedure is made.

A new user of SPECT or one who has just had new software installed will want to perform a number of tests to see how it behaves and to come to some conclusions about how the variables should best be set. There are several ways to proceed. The novice should probably start by using the reconstruction software with a series of standard images supplied with it by the manufacturer. All the major variables of the processing software should be tested: different slice thicknesses, interpolation methods, back-projection filter functions, values of the attenuation coefficient, projections, and ways of smoothing and manipulating the final images.

The user can do the testing reasonably expeditiously by making a list of the properties to be varied, with the range to cover for each one. Properties that require a new back projection are separated from those that do not, since back projection generally is the most time-consuming operation. One should try to get the most out of each set of back-projected images. It will quickly be seen that the number of maneuvers to be tried is still large, even if only a few values in each range are chosen. A matrix of experiments and a filing system for storing them can be established so that after all the processing is finished it will be possible to review the results. A record of the processing time for each step is helpful, because this may be a factor in deciding what methods to use. Hard copies of the results of the difficult decisions and of the set of values ultimately chosen for use with a particular kind of acquired data should be filed, so that the images may be referred to later. After the user has become more familiar with the system, a series of images of the cylindrical phantom can be substituted for those supplied by the vendor.

The software variables must start with those used by the computer before and during back projection. These will include, at the very least, the interpolation method used during back projection and the thickness of the transaxial slice to be produced. Slice thicknesses of 1, 2, or 3 pixels are reasonable, although images produced with thicker slices will be more uniform. There will probably be a choice of only two or three interpolation methods; the most common are nearest-neighbor, linear, and Nowak (Larsson 1980; Nowak and Eisner 1984). The differences among them in image appearance and in processing time should be appreciated. If information from opposite sides of the patient is averaged before back projection, one can try the linear and geometric averaging techniques. Bridging artifacts between one radioactive area and another in the transaxial images should be noted. Obviously, differentiation of the effects of the averaging technique cannot be performed on data acquired from the uniform section of a cylindrical phantom; there must be relatively hot areas in a colder background.

Filtering and attenuation correction can be accomplished before or after back projection. It will greatly simplify and shorten the testing process if they come afterward because new back projections will not have to be made for each change in a variable. The variables associated with filtering are infinite. Using techniques such as combining a softer filter with low count-density data and a harder, more ramplike filter with data of good statistical quality, one can choose images with which to test the filters. The filters must be re-examined from time to time to be sure the best combinations are being used. Methods of attenuation correction are various; users should explore the range available and examine the effect of the processing on the images.

Smoothing and image manipulation of the final images must be tried to be appreciated, but it should be relatively easy to run through a whole set of tests quickly. One must beware of making the results too smooth; the discriminating diagnostician needs to be able to see the detail. There is provision in some software packages for three-dimensional smoothing of the transaxial images; the effect of this must be tested on the images. Variable values should be tried. There are also specialized techniques for removing the most objectionable artifacts of back projection. The effects of these should be tested to be sure that they do not also remove valid linear structures in the images.

Those who want to become yet more intimate with the various properties should use images of the cylindrical phantom acquired under various circumstances as discussed in the next section. They may also want to get or create a set of simulated images whose properties have been determined. To the end of testing the software, quite a number of computer simulations have been performed that serve as phantoms in a sense. Very often the simulations consist of ideal data that have then had random error inserted into them. Thus all mechanical and electronic systematic errors of the camera and gantry can be avoided and properties of the software can be tested. This is most useful in testing the behavior of filters and projection algorithms (Chang 1978; Egbert and May 1980; Ramachandran and Lakshminarayanan 1971; Shepp and Logan 1974; Oppenheim 1974).

Acquisition Variables

The previous discussion of acceptance testing has brought the system to the point at which all the hardware and the processing software that was purchased seems to work. It now is time to test an operating system, but not yet with a patient unless everyone involved, except perhaps the patient, is prepared to become tired and confused. The patient has a relatively easy time, because he has only to lie on the table in a semi-comfortable position and allow the camera to go around him again and again.

The properties to be tested are the acquisition variables. Decisions must be made about the matrix size, angular increments, and dwell-time for the step-and-shoot system or rotational speed for the continuously rotating system, count density, patient activity and radiation dose, table motion and size of the circle of rotation, patient positioning, and whether to image for 180 or 360 degrees. Using the cylindrical phantom with a number of inserts, one makes decisions about the matrix size, angular increment and dwell-time variables, count density, and whether to image for 180 or 360 degrees. Depending on the patient organ to be imaged, the collimator to be used, and the possible range of appropriate doses of radioactivity, it will be possible to make some approximations to the patient situation with the phantom inserts. The patient will have certain kinds of motion that will degrade to some extent the quality of the information acquired. The images can be reconstructed according to the set of values decided upon in the experiments in the previous section. One must make hard copies of the images for examination in the diagnostic reading room. Of course, more activity in the patient and infinitely long imaging times would improve the images, but compromises must be made in favor of patient safety and comfort and completing the workload of the day.

228   *Chapter 7*

It helps to experiment with practical patient positions with the technologists, including the various possibilities for circle-of-rotation radius, table motion, and gantry control. These experiments should culminate in the imaging of some point sources placed firmly on the surface of the test model. The reconstruction of these point sources may well indicate difficulties that have not been encountered previously.

ROUTINE QUALITY CONTROL

At this point in development, paper and film records of the results of quality control testing and processing are relevant. These are kept at hand in notebooks for easy access. In the future, when a great mass of digital data will be stored, the quality assurance records will also be stored on magnetic or optical media for computer recall and comparison. Paper and film will be storage media of the past.

The previous sections of this chapter have presented discussions of the quality control of each section of the SPECT instrument. Here, the recommendations are turned around and classified by the interval at which they should be performed, so that the user can observe the grouping of tests using similiar equipment and plan the testing strategy.

Daily

1. Camera
    Energy and energy window:
        Present the system with a source, set the energy and the energy window. Take a Polaroid image. Record all camera settings.
    Sensitivity-correction percentage:
        Uniformity-flood source with collimator on or point source with collimator off. Record analog and digital images. If correction circuits are used, record corrected and uncorrected counts, images, times; record source activity, collimator. Calculate correction factor.
    Uniformity:
        Uniformity-flood source (use nondeformable one with this system all the time). Collect 3 M counts for daily checks to be sure 30 M-count image is still relevant.

Record digital and analog 3 M-count images. Record all relevant information as above, with special attention to reproducible energy peaking and window setting. Have computer do calculations on results. Be sure that numeric measurements of uniformity (i.e. a percentage) are always stated as a function of the counts in the image. Always use images as well as numbers to measure uniformity.

    Camera hard copy device(s):
        Examine the images to be sure dots are round and well focused and intensity is satisfactory.
2. Computer and interface
    ADCs—sensitivity:
        Make sure that camera and computer both record same number of counts in same time. Write this information down.
3. SPECT system
    Test safety devices:
        Test safety devices that prevent camera from harming patient and record fact that they have been tested and passed.

Weekly

1. Camera
    Uniformity correction image:
        Collect 30 M-counts for image to correct with, using nondeformable sheet source. Record digital 30 M-count image. Record all relevant information as above, with special attention to reproducible energy peaking and window setting.
    Resolution:
        Line source; image digitally with adequate statistics; calculate MTF and compare with standard for camera.
                OR
        Bar phantom backed by uniformity flood source, used in usual Anger camera quality control.
    Linearity:
        Orthogonal hole phantom or bar phantom backed by uniformity flood source. Collect statistically adequate sample. Look at image. Some systems base linearity correction on this image.

2. Computer and interface
    Center of rotation (x-axis offset) check:
        Use two point sources placed in field to test different parts of camera head. Make sure camera head is level. Acquire digital image at 0 and 180 degrees. Make a Gaussian fit to the data to find pixel positions. Calculate center of rotation (average position between the two images) for both sources. How close does it come to center of matrix?
3. SPECT system
    Hard copy device on computer:
        Use gray scale in computer and sample patient images to make test images. See how much detail is visible and remove dust from system. Reset if necessary.

Monthly

2. Computer and interface
    Distance calibration:
        Use bar phantom and uniformity-flood source, two well-defined point sources, or other measurable distance. Measure distance on collimator face. Find corresponding pixel positions accurately and calculate distance per pixel.
    Roundness of image in computer matrix:
        See uniformity test above. Look at digital image and see if it is correctly positioned and round.
3. SPECT system
    Levelness of camera head with rotation:
        To be sure camera head remains level during rotation, check it at 0 and 180 degrees. Devise methods for assuring correct angle with angled collimator. This might include imaging point source placed off axis of rotation to be sure it stays in same y position at all angles.
    Image cylinder phantom for sensitivity, uniformity, linearity, resolution, volume quantitation check, and correctness of ellipse for attenuation correction. Do not exceed camera's count rate capacity; use SPECT phantom filled with a known amount of water and radionuclide so microcuries per milliliter is known. Image phantom using SPECT acquisition and customary matrix size and angular interval; the total counts in the

test should be less than those used for uniformity correction or a new uniformity correction will be needed. Reconstruct images with and without attenuation correction. Form cine presentation.

Sensitivity:
    On attenuation-corrected transaxial slices, calculate the voxel size and find the counts per second-milliliters per microcurie. How does sensitivity vary over the slice and from slice to slice?

Uniformity:
    Examine uniformity of transaxial slices for all slices. Express nonuniformity as a function of counts in slice pixels and as a function of total number of counts acquired.

Attenuation correction:
    On attenuation-corrected images, is center of image more active or less active than the rest?
    To find attenuation coefficient, run a transect across center of uncorrected transaxial slice and calculate edge counts: center counts ratio. See how many pixels there are between center and edge and convert this to centimeters; $\mu = 2.303 \log(\text{edge counts}/\text{center counts})/(\text{distance from edge to center in cm})$

Patient ellipse and activity correspondence:
    Superimpose ellipse for attenuation correction over transaxial slice to see if they correspond.

Resolution:
    Image a line source in center of water-filled SPECT phantom with acceptable statistics. Calculate MTF on the transaxial slices. Vary filters etc., for amusement, always recording the variables used.

Linearity:
    Image cylinder phantom with straight structure inside and test for straightness in final image.

Volume threshold check:
    Image appropriate set of volumes in SPECT phantom under typical patient imaging conditions ("hot" or "cold," count rates, filters, etc.). Reconstruct. Using volume program and a range of thresholds, find volume of objects. Form ratio of each calculated volume to true volume at different thresholds and plot this as a function of threshold for each volume. Choose threshold that gives best match.

232 *Chapter 7*

Quarterly

2. Computer and interface
    Gantry control: angular interval and timing:
        Attach uniformity sheet source to camera head and rotate it. Are angles correct and does the gantry rotate 360 degrees exactly? Form activity-vs.-angle curves for total activity and for any suspect areas; are these acceptable to within statistical accuracy?
    Gating accuracy:
        Attach uniformity sheet source to camera head. Attach the ECG leads to a test source. Is heart rate on computer what it should be? After a gated acquisition, are counts in each of the beat intervals the same to within statistical accuracy?
3. SPECT system
    Uniformity as a function of angle:
        Attach uniformity sheet source to camera and rotate it, making 3 M-count images at 16 angles. Test uniformity as a function of angle by subtracting images from baseline image (from angle used for daily testing).

Semiannually

3. SPECT system
    Imaging technique:
        Place sources on human volunteer or rigid, elliptical test object and acquire 360-degree data. Form cine and sinograms of all sources. Reconstruct transaxial views of sources and examine images. Check cine for bumpiness. If technique is automatic, try to eliminate variables to isolate difficulties. If technique is manual, retrain technologists.

Annually

2. Computer and interface
    Check timing of computer:
        With stopwatch or good digital watch, check timing of camera and computer, all commonly used timing modes. Make sure they are the same and that they match stopwatch as closely as possible.

BIBLIOGRAPHY

Brookeman, V. A., et al. Analysis and correction of spatial distortions in gamma camera images. In *Proceedings of the Second Symposium on Sharing of Computer Programs and Technology in Nuclear Medicine,* CONF-720430. Springfield, Va.: National Technical Information Service, 1972, pp. 1–13.

Chang, L.-T. A method for attenuation correction in radionuclide computed tomography. *IEEE Trans. Nucl. Sci.* 25:638–643, 1978.

Egbert, S. D., and May, R. S. An integral-transport method for Compton-scatter correction in emission computed tomography. *IEEE Trans. Nucl. Sci.* 27:543–548, 1980.

English, R. J.; Polak, J. F.; and Holman, B. L. An iterative method for verifying systematic nonuniformities in refillable flood sources. *J. Nucl. Med. Tech.* 12:7–9, 1984.

Farrell, T. J.; Cradduck, T. D.; and Chamberlain, R. A. The effect of collimators on the center of rotation in SPECT (letter). *J. Nucl. Med.* 25:632–633, 1984.

Gray, J. E., et al. *Quality Control in Diagnostic Imaging.* Baltimore: University Park Press, 1983.

Greer, K. L., et al. Quality control in SPECT. *J. Nucl. Med. Tech.* 13:76–85, 1985.

Greer, K. L.; Coleman, R. E.; and Jaszczak, R. J. SPECT: a practical guide for users. *J. Nucl. Med. Tech.* 11:61–65, 1983.

Greer, K. L.; Jaszczak, R. J.; and Coleman, R. E. An overview of a camera-based SPECT system. *Med. Phys.* 9:455–463, 1982.

Harkness, B. A., et al. SPECT: quality control procedures and artifact identification. *J. Nucl. Med. Tech.* 11:55–60, 1983.

Johnson, T. K., et al. Spatial/temporal/energy dependency of scintillation camera nonlinearities. In *Emission Computed Tomography: Current Trends,* ed. P. D. Esser. New York: Society of Nuclear Medicine, 1983, pp. 71–80.

LaFontaine, R.; Graham, L. S.; and Stein, M. A. Effects of asymmetric photopeak windows on flood field uniformity and spatial resolution for scintillation cameras (abstract). *J. Nucl. Med.* 25:P22, 1984.

Larsson, S. A. Gamma camera emission tomography. *Acta Radiol.* (Suppl.) 363:1–75, 1980.

Macey, D. J., et al. A calibration phantom for absolute quantitation of radionuclide uptake by SPECT (abstract). *J. Nucl. Med.* 25:P105, 1984.

Muehllehner, G.; Wake, R. H.; and Sano, R. Standards for performance measurements in scintillation cameras. *J. Nucl. Med.* 22:72–77, 1981.

National Electrical Manufacturers' Association. *Performance Measurements of Scintillation Cameras,* Standards Publication No. NU 1–1980. Washington, D.C.: National Electrical Manufacturers' Association, 1980.

Nowak, D. J., and Eisner, R. L. Distance weighting for improved tomographic reconstructions (abstract). *J. Nucl. Med.* 25:P54–55, 1984.

Oppenheim, B. E. More accurate algorithms for iterative 3-dimensional reconstruction. *IEEE Trans. Nucl. Sci.* 21:72–77, 1974.

Oppenheim, B. E., and Appledorn, C. R. Uniformity correction for SPECT using a mapped cobalt-57 sheet source. *J. Nucl. Med.* 26:409–415, 1985.

Powers, T. A., et al. The effects of gating delays on ejection estimates: concise communication. *J. Nucl. Med.* 23:15–16, 1982.

Raff, U.; Spitzer, V. M.; and Hendee, W. R. Practicality of NEMA performance specification measurements for user-based acceptance testing and routine quality assurance. *J. Nucl. Med.* 25:679–687, 1984.

Ramachandran, G. N., and Lakshminarayanan, A. V. Three-dimensional reconstruction from radiographs and electron micrographs: application of convolutions instead of Fourier transforms. *Proc. Nat. Acad. Sci.* 68:2236–2240, 1971.

Rogers, W. L., et al. Field-flood requirements for emission computed tomography with an Anger camera. *J. Nucl. Med.* 23:162–168, 1982.

Shepp, L. A., and Logan, B. F. The Fourier reconstruction of a head section. *IEEE Trans. Nucl. Sci.* 21:21–43, 1974.

Spector, S. S., et al. Analysis and correction of spatial distortions produced by the gamma camera. *J. Nucl. Med.* 13:307–312, 1972.

Williams, D. L., et al. Preliminary characterization of the properties of a transaxial whole-body single-photon tomograph: emphasis on future application to cardiac imaging. In *Functional Mapping of Organ Systems and Other Computer Topics*, ed. P. D. Esser. New York: Society of Nuclear Medicine, 1981, pp. 149–166.

8

Clinical Uses of SPECT

This chapter opens with a general discussion of clinical technique so that every detail need not be repeated in each section. Details of other chapters are recapitulated to the extent that they bear directly on clinical practice. The sections are arranged as they might be in any clinical nuclear medicine book; details of the illustrated clinical material are to be found in the figure legends.

GENERAL TECHNICAL DETAILS

Before launching into a welter of clinical details and the contemplation of the human body sliced transaxially like Swiss cheese, let us consider the choices and decisions to be made when devising a SPECT protocol.

Consider the rationale for using SPECT in a particular diagnostic setting: it gives three-dimensional information, separates overlying structures, and may provide better contrast and quantification. On the other hand, the time course of radionuclide decay or distribution of the radiopharmaceutical in the body may make SPECT inappropriate. Can the same information be obtained more easily or inexpensively by another modality? Tomography, either SPECT or x-ray-transmission, is not the automatic answer to all imaging situations, just as imaging of any kind does not provide the answer in all diagnostic situations.

Patient and Instrument Preparation

Careful patient selection will ensure that the examination is performed for those whose medical conditions might benefit from it, and not for persons whose disease is not amenable to diagnosis by SPECT or who would not be able to undergo the procedure. Patients who are too heavy for the imaging table, those whose organ of interest is too large for the Anger camera's field of view, and those unable to remain motionless or to lie flat for the required period of time should be excluded. Patients with many intravenous lines, drain tubes, and monitor wires may be difficult to image. Technologists skilled in positioning and in patient psychology will often facilitate the examination with such borderline patients. Beyond these limitations, patients in whom accumulation of radioactivity is not adequate or in whom the peak of activity is long past may present problems, although SPECT may be successful when other imaging procedures would fail.

The radiopharmaceutical to be used depends not only on the differential diagnoses being entertained but on the optimum use of the Anger camera. If possible, one should always choose a radionuclide with an energy between 100 and 180 KeV, and with a half-life no longer than the time it will take to perform the examination. One should avoid radionuclides with higher-energy emissions that must be collimated even if they are not being imaged and those with beta radiation that raises the radiation dose without any diagnostic gain. None of these ideas is new, but they are especially important for SPECT, because it is necessary to maximize the counts acquired in a reasonable period of time. One should inject as large an amount of radioactivity as the risk-benefit ratio suggests is sensible based on the patient's disease and the diagnostic information to be gained. More counts can always improve a scintigraphic image, but only if they are acquired over a time period in which patient movement is not significant. The route of administration of the radiopharmaceutical is usually intravenous, but for certain examinations special consideration should be given to the use of catheters, intra-arterial administration, and other special maneuvers. During the formative stages of a protocol, it may be desirable to use two radiopharmaceuticals, one for the organ of interest and the other to outline the anatomy. Often the second dose may be eliminated after sufficient experience has been gained and such highlighting is no longer necessary. Attention should be paid to the proper time for imaging; several standard nuclear medicine imaging protocols call for scintigraphy at such a time as the background has cleared in order to achieve the best contrast on planar imaging. The count rate in the organ of interest may also have fallen from previous levels, but the ratio is most important in planar work; for SPECT, the ratio matters less and count rates in the organ of interest matter more, so imaging should be performed when the organ's localization of the radiopharmaceutical has the highest reasonably stable count rate. A 20:1 target:background ratio in an organ with 800 counts per second (cps) will not provide the handsome SPECT images that a 5:1 ratio with 10,000 cps will.

The instrument and the examination should be properly quality controlled, including uniformity images of the radionuclide at the window and energy settings used for the patient. The energy window should be symmetric about the peak, unless the laboratory protocol determines otherwise, and it should be as narrow as possible to avoid scattered radiation. Incorrect energy peak and window settings contribute to fuzzy, nonuniform images and, furthermore, do not collect all the available counts. The patient area to be imaged must be located and the patient positioned so that the area falls in the middle of the camera's field of view. The protocol should specify where markers are to be placed and what their activity range should be, so they will provide anatomic landmarks and information about the constancy of the patient's position throughout the examination. Data acquisition protocols involve choices of numbers of angles, matrix size, and 180– or 360–degree rotation, as well as time to be spent acquiring data at each angle. The variables are to be optimized to create the least noisy image, with the required accuracy, in a total time consonant with patient position and constancy of radioactivity distribution. Particular examinations may require the precollection not only of uniformity images but of views of the patient, such as transmission or background images. Reconstruction protocols should be specified for each SPECT imaging situation, including attenuation correction, filtering, slice thickness, and standard or computer selection of section orientation.

The specification of a certain product (films, numeric results, and so forth) at the end of the examination is important. Images processed and photographed in a particular way make possible the comparison of results and mean the technologist will not have to guess what the most diagnostic information is. Besides images, numeric values may be calculated. One should consider carefully what information should be archived, what should be stored for short periods of time, and what is necessary only until the hard copy is produced.

Conducting a Typical Study

As mentioned earlier, and especially in Chapter 5, decisions have to be made in the course of setting up a protocol for a SPECT examination. Sometimes less than perfect situations are unavoidable, but every effort should be made to minimize difficulties.

The typical SPECT examination involves imaging for 20 to 30 minutes, acquiring 60 to 100 angular increments of 64 x 64 or 128 x 128 data, either in a 180–degree half-circle or a full 360–degree circle. Count rate limitations may be addressed by increasing the imaging time, increasing the radionuclide dose, or using special collimators. Special collimators may also be used to allow the camera collimator face to approach the patient as closely as possible, although a differently shaped Anger camera head would do this as well.

In general, the patient should be positioned as comfortably as possible and in such a way that the camera collimator face will come as close to him as possible. Arms should be over the head for any torso images, because their attenuation is detrimental to the images. Patient restraint must also be consistent with the short distance to the camera face. Elaborate restraint devices and binders that add bulk to the patient and imaging table are not helpful. Patient movement during the examination, to remove the arms from the path of the camera, for example, may also move or change the shape of the organ being imaged. The organ or the center of the body should be placed on the axis of rotation, if possible. Since the imaging table may not be very steady under a bouncing patient, it may be desirable to design a prop that can be used whenever the camera is not under the table. Some imaging tables may have areas with metal or another significant attenuator included; these areas must not come between the patient and the camera. Even snaps on the table cover can cause problems, and one table has a metal end that cannot be between the patient's head and the camera. In this case, a special head holder must be used; such a device can be purchased from the manufacturer or fashioned from a plastic infant-restraint device available in every radiology department. In circumstances where repeated imaging of the same patient's head is anticipated, a head holder molded for the patient may be useful (Kearfott, Rottenberg, and Knowles 1984).

Markers placed on the patient outside the field of the organ of interest will help in finding and solving motion difficulties. These markers should be of such activity that they do not dominate the images or interfere with their contrast.

Before reconstruction, the cine presentation and sinogram of the images should be examined to see if they show patient motion or other difficulties. The correct filter must be chosen for reconstruction; if the count rate is low, the high frequencies must be eliminated. During reconstruction a choice must be made about the thickness of the slice; naturally, the area of the body, the organ being imaged, and the number of counts collected will influence this choice, but the usual slice thickness is 6 to 12 mm. Since there is no need to reconstruct areas that are not of interest, one should do only the necessary images. The typical reconstruction for a technetium-99m–based radiopharmaceutical involves attenuation correction; in the future, methods for correction for all parts of the body will be developed. Once the transaxial images are produced, they should be photographed using an exposure time and contrast that will display as much of the gray scale as possible. Coronal, sagittal, and oblique slices may be created according to a standard protocol. The films and cine presentation should be available to the diagnostician.

Quality Assurance for Clinical SPECT

Chapter 7 contains a series of recommendations for routine quality assurance. This is very important, because the clinical images are only as good as the quality assurance program. What is really required is that someone who understands the system and cares about the quality of the images be responsible for the condition of the instrument.

Troubleshooting

Naturally, quality control measures using phantoms are only part of a quality assurance program. The patient images themselves may contain clues about the condition of the instrument: Are there rings in the images? Is there a bull's-eye in the center? Perhaps the flood correction was not done correctly or the wrong uniformity flood image was used in the correction. Fixing this requires quick work to collect a flood image with the same settings that were used in the patient images. Does part of the patient organ seem to be cut off in the transaxial images or in the cine? Perhaps the patient moved after the attenuation correction ellipse was determined or maybe the organ was not visible to the camera at all angles. Does the cine image seem to "bounce" or the sinogram seem broken? The patient may have moved during data acquisition, in which case perhaps the planar projection images can be repositioned before the tomographic reconstruction; or the contour-following mechanism may not be working correctly. Is a low count rate area visible in the cine presentation during part of the rotation? Perhaps the table has some hidden high-attenuation material or the patient put his arm in the way. Does a "hot" spot appear off to the side in some of the images in the cine? Perhaps the injection site in the arm is in the image; this problem is not bad because the reconstruction correctly places this activity outside the patient's body. Do the images seem very contrasty? Maybe someone has tampered with the settings on the formatter. Do the images seem oversmoothed or undersmoothed? Perhaps the wrong filter has been used or too much smoothing was performed before photography.

HEAD

The first significant SPECT imaging was done in the head (Kuhl and Edwards 1964). Instruments, usually multiprobe-based, were created to perform SPECT brain scintigraphy. Statistical precision was poor and computers and reconstruction methods were primitive, so the results could be disappointing.

The specialized instruments designed to image the head proved to be useful in their place, but did not satisfy the need for a general-purpose SPECT instrument. In its turn, the Anger-camera-based general-purpose SPECT unit has slowly been evolving into an instrument suitable for head imaging. The problem, pure and simple, is that patients have shoulders; the adult human cross-section broadens rapidly at the shoulder. To make the unimageable zone for well-resolved SPECT imaging as small as possible, some method for circumventing the shoulders, such as a specially angled collimator (Esser et al. 1983) or a specially shaped Anger camera (Larsson et al. 1984)(see Fig 3–3) must be used. The special collimator (Esser et al. 1983, 1984) is built with parallel holes on a 30–degree angle, so that most patients' shoulders will be passed (Esser et al. 1984). In use, it is angled at 30 degrees from the axis of rotation so that acquired data permit the reconstruction of transaxial slices (see Fig 3–5). The average minimum radius of rotation with the collimator is 13 cm compared to the 25 cm expected when shoulders must be cleared; the decrease in rotational radius allowed with the angulated collimator permits a decrease in full width at half maximum (FWHM) of 0.4 cm. Experiments with phantoms involving small nonradioactive spheres showed the improved resolution of the angulated collimator. (Note that the collimator is being used mostly for sinus work with bone-imaging agents, discussed in "Bone" section of this chapter.) All of the head and neck lie within about 7 cm of the collimator face.

An Anger camera specially designed to image heads would have at least one flat side with less than the usual thickness of material between the active area of the collimator and the edge of the whole assembly. The customary Anger camera design has a row of photomultiplier (PM) tubes as well as shielding measuring about 12 to 15 cm outside the active area of the collimator. Thinning and flattening one side requires re-engineering.

Once the shoulder problem is solved, the question of how to make the most of the counts coming from the human head should be addressed: the head does not subtend much of a solid angle compared to the angle of acceptance of the camera (Coleman, Drayer, and Jaszczak 1982). For the camera to receive more counts from the head, it must direct more of its attention toward the head, that is, more of the crystal must be aimed at the radioactivity. A special converging fan-beam collimator (Jaszczak, Chang, and Murphy 1979) accomplishes this. The collimator has a converging fan-beam acceptance in one direction and a parallel-hole configuration in the other, so that the transaxial slices still receive data from the same planes, as they would in the case of a straight parallel-hole collimator (see Fig 3–4).

Careful attention should also be paid to the patient couch. A special narrow head holder, probably with a positioning strap, should be used so that the couch does not interfere with attempts to bring the collimator face close to the patient. Molded head holders may also be useful for patients having repeated examinations (Kearfott, Rottenberg, and Knowles 1984).

The head is a small body part that is not affected by respiratory motion, so greater resolution should be possible there than in the larger parts of the body. Constant and intelligent attention to quality control is necessary to achieve good resolution. Lack of attention to center-of-rotation quality control can cause minimal lesions to be invisible (Jaszczak, Greer, and Coleman 1983). The head contains bone and soft tissue. Ordinarily, attenuation corrections should be made under such circumstances. An experimental attenuation coefficient a bit higher than that for soft tissue in the body, or a correction scheme that iterates to correct the transaxial images by comparison to the planar projections, might be preferable to the use of an attenuation coefficient of 0.12 reciprocal centimeters for 140–KeV gamma rays (0.12 per centimeter includes both attenuation and scattering effects [Larsson 1980]). A model for brain and bone in the head would help with attenuation corrections (Carril et al. 1979).

A strategy for obtaining accurate images with the desired orientation is necessary. One must decide whether, for example, a Townes position with its angled slices or a Caldwell position with its straight slices would be better, and then stick with the position and learn the appearance of the normal anatomy when imaged this way. Most SPECT and x-ray CT work uses the Townes position; the Caldwell position is used for sinuses.

The brain can be imaged in many ways: blood-brain barrier, cerebral blood flow, receptor binding, cisternography, and pituitary imaging. Various radionuclides and radiopharmaceuticals are employed in the search for accurate descriptions of disease and function in the brain (Holman 1985). X-ray CT gives a good image of cerebral anatomy, with much better resolution than any scintigraphic technique can hope for. Because cerebral function often does not follow anatomy, or vice versa, there is a distinct place for radiotracer brain imaging. In the head, SPECT permits the separation of structures, the creation of a transaxial slice to compare with x-ray CT images, and perhaps quantification of radioactivity distribution for a measurement of cerebral function (Kuhl et al. 1976; Hill 1980; Coleman, Drayer, and Jaszczak 1982).

Because there are so many facets to cerebral imaging, SPECT and the radiopharmaceuticals may be combined in different ways. At some times the diagnosis is based on areas with the greatest radioactivity, at others on those with least activity; at yet other times the difference or washout is crucial. No one technique or method of analysis and presentation will do for all. It will soon be possible to use images from x-ray CT, SPECT cerebral blood flow, and NMR (MRI) to complement and supplement each other.

Blood-Brain Barrier

For quite a number of years, brain scintigraphy consisted of looking for blood-brain barrier deficits in a varied patient population. Even the conventional examination, whether by rectilinear scanner or Anger camera, was fairly time consuming and the yield of positive examinations was low. Early SPECT brain studies took even longer than conventional studies or were limited to one or two selected slices with the same low yield. This did not stop instrument development or its application to blood-brain barrier imaging by investigators who praised the success of SPECT in this endeavor (Kuhl and Edwards 1964; Kuhl and Sanders 1971; Keyes 1976; Kuhl et al. 1976; Dendy et al. 1977; Jaszczak et al. 1977; Keyes et al. 1977; Hill et al. 1978; Burdine et al. 1979; Carril et al. 1979). When x-ray CT burst upon the scene, however, interest in and performance of blood-brain barrier imaging decreased greatly.

Statistics on the efficacy of SPECT in blood-brain barrier imaging are few but favorable, even with older scanner-based equipment and methods; however, the technique is doubtless widely used. Statistics were often based on a single slice image, taken at the level most likely to give a result, because of time and instrumental constraints. Carril and co-workers (1979) chose the level for SPECT imaging from the conventional views, the patient's history, or, if neither of these suggested a level, the basal zone, in which conventional imaging might be the most difficult. They compared SPECT with x-ray CT imaging in 512 patients for whom there was a final diagnosis. The 140 positive results were mostly infarcts (59) or brain tumors (50), with 16 extracranial lesions. Four of the tumors detected only by SPECT were in the basal zone of the brain; basal infarcts were similarly rendered visible by SPECT. These authors felt the greatest merit of SPECT was in providing further information about any area of suspicion, thus improving diagnostic confidence (Table 8–1).

Hill, Lovett, and McNeil (1980) reported statistics on 200 patients in whom the 62 positive findings represented mostly strokes (31) and metastases (15). Eight tomographic slices were acquired for each patient on the Harvard Head Scanner. The effectiveness of SPECT in their study was much the same as it was in the work of Carril and co-workers (1979). N. E. Watson and colleagues (1980) used the same instrument; SPECT and conventional brain scanning yielded very similar results (Table 8–2). They felt that SPECT was helpful in dis-

TABLE 8–1.—COMPARISON OF THE ACCURACY OF BRAIN IMAGING WITH AND WITHOUT SPECT

	SENSITIVITY	SPECIFICITY	ACCURACY
Without tomography	83/140 (59%)	363/372 (98%)	446/512 (87%)
With tomography	107/140 (76%)	367/372 (99%)	474/512 (92%)

From Carril et al. 1979.

TABLE 8–2.—BRAIN SCANNING ACCURACY COMPARED WITH SPECT

	SENSITIVITY	SPECIFICITY	ACCURACY
Conventional	42/62 (68%)	133/138 (96%)	175/200 (88%)
SPECT	48/62 (77%)	137/138 (99%)	185/200 (92%)

From Hill, Lovett, and McNeil 1980.

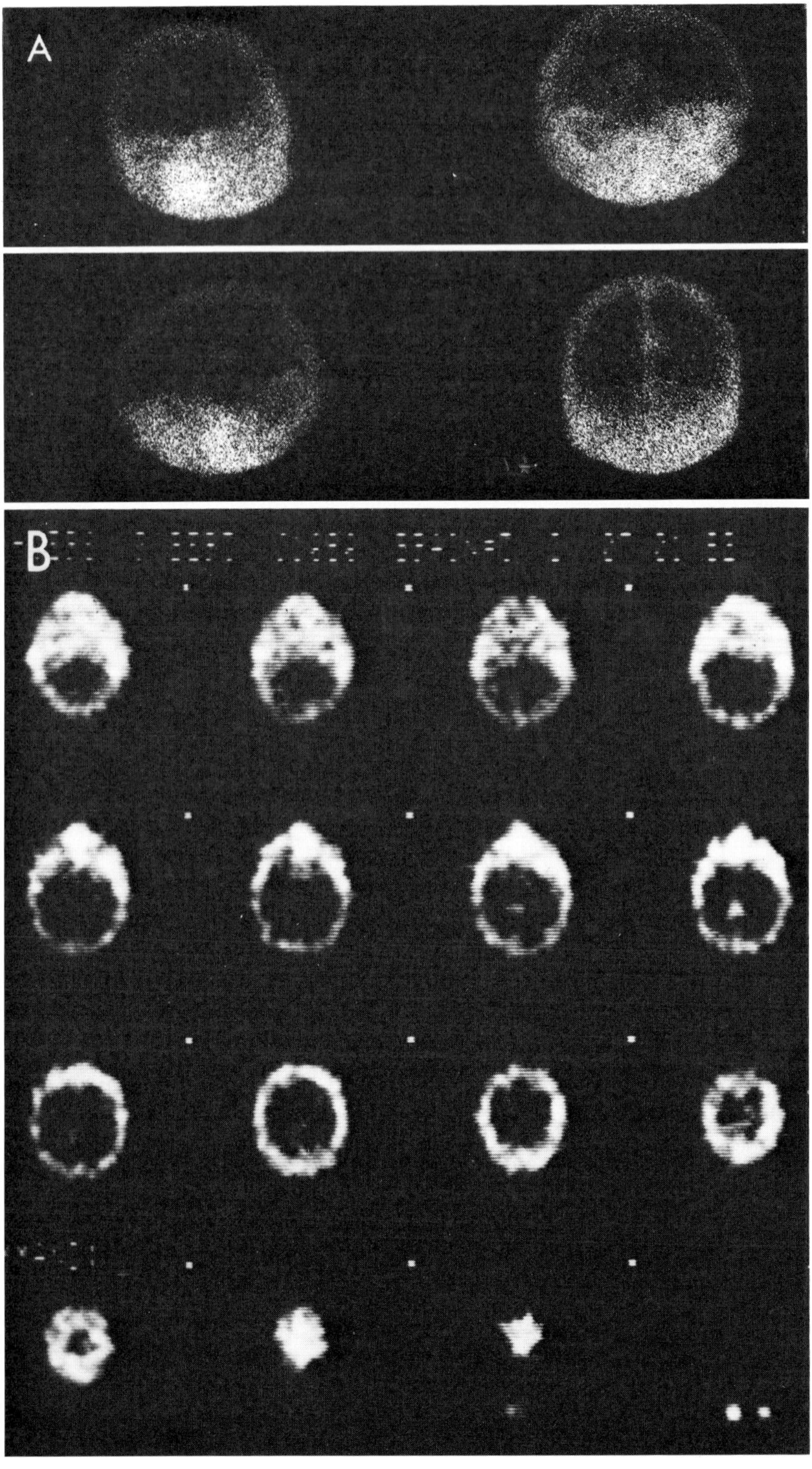
A
B

tinguishing between brain and skull metastases, defining the depth of a lesion, and increasing their own confidence in the diagnoses.

It is possible for SPECT to image a brain lesion in three dimensions so that it need not be localized by reference only to two or three images. It separates structures so that activity seen on conventional images may be accurately called normal or abnormal (Fig 8–1). Normally, SPECT does not suffer from that problem of x-ray CT wherein great disparities of attenuation coefficients between the skull and brain tissue cause artifacts on the brain surface. Small metal objects such as surgical clips are not such a problem in SPECT images as they are in x-ray CT images. Blood-brain barrier imaging taught the early users a great deal about the benefits of SPECT, so that clinicians and experimenters are prepared to image with other cerebral agents as they come along.

Cerebral Blood Flow

The blood-brain barrier study was often accompanied by a radioangiogram or vascular sequence that imaged the first pass of the radiopharmaceutical through the head. Crude information was obtained about blocked arteries, arteriovenous malformations, subdural hematomas, and tumor vascularity. Positron-emission tomography (PET) showed the value of a better-resolved image of tissue perfusion in the brain, with a number of diffusible and metabolic tracers. Kuhl and associates (1976) quantified local cerebral blood flow with the Mark IV multiprobe scanner SPECT using technetium-99m–labeled red blood cells; however, an agent that diffuses into the brain so that its distribution reflects blood flow can give a higher concentration and better images than red blood cells. Marvelous PET images were obtained of brains at rest or engaged in sensing or directing various kinds of activity (Phelps, Kuhl, and Mazziotta 1981) as well as of epileptics showing seizure foci. These results have been a continuing inspiration to develop methods exploiting single-photon-emitting radiopharmaceuticals to delineate regional cerebral blood flow.

Diffusible tracers for visualizing and measuring cerebral blood flow must be soluble in brain tissue, often by virtue of being lipid soluble. If the distribution of radioactivity is to be measured with

---

Fig 8–1.—Images of head with Tc-99m glucoheptonate. The patient, a 59–year-old male, had left facial pain. On the **top** are the four planar views, while on the **bottom** are the transaxial SPECT images. X-ray CT scans showed an intense enhancing rounded lesion in the posterior corpus callosum mainly on the right side.

Anger-camera SPECT, the distribution must be fixed in time in some way, either by continuous infusion or by some chemical or biochemical interaction in the tissue. Distributions that change rapidly must be studied with faster instruments.

Radioactive gases, soluble in body fat, were first employed to help map regional cerebral blood flow. The gas was either injected intraarterially or rebreathed until a sufficient brain tissue concentration was reached. Counting or imaging of gas washout was begun at maximal tissue concentration and carried out with systems with a short time constant in order to freeze the rapid changes in gas concentration with a sufficient number of frames. Typically, xenon-133 is used in this examination, although it has unfavorable energy and emission characteristics. Anger-camera-based SPECT systems are not fast enough for such imaging, but many of the multiprobe-based systems will do acceptably. A special system (Stokely et al. 1980; Bonte and Stokely 1981; Lassen, Henriksen, and Paulson 1981) was built to create transaxial functional images from xenon-133 data, monitoring uptake and washout of the gas. The instrument records three 2–cm slices (separated by 2 cm) simultaneously after the patient begins rebreathing gas for one minute from a xenon-133 reservoir containing 10 mCi per liter. Each slice is 1 to 2 cm thick; the whole head cannot be imaged at once. A series of four one-minute images is collected and from them is created a functional map of the washout half-times in the transaxial plane. Realizing that information was needed about other planes, a new collimator (Stokely 1982) was designed for this instrument to create six slices with an intrinsic resolution of 1.3 cm in the axial direction. Although this special-purpose instrument is available commercially as the Tomomatic 64, its popularity is not great because only heads can be imaged with it. Other models are being developed for body imaging.

Measurements of cerebral blood flow can be helpful in a variety of diseases such as arteriovenous malformations (Bonte et al. 1983), cerebrovascular disease (Buell et al. 1983a; Rezai et al. 1984), and mental illness (Devous et al. 1984). It may not be necessary to have a special-purpose instrument, since some (Patton, Cardell, and Woolfenden 1983) use the conventional Anger camera and the same rebreathing technique for xenon-133 cerebral blood flow studies in the vertex projection.

The xenon-based methods for imaging regional cerebral blood flow require that an instrument be sensitive and that it be able to complete an image of a slice in a minute or less, because the distribution of radioactivity changes rapidly. It has been suggested that xenon-127 would improve the examination (Budinger 1981) because of its more favorable emanations, but there are no published results of this technique.

Krypton-81m (half-life, 13 seconds) may be infused constantly into an artery (Fazio et al. 1980; T. Maeda et al. 1981); radioactive decay is in equilibrium with blood flow, so images are of the regional arrival of the radioactivity and may be acquired over two to 20 minutes during the infusion. Only one hemisphere is visualized since only one artery is used for perfusion at a time. A superposition of selective artery perfusion examinations (Higa et al. 1983) combined with anatomic outlines derived from x-ray CT images provides landmarks for the functional images. Advantages are high count rates, low radiation dose and waste, ability to reimage immediately, and the practicality of use with any SPECT instrument. Disadvantages are the invasiveness of arterial infusion and rubidium-81 parent half-life; also, a new generator must be received at least once a day. Krypton-81m could become popular, but the rubidium-81 parent half-life is too short to make this nuclide practical.

Anger-camera SPECT requires a distribution of radioactivity that will remain fixed over a period of 20 minutes to one hour, preferably without complications such as constant infusion. One useful agent is N-isopropyl I-123 p-iodoamphetamine (IMP) (Fig 8–2). It is lipid soluble and has a high extraction fraction in the brain, where it seems to stay fixed by virtue of a combination of pH differences between extravascular and intravascular spaces (Winchell, Baldwin, and Lin 1980), metabolism, and receptor binding (Holman, Hill, and Magistretti 1982). Initial SPECT imaging (Kuhl et al. 1981; Lee et al. 1982a, 1982b; Hill et al. 1982) showed its great promise: cerebral uptake patterns seemed to be related to gray matter perfusion and could be correlated with stimuli presented to the patient at the time of injection (Hill et al. 1982). Seizure foci are visible (Magistretti et al. 1982) as areas of less than normal perfusion when no seizure activity is present and greater than normal perfusion when there is seizure activity.

The original SPECT images of IMP were made with the Mark IV scanner (Kuhl et al. 1981) and the Harvard multiprobe scanner, itself an updated Cleon 710 imager (Hill et al. 1982). The iodine-123 was made by the (p,2n) reaction, which means it had 2% to 5% iodine-124 contamination, leading to a high background at higher energies; this must be carefully collimated and compensated for. Radiation doses for the contaminated material were estimated to be 0.7 rads to the brain, 4.9 rads to the lung, 4.1 rads to the liver, and 0.45 rads to the whole body, for 5 mCi of iodine-123 IMP contaminated with 5%

248 *Chapter 8*

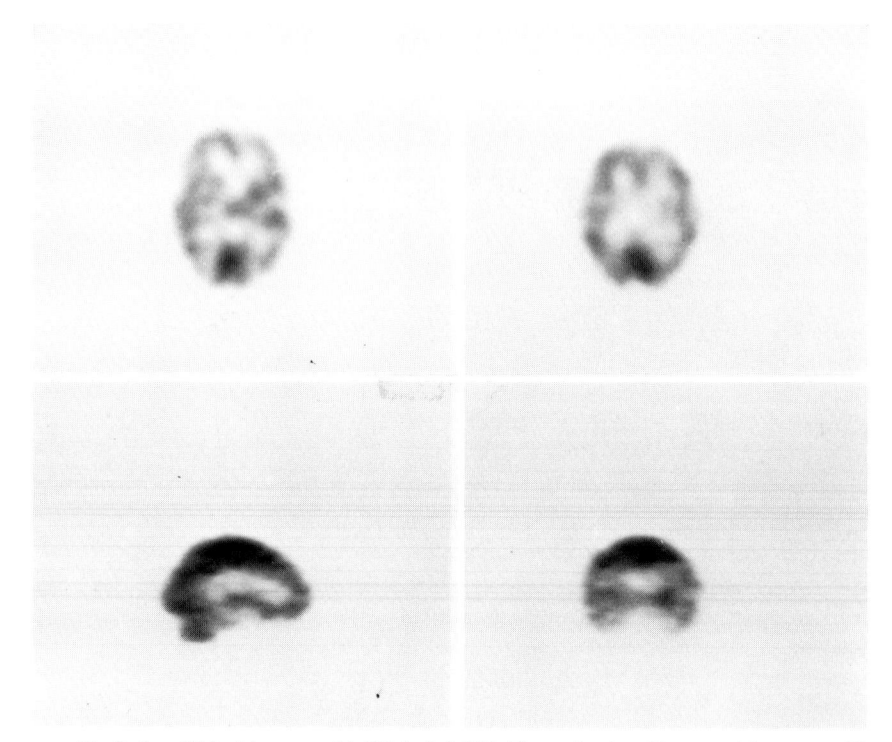

Fig 8–2.—Clinical images of I-123 (p,2n) IMP. The patient, a 23–year-old woman with a known history of temporal lobe epilepsy, was injected with 5 mCi of I-123 IMP in the ictal state. Tomographic imaging was begun 45 minutes after injection; 20 minutes of continuous rotation was required for imaging with a medium-energy collimator. The reconstruction was performed with a Shepp-Logan filter with a roll-off of 0.75 times the Nyquist frequency. The Chang method was used for attenuation correction. The upper images are transaxial slices at two levels, while the lower images are a sagittal on the left and a coronal on the right. (Courtesy of T. C. Hill, New England Deaconess Hospital, Boston, Mass.)

of iodine-124 IMP (Kuhl et al. 1982); half of the estimated dose is caused by the iodine-124. The IMP should be made with uncontaminated (p,5n) iodine-123.

The SPECT technique and IMP form an ideal combination for cerebral blood flow imaging and quantification. Experience gained with the compound will elucidate its utility and quirks. To validate its use as a quantitative blood flow agent, IMP was compared to carbon-14 iodoantipyrine with autoradiography in rats (Kuhl et al. 1982); the distributions were very similar except for greater choroid plexus activity, especially on the radiograms soon after injection. The IMP images were compared to labeled microsphere flow in dogs (Kuhl et al.

1982); the two methods related in a linear fashion for flows from 10 to 50 ml per 100 gm per minute. Lassen and co-workers (1983) directly compared (p,5n) iodine 123 IMP to xenon-133 for cerebral blood flow imaging using the multiprobe instrument. The xenon-imaging protocol was described above. Two millicuries of iodine-123 IMP were injected and a series of ten-minute images was acquired over the first hour after injection. Eleven subjects were examined; excellent agreement was found between the xenon-133 flow studies and the IMP images at ten minutes after injection. For the IMP images at later times, there was some tendency for the contrast between diseased areas and the normal brain to decrease, although even these later pictures were acceptable. Lassen does not feel that high-quality cerebral blood flow images are possible with Anger-camera–based SPECT instruments because their sensitivity is not adequate. Improved collimators, decreased collimator-to-head distance, and the possibility of imaging for more than ten minutes might well make the images acceptable (Lassen 1983). More recently, von Schulthess and co-workers (1985) measured cerebral blood flow with iodine-123 IMP in 51 patients compared to ten normal individuals; they began imaging at 30 minutes after the injection of 4 to 6 mCi (150 to 225 MBq) of activity. The technique seemed most useful in cerebral vascular disease, although the quantification suffered because of variability in lung uptake of IMP. On the other hand, Buell and associates (1985) compared IMP measurements made with SPECT over different time intervals after injection with xenon-133 flow measurments and found the best congruence when the IMP imaging was done between 13 and 27 minutes.

Lee and associates (1983) evaluated IMP for use in patients suffering acute stroke. The agent's distribution did reflect cerebral perfusion, but the deficit size did not correlate well with clinical progress. Moretti and co-workers (1983) imaged IMP in epileptics and cerebral ischemics; in the epileptics, lesions detected by electroencephalogram and x-ray CT were demonstrated by SPECT. In patients with cerebral ischemia, the poorly perfused area was often greater on SPECT than on x-ray CT; in two of 22 patients, SPECT showed ischemia while the x-ray CT was normal. SPECT of iodine-123 IMP also was more sensitive in demonstrating middle cerebellar artery stroke.

Iodine-123 IMP has been accompanied into the field of blood flow imaging by another amine, N,N,N'-trimethyl-N'-(2–hydroxy-3–methyl-5–(I-123)iodobenzyl)-1,3–propanediamine (I-123 HIPDM), which exhibits less brain uptake, more liver uptake, and slower lung clearance than IMP (Holman et al. 1983), making it a less useful agent for cerebral imaging. When HIPDM was studied in the human brain it performed adequately (Fazio et al. 1983 a,b, 1984). The concentration of HIPDM in the brain appears fixed over at least four hours. Gelfand and co-workers (1984) quantitated the uptake of HIPDM in normal individuals; their work showed at least one site of significantly decreased uptake in the 13 of their 18 subjects who evidenced decreased uptake.

The patient is injected with 5 to 10 mCi of iodine-123 IMP and imaged between 15 and 60 minutes later. If IMP is imaged with an Anger-camera–based SPECT system, the question of proper collimation is not automatically solved by using (p,5n) iodine-123. Iodine-123 has a principal energy of 159 KeV and a small emission at higher energies, even if uncontaminated by iodine-124. Coleman and co-workers (1983) demonstrated that low-energy high-resolution or fan-beam collimators were superior to medium-energy collimators for (p,5n) iodine-123. Low-energy all-purpose collimators should, however, be tested for their septal penetration characteristics before use with iodine-123 (Graham and Zielinski 1979). Some of the technetium-99m collimators are not suitable.

Research continues into lipophilic agents with technetium-99m labels to penetrate the blood-brain barrier and yield high activity in static images of blood flow (Troutner et al. 1983; Epps et al. 1983; Ravert et al. 1983; Kung et al. 1983). A good technetium-99m agent prepared with a kit would be a radiopharmaceutical incentive to improve the instrument for brain work. In addition, PET research into compounds to image cerebral metabolism is being continued (Kuhl 1984); of necessity, there must be blood flow for metabolism, but the presence of an adequate blood supply does not guarantee metabolism and proper function. The PET research will spawn single-photon analogs or substitutes in the metabolic area, too.

Receptor Binding

The brain can also be approached from the point of view of receptor binding. Iodine-123 quinuclidinyl-(3–iodo-4–hydroxy-benzilate) (I-123 QNB) was synthesized in an attempt to visualize the muscarinic cholinergic system (Drayer et al. 1982) and tested in calves. The study pointed out that receptor imaging will be difficult even with ideal agents because changes in binding between health and disease are small, and the gray matter and white matter are mixed in SPECT voxels, while only the gray matter contains specific binding sites. Partial voluming is hard to avoid under these circumstances. Gibson and co-workers (1984) concluded that washout of the tracer may be the measurement to make; if so, radiopharmaceutical receptor affinity may be tuned to the response time of the imaging instrument. Kilbourn and Zalutsky (1985) have written a thorough review of receptor-based radiopharmaceuticals.

Cerebrospinal Fluid Space

Radionuclide cisternography permits imaging the cerebrospinal fluid space and its dynamics. Indium-111 pentetate (DTPA) and ytterbium-169 DTPA are commonly used today if cisternography is to be carried out beyond 24 hours, while technetium-99m DTPA may be employed in shorter studies. The Anger camera and its collimators are well suited for low-energy gamma emitters. Published work on SPECT cisternography (Kuhl et al. 1976; Wooley, Williams, and Venkatesh 1977; Rothenberg, Devenney, and Kuhl 1976) has been done on multiprobe scanning SPECT instruments, which are more tolerant of higher energies than the Anger camera. If the statistical precision is adequate, very nice correlation with anatomy can be made (Kuhl et al. 1976). These examinations may be especially important in children.

At the proper time after intrathecal injection of 500 µCi of ytterbium-169 DTPA, the patient is carefully positioned to image as much of the head as possible, in as tight an orbit as possible (Fig 8–3). A source should be positioned off the top of the patient's head for positioning quality control; sources may be used for other positioning information if their activity is carefully controlled so that they are just visible and do not dominate either the planar image or the transaxial image. Data are acquired into a 64 × 64 or 128 × 128 matrix at 60 to 100 angles for 15 to 20 seconds each or 20 to 30 minutes for the whole examination. A total of 500,000 counts may be collected during the examination. Transaxial slices 1.2 cm thick are reconstructed after filtering with a smooth filter. To the extent that the SPECT instrument can be adapted to overcome the problems posed by shoulders, confusing cisternographic patterns in the midbrain will be resolved, as will those at the base of the brain.

Pituitary Gland

It is possible to image the pituitary gland and to separate it from overlying structures with SPECT (Britton and Shapiro 1981; Britton 1982). The patient is injected with 15 mCi of technetium-99m pertechnetate after having been premedicated with potassium perchlorate. After 40

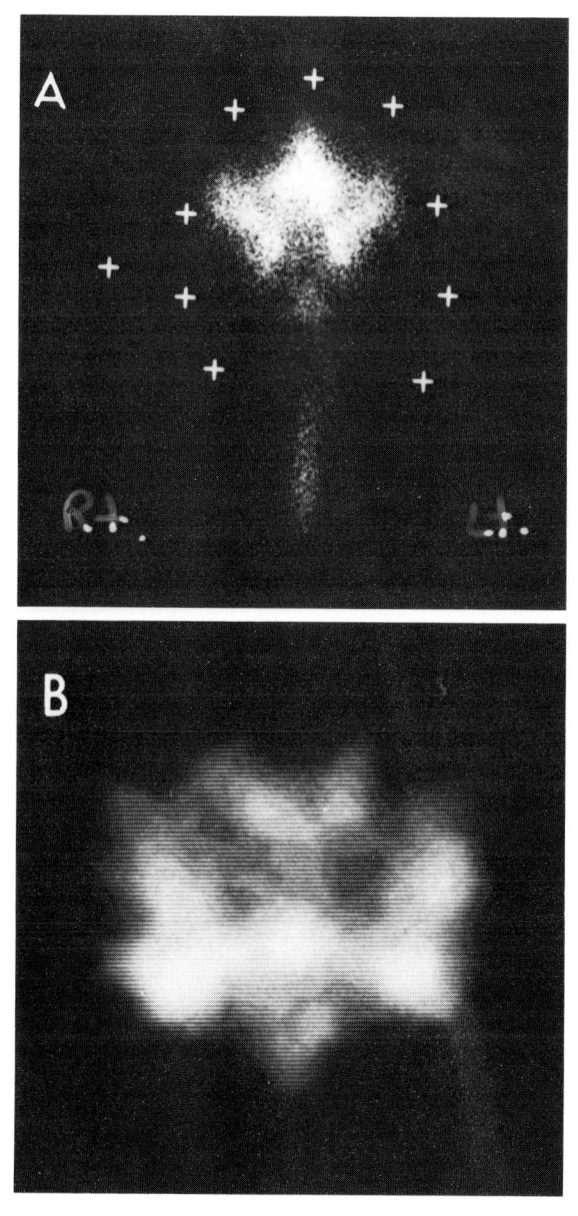

Fig 8–3.—Clinical images of Yb-169 DTPA cisternography. The patient was an 81-year-old male with a three-month history of ataxia and dementia. The X-ray CT scan showed enlarged lateral ventricles; a diagnosis of normal pressure hydrocephalus was being considered. The patient was injected with 0.460 mCi of Yb-169 DTPA intrathecally. He was imaged at 6 and 24 hours post injection, with SPECT imaging at 24 hours. Sixty-

minutes (Britton 1982), the patient is imaged with SPECT, with great care given to positioning the head to have the outer canthal-meatal line in the vertical plane. The pituitary is perfectly centered in the transaxial image either through the outer canthal-meatal line or the next image above it. The activity may be quantified (Britton 1982) by comparing the activity per pixel in a tight region of interest (3 × 3 or 4 × 4) around the pituitary with a background region of interest chosen to surround the pituitary but excluding counts from the gland region itself. Ratios of pituitary counts to background higher than 1.27 are positive for pituitary adenoma. Accuracy of SPECT was compared with that of x-ray CT in 21 patients, of whom 19 were known and two were suspected to have pituitary adenomas; SPECT was 81% accurate and x-ray CT 47% accurate.

LUNGS

The lungs would certainly seem to be a natural clinical target for SPECT, especially in view of the often-recommended six or eight views for conventional lung scintigraphy. On the other side of the argument is the complex anatomy of the chest, which is not simplified on transaxial section. The lobes of the lungs are not arranged in the chest in the manner of blocks stacked in a box. X-ray imaging ordinarily does not differentiate the lobes and x-ray CT does not give an appreciation for the relationship of the parts of the lung to each other. When lung perfusion agents were first imaged with SPECT (Burdine, Murphy, and DePuey 1979), the information on the transaxial slices was too difficult to assimilate. This may remain the position of most clinicians, but it has not hindered a few groups from doing clinical work in the chest with special emphasis on the lungs (Khan et al. 1981; Osborne et al. 1983; LeJeune et al. 1982; Biersack et al. 1982; Donaldson et al. 1982), as well as experimental work in this area (Osborne, Jaszczak, and Coleman 1983).

The usual observation about the utility of SPECT, that it allows the separation of overlying structures, is made about pulmonary

---

four angular images were acquired into a 64 × 64 matrix for 20 seconds per angle. The transaxial image was formed with lowpass filter and no attenuation correction; each slice was 1.2 cm thick. The 24–hour anterior view is seen on the **top** and a transaxial SPECT view on the **bottom**. There was marked early ventricular entry which persisted in the delayed views, as well as delayed flow over the convexities, all consistent with normal pressure hydrocephalus.

SPECT. The procedure eliminates shine-through and questions about defects that may really be cardiomegaly. The difficulties to be overcome are respiratory motion and the decreased attenuation of lung tissue compared to the rest of the body. The lung is about one third as dense as water. The chest is therefore very nonuniform in attenuation. For ordinary images this does not cause a problem, but if quantification is desired, some accommodation must be made. An average attenuation coefficient of about 0.09 per centimeter (Osborne et al. 1982) may be used, although this might profitably be changed in the lower part of the chest where the heart contributes more tissue and more attenuation. Clearly, better accuracy in the chest could result (Osborne et al. 1982) from an iterative procedure in which the reprojected transaxial slices are compared to the acquired planar projections and corrections to the image are calculated. Another way to proceed with attenuation correction in the chest is to collect a set of transmission images, perhaps rapidly, to give an idea of the major features, and to use them as a guide to fitting that patient with a suit of standard attenuation coefficients for heart, lung, and so forth, which were previously determined (W. J. MacIntyre, personal communication, 1982). H. Maeda and co-workers (1981) suggest the use of SPECT transmission imaging to delineate lung margins. These images can be laid over the technetium-99m macroaggregated albumin (MAA) images to detect hypoperfusion at the lung margins.

The group at Duke has been working on lung quantification for several years (Osborne et al. 1981, 1982, 1983; Osborne, Jaszczak, and Coleman 1983; Osborne et al. 1985), with most of the research performed in dogs to measure regional perfusion. It is well to remember that 20– to 25–kg dogs are really much smaller than people, thus lessening problems of attenuation, scatter, and resolution; also, larger amounts of radioactivity can be given to dogs, which improves statistics. Work involving quantification of an esophageal line source (Osborne et al. 1982) could well be repeated in consenting humans; it resembles the clinical technique (Hattori et al. 1983) used to determine the position of gallium-67 accumulation in esophageal tumors relative to the esophageal lumen. The most recent research (Osborne et al. 1985) involved quantification of technetium-99m microspheres; the work of validating quantification is very difficult.

There are several ways to approach respiratory motion. One is to ignore it and be satisfied that only small structures will be completely blurred out. The second way is to gate the respiratory motion, either teaching the patients to breathe regularly while watching a monitor so that the volumes match from one cycle to the next or by having them breathe normally while data are gated according to volume rather than respiratory cycle (Line et al. 1980, 1981). This last is more difficult given the discipline that SPECT already imposes, but it may be easier than controlling the patients. If the SPECT system can acquire and process gated cine and gated transaxial images in the heart, it could also be used for gated pulmonary perfusion imaging.

The question of pulmonary ventilation SPECT imaging is still open. What is needed is a technique that gives a distribution of radioactivity that will be stationary over 30 minutes and have enough activity to image. Aerosols are not stationary and the xenon-gas–based methods do not give a correct picture of ventilation if rebreathing is continued for long periods of time. Krypton-81m with its 13–second half-life gives an image of the equilibrium between ventilation and decay and has a suitable gamma ray energy for Anger camera imaging. Lavender, Al-Nahhas, and Myers (1984) present data on krypton-81m ventilation imaging of normal subjects, compared to technetium-99m perfusion imaging. They also tried krypton-81m for perfusion imaging; ventilation alters the krypton-81m image compared to the technetium image.

The variation of lung density or attenuation can be used to diagnose lung edema and other difficulties related to density change, such as tumor and emphysema. Transmission imaging or Compton scatter imaging (Pistolesi et al. 1978) is a way to approach differences in lung tissue density. There are no published Compton scatter images.

Osborne, Jaszczak, and Coleman (1983) suggested that lung metabolism is an area in which SPECT might be helpful. Quite a number of radiopharmaceuticals, such as iodine-123 IMP when used to study cerebral blood flow and metabolism, localize in the lungs. Iodine-123 HIPDM does the same. These agents might be used for lung imaging (Touya et al. 1983; Pistolesi et al. 1983) with the suggestion that their distribution or kinetics may reflect pulmonary cellular damage.

The technique for clinical lung perfusion SPECT imaging is to inject about 2 to 3 mCi of technetium-99m MAA or microspheres amounting to at least 60,000 particles for acceptable images. The patient is placed in a supine position, with the arms over the head, and body contour data are acquired if necessary. Two to four sources are placed on the patient for localization and quality assurance. The sources should be no more active than the patient and not actually in the field of the lungs if at all possible. A 64 × 64 matrix of 64 angular increments and a total imaging time of ten to 20 minutes leads to the acquisition of 2 to 4 M total counts. Images are corrected for nonuniformity using a previously acquired uniformity image, and for attenuation using an average attenuation coefficient of 0.09 per centimeter or a more sophisticated method. Initial transaxial slices may be 0.6 to 1.8 cm thick; for interpretation, a balance should be struck between slice thickness and statistical precision. If sagittal and/or coronal slices are to be prepared from the transaxial images, slice thickness should be 0.6 cm to allow the preparation of uninterpolated coronal and sagittal images. The filter applied should not have much high-frequency bandpass because the statistical precision of the data does not warrant the inclusion of high frequencies. The resulting transaxial slices may well be smoothed again before diagnostic reading. Cine presentation and sinograms of the sources should be made.

The use of SPECT in lung imaging does seem to improve clinical accuracy. LeJeune and associates (1982) reported that in nine of 23 cases of suspected pulmonary embolism, conventional scintigraphy gave ambiguous results; in five of these, SPECT images showed clear defects, while in the other four, defects suspected on planar images were not borne out by SPECT. Three of these four had cardiomegaly, which seemed to account for the decrease in activity. The same authors also reported that in two bronchopulmonary malignancies, SPECT gave more useful information about the site and extent of the tumor. Biersack and colleagues (l982) reported a total of 41 patients, in six of whom SPECT improved diagnostic accuracy. In three of the 18 healthy patients the normal variant recessus retrotrachealis was visualized, while two of the five patients with emphysema had mediastinal hernias nicely visualized with SPECT. The article gives images of each of these interesting cases. Donaldson and co-workers (1982) reported 84 cases of suspected pulmonary emboli. All the patients were imaged both with conventional planar six-view Anger camera scintigraphy and with SPECT, either by Cleon 711 mulitprobe scanner or by GE 400T rotating camera. Twelve of the patients also

TABLE 8–3.—Suspected Pulmonary Emboli (N = 155)*

	ABNORMAL	NORMAL	UNDETERMINED
Conventional	88	44	2
Additional information on SPECT	18	9	...

*The number of cases included in the table adds up to more than 155 because some patients were correctly identified as to presence or absence of disease on conventional image, but additional information was learned on SPECT.
Pooled data from LeJeune et al. 1982; Biersack et al. 1982; Donaldson et al. 1982.

had angiography within 48 hours. Shine-through from normal areas seemed to be the major reason for the lack of sensitivity of the planar technique. There was good correlation between the SPECT images and the pulmonary angiography (Table 8–3), leading the authors to suggest that SPECT could be used to measure lung volume in assessing affected tissue and to quantify more accurately the success of pulmonary embolic therapy (O'Donnell et al. 1984a).

HEART

Nuclear medical techniques are addressing a number of questions of heart disease, ranging from valvular dysfunction and congenital malformations through coronary vessel stenosis, transient ischemia, and infarct damage assessment to long-term follow-up and prognosis for life and quality of life without or after surgery. A great deal of human emotional energy, as well as medical resources, is invested in cardiac problems. This discussion is as clinical and factual as possible, but it should be realized that emotional issues may divide practitioners of cardiology and cardiac nuclear medicine into camps.

For a number of reasons, the heart is not an easy organ to image. It is deep in the body, asymmetrically placed, and surrounded by tissue of varying density that itself expands and contracts with respiratory motion and rhythm. Beyond this, the heart moves, not just in an elastic pumping motion but with a rotational motion and in response to respiration. Action of the cardiac chambers is not in concert but in series during a cycle. The cycle is normally very repetitive. If this were a description of the rivers and mountains of Tibet in snowfall, spring thaw, and low flow, the reader would now be thoroughly confused, in unfamiliar terrritory; the heart is more familiar but this is a great deal to keep in mind at once, so simplifications are necessary. Attempts will be made to point these out explicitly where they occur.

A jump into the functional realm shows the heart reacting to external stimuli, beating faster or slower, metabolizing, receiving chemical messages, and getting, or not getting, enough blood in its own circulation to perform the work asked of it.

A good radiologist can read a great deal of a person's history (or fortune, if you like) from a chest x-ray. The same could be said for a thorough examination of just the heart, even by noninvasive means.

Cardiac imaging has been as important a stimulus to SPECT development as it has been to planar nuclear medicine. For SPECT, thallium-201 coronary imaging without gating is more easily practiced than a technique requiring gating, although the issues of thallium-201 imaging are complex and by no means settled. Thallium imaging, after stress and with observations immediately and later to observe any redistribution, is an attempt to view the perfusion of the heart while the spatial motion is blurred out. Typical plane-projection imaging, carried out after exercise to some predetermined stress level and after the injection of 1 to 2 mCi of Tl-201 thallous chloride, involves a set of three images (anterior and 45–degree and 70–degree left anterior oblique views) begun five or ten minutes after injection and a set of three delayed images in the same positions 1.5 to 4.0 hours later. The images are analyzed by computer, which subtracts background and repositions them to match; comparisons are made of the relative activities in different parts of the image, and at different times for the same parts of the image. The left ventricle projects as a ring bringing into silhouette the edges visible in that projection. Viewing from different angles brings different edges into view. Given the low energy of thallium-201 and the position of the heart in the body, it is impossible to bring all the edges into position for imaging; the right heart also contains activity that forms a general background or absorbs radiation in some projections. In spite of the obstacles of blurred motion and incomplete sampling, through animal experiments and comparison of clinical examinations with x-ray cardiac catheter images (themselves planar but resolving the heart motion and with vessels highlighted by contrast agents), maps and diagrams of the parts of the heart supplied by each major vessel have been worked out. Standard normal, normal variant, and abnormal thallium examination results have been much discussed and written about. There is a great deal more argument about the meaning of the images in terms of the patient's prognosis than about their production. The computer's part in the examination is to subtract background according to what one hopes is a standard convention, to quantify the relative uptake of thallium-201, to reposition later images to match the earlier ones, and to compare images, perhaps in a series of curves or in a set of functional images portraying "absolute" uptake, relative uptake, and changes as a function of time. Animal experiments comparing thallium-201 images with thallium-201 tissue counts and labeled microsphere tissue counts, as well as cardiac catheterization, have validated the planar technique.

What then might be the place of SPECT in coronary perfusion imaging? Is there any need for three- (or really four-) dimensional information? What can SPECT add that is not already present? These questions could be turned around to ask what it is that the planar imaging technique is aiming for and not quite managing to achieve by the series of angled views. Tomography allows the back of the heart to be seen almost as well as the front, integrating information from the three standard views with that from the other angles in between and beyond; it does not require exacting positioning for later comparisons and it automatically separates right heart from left, background from heart muscle, and edge from projected tissue (Berger et al. 1984; Go et al. 1985). Because SPECT is not immune to partial voluming, there can be problems with correct assessment of thallium-201 distribution differences because of slice thickness. Other problems are that thallium-201 is not an obliging nuclide; its energy is too low either for good Anger camera resolution or for good tissue penetration, and the amount that is normally given (because of the half-life's effect on radiation dose) does not produce a high photon flux. The concentration decreases with time so that later views are even more photon poor than the earlier ones. The nonuniformity of the chest tissue makes attempts at attenuation correction difficult although not impossible. Finally, SPECT still blurs the spatial motions and to some extent blurs the time function as well, because the collection of an acceptable number of counts takes at least 20 minutes.

A SPECT examination of cardiac perfusion with thallium-201 may involve the injection of more activity (3.0 to 3.5 mCi) than is used for planar imaging. The radiation dose to the kidney, the target organ, is 1.17 rads per mCi (Atkins et al. 1977); the gonads have been implicated as a possible target organ with an estimated dose of 1.5 rads per mCi (Hosain and Hosain 1981). Imaging is started five minutes after thallium-201 injection (at maximum stress if desired) and continues for 20 to 30 minutes using a 64 × 64 matrix and 30 to 60 projections over 180 to 360 degrees. The sequence is repeated two to four hours later. The planar data acquired for tomographic processing must be the best available. All the tricks for ensuring good data must be used: keeping the collimator close to the patient, either by off-centering him in the circle of rotation or by moving the bed and/or camera to maintain closeness; quality control of patient positioning by placement of sources cranial or caudal to the heart region but in the camera's field of view (Friedman et al. 1984); using light restraint and having the technologist keep a close watch on the patient; and focusing the patient's attention on something other than his heart or his position on the table.

There are substantial questions about whether to acquire data for a full 360 degrees around the patient or rotate only 180 degrees to cover the heart on the left side from right anterior oblique to left posterior oblique (Fig 8–4), where two-thirds of the counts from the heart arise (MacIntyre et al. 1982). The body blocks the rays on the far side; this effect is most pronounced for low-energy photons, such as thallium's (Hoffman 1982). The proponents of 180–degree imaging include a number of current practitioners (Tamaki et al. 1982; H. Berger, personal communication, 1984; Chang and Henkin 1983; Caldwell et al. 1983; Garcia et al. 1983; Pettigrew et al. 1983a; Summerville et al. 1984b), while those on the other side represent some laboratories with a number of years' experience with SPECT performing serious and telling experiments in this area (MacIntyre et al. 1982; Lewis et al. 1982; Coleman, Jaszczak, and Cobb 1982; Kirsch et al. 1983; Go et al. 1984; Eisner et al. 1984). The decision about the efficacy of 180– vs. 360–degree imaging hinges on the issue of the object of thallium-201 imaging (Hoffman 1982): is it to determine the location and volume of ischemic or infarcted areas, or is it to quantify the amount of thallium-201 in those areas in three or four dimensions? If location and volume are the goals, 180–degree imaging may be sufficient if care is taken to ignore streak artifacts in the diagnosis, especially for thallium-201 (Maublant 1983; Tamaki 1983). If quantification of thallium-201 is the goal, many of the proponents of 180– degree imaging will concede that 360 degrees' worth of data are re-

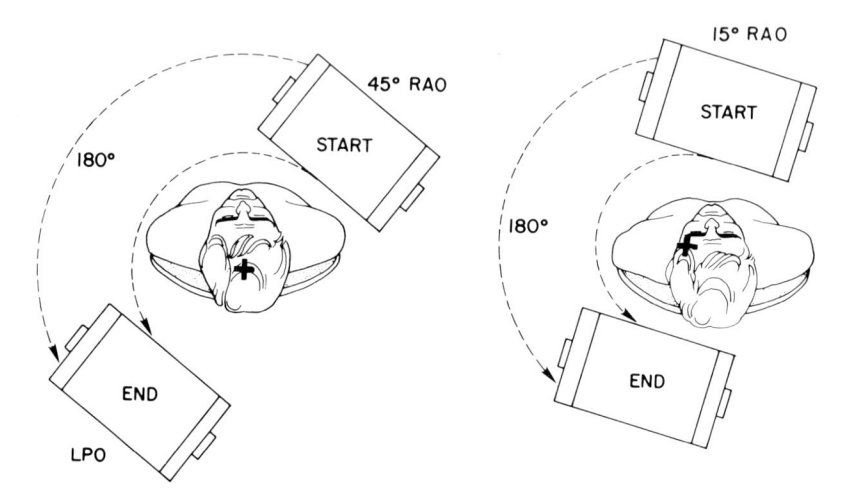

Fig 8–4.—On the left is a schematic drawing showing the path of the Anger camera during a 180–degree SPECT scan of the heart. On the right the patient is off-centered to enable the heart to be closer to the camera face during the 180–degree rotation of the camera. A + sign marks the center of rotation.

quired (Maublant 1983; Tamaki 1983). Quantification must be viewed as a goal, not a sure consequence of 360–degree imaging, because absolute quantification of SPECT images is still the object of a great deal of research. Coleman and Jaszczak (1983) pointed out that quantification of variations in concentration in the heart muscle is not possible until it can be shown that the situation of constant activity in the object (a heart or heart phantom) yields constant activity in the image. Only 360–degree acquisition allows equalization of resolution over the whole section; semicircular data have good resolution at the surface and very poor resolution at depth inside the chest.

Since the verdict is not in, even for thallium imaging of the presence or absence of affected tissue and perhaps an estimate of the amount of involvement, each clinician should keep an open mind and be willing to try 360–degree imaging when the SPECT system is first used for thallium imaging, and afterwards at intervals whenever improvements are made in hardware or software. When a radiopharmaceutical with a more suitable photon energy appears on the scene, a complete switch should be made to 360–degree imaging because the tomographic reconstruction requires information from both sides of the patient, if any information is coming through. Attenuation corrections, unless based on a very carefully constructed model cleverly adapted to each patient, must be applied to 360 degrees' worth of data.

Attenuation correction, filtering, and the projection to use for diagnostic reading are all issues in thallium-201 SPECT imaging. Attenuation correction for 180–degree thoracic data can only be done by an empiric or modeled scheme because the standard methods require averaging of data from both sides of the patient and approximate the tissue column as homogeneous, which the chest surely is not. Under certain circumstances (Osborne et al. 1982), one may be able to get by with assuming a constant, lower attenuation coefficient than solid tissue would require, but this is taking a chance. A method for empiric correction of attenuation (Chang and Henkin 1983) has been devised. A lifelike cardiac phantom was built and imaged both in air and in a phantom chest (the chest lacked a real rib cage or surface musculature and fat, but did have spine, sternum, and "lungs" of an average density of 0.3 made of a mixture of Styrofoam pellets and water) with a right heart made of water. Both the air and chest images were reoriented along the long and short axes as human images are, as will be described. Then difference images between the phantom in the mock thorax and the phantom in air were created and normalized to the air images; the new image is attributed to the effect of the mock thorax and can be called an attenuation image. The attenuation correction or compensation image is the inverse of the attenuation image and can be applied as a correction factor to clinical examinations in which there is gross similarity between the patient and the mock situation. Garcia and co-workers (1984) have devised a similar method. With an appropriate library (Chang and Henkin 1983) of phantom measurements and corresponding attenuation images, this method can be extended to all patients. Attenuation in the chest may also be examined, in clinical situations, by a fast SPECT transmission image to position roughly the heart and lungs, so that model-based attenuation corrections can be carried out.

The filtering applied to thallium-201 SPECT images depends on the number of counts in the image. The statistical quality of thallium-201 cardiac perfusion images only warrants the use of smoothing filters; any filter with too much high-frequency bandpass produces a very noisy image. Users should experiment with filters to achieve a smooth, but not oversmooth, image; the correct filter will probably be between the middle and the smoothest filter. Prefiltering statistically poor data with the customary filters (Gilday et al. 1984) or with those developed especially for the data (Raff, Nelson, and Ritenour 1984) can improve the quality of the reconstructed image and reduce the noise and background levels without degrading resolution.

Not only is the heart not symmetrically placed in the chest, it is not positioned the same way in everyone and its major and minor axes do not coincide with parallels to or perpendiculars to the axis of rotation. Therefore the usual transaxial, coronal, and sagittal slices are not very helpful, even for comparison with planar images, and especially for thinking about heart muscle perfusion. Each individual heart itself is a better frame of reference that is more reproducible from visit to visit as well as from early to later views. Computer programs have been written to find the long and short axes of the heart in three dimensions and to turn the heart upside down so that the apex points up (Han and Song 1983; Borrello et al. 1981; Olson et al. 1981) (Fig 8–5). A problem that does not seem to bother anyone is that a set of coordinates based on the long and short axes of the left ventricle does not have any particular relationship to the images of x-ray coronary angiography or even to planar thallium images. The areas of perfusion of the coronary blood vessels are related to the heart's own shape. O'Donnell and colleagues (1984b) concluded that the short axis display was sensitive, specific, and reproducible.

The first reconstruction of planar projection data is always transaxial. If a series of angular rotational maneuvers is to be performed

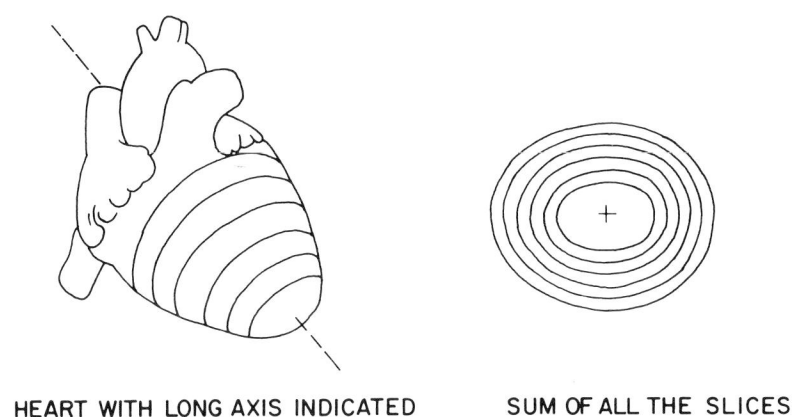

HEART WITH LONG AXIS INDICATED   **SUM OF ALL THE SLICES VIEWED END-ON**

Fig 8–5.—After creation of the transaxial images, a set of images of left ventricular slices perpendicular to the long axis of the ventricle is prepared. These may be stacked up as shown on the right, to present the data from all the slices in one image.

using the transaxial images before they are presented for diagnostic viewing, the transaxial slices must have the finest resolution possible in the on-axis direction, which is one pixel wide. The rotational maneuvers have the possibility of employing angles whose obliquity could cause great distortion if thick slices are used to make interpolated images.

The preparation of thallium-201 SPECT images for diagnostic interpretation involves two processes: one is the preparation not only of the long- and short-axis sectional images, but of combinations of these images designed to make the information more compact and less diffuse and confusing both in spatial and time domains; the other is the interaction of the computer and the formatter's contrast with the film to produce acceptable diagnostic images. One means of simplifying and combining the information is to put the short-axis slices together in a "stack" and look at them end-on. The stack can be divided into segments to correspond to areas of perfusion of the coronary arteries. Stacks can be compared for redistribution, changes between one examination and the next, and so forth. Once all the images have been prepared, photography begins. The computer can make adjustments in the gray scale and its relationship to the counts, since the photographic process and the eye may appreciate better the differences in activity if the scale is not linear (D. D. Watson et al. 1980). Just as in rectilinear scanning in the days of yore, the images should not be rendered with too much contrast enhancement; there should be a bit of background and always some visible trace in all parts of the heart, as well as numerous shades of gray; otherwise the reader is being cheated out of some of the information. The photographic process usually enhances contrast (hence images in published materials, being at least twice photographed, may have more contrast than what the technologist and physician saw and liked on the oscilloscope screen). The enemy you can see is much better than one you can't see; what has been eliminated by contrast enhancement is just not available for diagnostic consideration.

It is a natural step to quantification of these images. Work previously mentioned as well as other articles and abstracts (Keyes et al. 1981; Kirsch et al. 1981; Caldwell et al. 1982; Holman et al. 1982), mostly done with phantoms and dogs, has suggested that the quantification riddle is not solved yet. The first level of quantification involves determining the mass of affected and normal tissue, a measurement very sensitive to the threshold and therefore to the reconstruction method (Holman et al. 1982). Keyes and colleagues (1981) assumed the dog heart had a doughnut shape; their program flagged as "infarcted" the missing parts of the doughnut. Caldwell and associates (1982) injected technetium-99m microspheres into coronary arteries in dogs and used a computer program that analyzed a circular section of tissue in 60 six-degree segments. Dog hearts were analyzed in living and dead animals, in air, and as slices. The live hearts and the slices correlated well except that SPECT gave more counts for the infarcted tissue than were present in the in vitro slices. Explanations included partial voluming, scatter, and resolution difficulties in the dog heart. In addition, PET studies in dogs have suggested that abnormal wall motion connected with infarction may itself cause defects (Parodi et al. 1984); gating could aid in the elucidation of the dual effects of infarction. A study of empiric attenuation correction (Chang and Henkin 1983) using thallium-201 found that the phantom results gave an apparent 31% of apex concentration even when there was no activity present at all. They explained this on the basis of a number of factors: one-third of the effect resulted from an artificial bias level in the reconstruction software and two-thirds resulted from scattering. Clearly, the effects of the calculation and those of scattering should be separated and the calculation cleaned up.

There has been more recent work along the lines of developing automatic programs to analyze SPECT thallium images (Garcia et al. 1985), comparing values calculated to those of pooled normals.

Those using SPECT clinically for thallium imaging have found it to be helpful (Fig 8–6), either in stress and redistribution studies (Tamaki et al. 1983, 1984; Garcia et al. 1985; Prigent et al. 1983, 1984; Go et al. 1982) or in resting studies (Kirsch et al. 1983; Maublant et al. 1982; Tamaki et al. 1981) (Table 8–4). A great deal of the eagerness about SPECT in thallium studies comes from experienced users; those not familiar with it (Smalling 1983; Gould and Mullani 1984) do not see it in such a friendly way. Even they admit that the evidence suggests that diagnostic improvements are being made with SPECT, although they deny that such an instrument could be of enough benefit in the noninvasive cardiology laboratory to justify its presence there. Such a unit might be shared for cardiac imaging in-

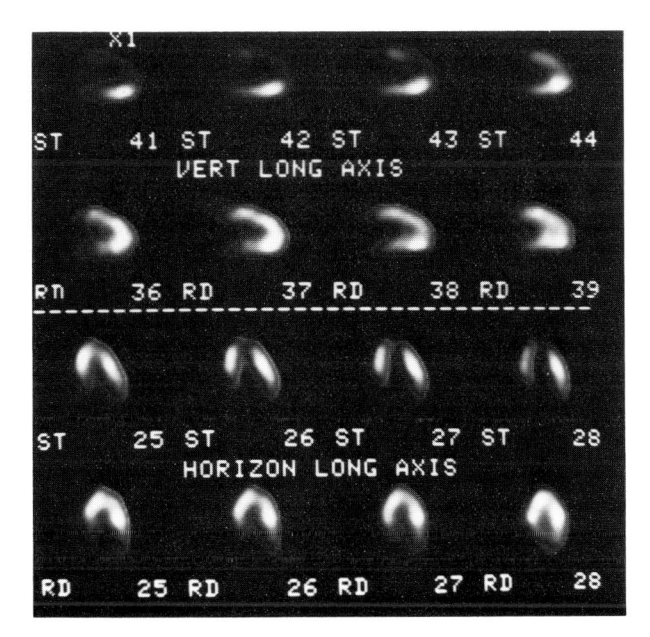

Fig 8–6.—Clinical SPECT images of Tl-201 distribution in the heart. The patient was injected with 3.5 mCi of Tl-201 after stress to 85% of maximal predicted heart rate. Tomographic imaging was carried out immediately and after 4 hours, using thirty-two 40–second views around 180 degrees starting at the right anterior oblique. Axes were chosen by the computer operator after the transaxial reconstruction. The images in the top row are vertical long-axis images from the stress (ST) study. There is a perfusion defect in the anterior wall extending from the base to the apex. The second row shows images from the redistribution study (RD), which is normal. The third row contains long axis images after stress (ST) which show an apical perfusion defect. The fourth row shows the corresponding images after redistribution which are normal. These findings indicate myocardial ischemia in the anterior wall and apex. (Courtesy of H. Berger and E. C. McClees, Emory University School of Medicine, Atlanta, Ga.)

TABLE 8–4.—THALLIUM-201 CLINICAL STATISTICS

	SENSITIVITY	SPECIFICITY	ACCURACY	REFERENCES
Stress Imaging				
Conventional	10/14	5/11	15/25	Go et al. 1982
SPECT	48/52	21/24	69/76	Go et al. 1982; Tamaki et al. 1982
Resting Imaging				
Conventional	136/177	44/57	180/234	Kirsch et al. 1983; Maublant et al. 1982;
SPECT	169/177	46/57	215/234	Tamaki et al. 1981

cluding thallium and other nuclear medicine imaging of a department. Once the instrument finds its way in, however, it is very useful and has supplanted planar imaging for diagnosis in some laboratories.

Quantification of the total amount of viable left-ventricular mass is possible with SPECT. The mass measured with SPECT has been correlated with that from cineangiography in patients (Wolfe et al. 1984) and with values created in the Iowa heart phantom (Summerville et al. 1984a).

Smaller areas of decreased or absent perfusion or parts of the heart lost in background or overshadowed become visible with SPECT. Inferior and nontransmural infarcts may be more visible. Details such as the so-called papillary muscle, breast shadows, and defects in perfusion of the posterior heart can be seen. In addition, the automatic processing of SPECT decreases the amount of subjectivity in the diagnosis.

Human albumin microspheres (HAM) labeled with technetium-99m have been used to assess regional coronary blood flow during cardiac catheterization. Liu and co-workers (1984) found that SPECT imaging of HAM labeled with technetium-99m before intervention and with indium-111 after intervention provided a sensitive method for assessing the changes in coronary blood flow caused by intervention.

It is expected that SPECT will be used in testing of new technetium-99m–labeled radiopharmaceuticals designed to replace thallium-201 as a myocardial perfusion agent. The most recent of these agents to appear promising is hexakis (*t*-butylisonitrile) Tc(I) (TBI) (Holman et al. 1984). It may be necessary to compare the results after two injections of this material, at rest and during exercise, because there does not seem to be any redistribution into ischemic areas.

The gated blood-pool SPECT examination is no more trouble than an ordinary gated blood-pool examination or an ordinary SPECT examination if the hardware and software are available to accommodate the combination and display it to greatest advantage. This is a big "if." Consider the quantity of data to be acquired: sixty-four 64 × 64 images (or some might even want one hundred twenty-eight 128 × 128 images) times 16 gated frames, all stored at once and accessible at once. A few years ago the size and cost of computer core memory, disk memory, and input/output speed ruled out such large data volumes. Many laboratories still have older computers that are incapable of such work. Compromises have been struck during the research phases, but the desire to do gated cardiac SPECT will stress the computer budget and/or be limited by it now that the hardware is available.

In an early attempt (Moore, Murphy, and Burdine 1980) at gated SPECT, data were collected in list mode and dumped immediately to magnetic tape. The dual-camera SPECT system could accommodate 8,000 cps for a total of 14 M counts; 2–degree angular intervals were used and data collection took 16 to 20 minutes. The camera faces were masked to restrict the data rate. Taped data were reformatted into eight to ten frames per beat. There was inaccuracy at the end of each angular sample because sampling did not end at the end of a beat; typically, six to ten beats were included at each angle. In spite of the severe limitations the computer placed on the examination, the group was enthusiastic about the results.

Data handling and storage restrictions continue to hamper anyone doing gated SPECT. The typical examination has involved 16 angular increments over 180 degrees and two to ten segments per heartbeat after the injection of technetium-99m albumin or technetium-99m pertechnetate after a tin-phosphate agent for the labeling of red blood cells (Phillippe and Itti 1981; Phillippe et al. 1983; Alcidi et al. 1983; Van Herk et al. 1983; Doherty, King, and Schwinger 1984). Although there is enthusiasm among users of the technique (Lazewatsky and Tow 1983; Maublant et al. 1983; Mukai et al. 1982; Barat et al. 1984; Underwood et al. 1984), a great deal of development still must be accomplished. The examination does require a computer with large capacity and high speed so that 360–degree acquisition at standard data rates and acceptable spatial and temporal resolution can be accomplished. The software to implement such new hardware must also be written. The desired output is (1) gated cine so that one can observe a rotating beating heart; (2) reconstructed views at any obliquity, either to match standard thallium-201 long- and short-axis images or for other views, because transaxial images will be no more useful for gated ventriculography than they are for coronary perfusion images; and (3) automatic chamber volume calculations that may be based either on the outline of the chamber or on the counts encompassed (Graham and Caputo 1983). Extra features include Fourier analysis of the whole heart to highlight dysfunctional areas (Nakajima et al. 1984). Gated cardiac SPECT must finally bring us to terms with the rotating and moving heart; the rotation movement can be removed before questions about the behavior of the ventricular walls are answered.

As gated SPECT matures, the difficulties of quantification will become apparent and will need to be solved (Barat et al. 1984; Hutton et al. 1985). An added problem is the lack of an adequate "gold standard," since x-ray ventriculography is not perfect. Partial volume effects appear to limit x-ray CT gated ventriculography in experimental circumstances (Guthaner et al. 1985).

The latest wrinkle is the performance of gated blood-pool studies with gold-195m between thallium-201 views so that the patient is actually imaged in the same state and position for each examination (Wackers et al. 1983; Mena et al. 1983). One stress test serves for both perfusion and blood-pool imaging. Performance of both of these by SPECT naturally uses yet more computer space and time, but with results that can be compared. Gold-195m has a 30.5–second half-life and is used as a continuous infusion; once the infusion is stopped, the residual activity decays away quickly, allowing thallium-201 imaging. A special collimator (Kipper 1984) has been developed to allow imaging the two nuclides in rapid succession; half of the collimator is designed for thallium-201 and half for gold-195m, and it is rotated for use of the proper half. This maneuver is only practical for small organs.

Infarct-avid imaging with technetium-labeled phosphates is more popular and more successfully practiced at some centers than at others. Use of technetium-99m pyrophosphate with SPECT in the diagnosis of acute myocardial infarction has been more or less successful in different hands (Holman et al. 1980; Pettigrew et al. 1983a; Lewis et al. 1983) and has not been the subject of a major review. Thallium-201 and technetium-99m pyrophosphate for imaging the extent of infarct have been compared in dogs (Lewis et al. 1983); the technetium-based method gave the best estimate of infarct volume. It is important that experiments with induced myocardial infarctions imaged with technetium-pyrophosphate (Kirsch et al. 1981), thallium-201 (Keyes et al. 1981), or technetium-labeled antimyosin antibodies (Yasuda et al. 1983) be conducted and the infarcted tissue removed, weighed, and counted to validate tomographic volumetric measurements. The technique may be difficult to scale up to human size, especially when activity doses are scaled down to human size. Because SPECT increases the sensitivity for subendocardial infarcts (Ashburn 1984), it may prove to be just the method for stripping the overlying activity away from the concentrations in the heart so that the infarct-avid imaging will begin to live up to its early promise. Imaging of antibody-based infarct-avid agents would seem to benefit greatly from SPECT because of the high background so far associated with antibody imaging (Yasuda et al. 1984).

Imaging aerobic cardiac metabolism with labeled fatty acids has been almost exclusively performed with positron emitters and PET imagers. Fatty acids can be labeled with iodine-123 for single-photon imaging; phenylpentadecanoic acid (Reske et al. 1982) and heptadecanoic acid (Britton 1982) have been tried thus far. The rate-limiting step in iodine-123–labeled fatty acid clearance from the heart may well be the iodide's exit time (Gatley et al. 1983), in which case carbon-11 acids and iodine-123 acids are not the same at all; the label should stay with a metabolite, not be turned loose as iodide. Visser and associates (1983) reported conventional imaging of iodine-123 heptadecanoic acid in patients with thrombolysis; this material does yield iodide as a metabolite. Dog research with iodine-123 phenyl pentadecanoic acid (Rellas et al. 1983) showed good correlation with blood flow in infarcted areas; initial uptake of this material is related to blood flow directly (Reske et al. 1983a). Patient examinations by this group (Reske et al. 1983b) back this interpretation. Again in the heart, we are looking at the meaning of the separation of perfusion and metabolism. Iodine-123 in its (p,5n) purity offers shorter half-life and higher photon energy than thallium-201 and thus has obvious advantages of better resolution, decreased attenuation, and higher administered activity for better count rates (Biersack et al. 1983). There are no approved iodine-123 fatty acids on the market, and the isotope suffers from severe logistic and cost problems.

LIVER AND SPLEEN

The liver is a large (about 1,000 cc) organ, imaging of which has proved a mainstay of nuclear medicine practice. The procedure is not without difficulties, however. Reticuloendothelial (RE) cell imaging in the liver presents an almost ideal situation for SPECT to show its capabilities (Strauss et al. 1982). It is ideal in the sense that (1) the liver and spleen are hard to image using other than radiotracer techniques; (2) the liver presents a complicated three-dimensional situation that proves amenable to solution by tomographic methods; (3) lesions may be hidden in the interior of the organ and may be elucidated by SPECT; (4) the colloid radiopharmaceuticals are deposited in the liver, spleen, and bone marrow, giving a high contrast between target organ and background; (5) the colloid, once deposited, does not redistribute, so the distribution remains fixed over a long enough time for many counts to be accumulated; and (6) the colloid may be tagged with technetium-99m, which has a very good energy for Anger camera collimation and detection. The SPECT imaging of the liver, and indeed all radiotracer liver imaging, is less than ideal, both because of respiratory motion, which causes an irregular plastic liver motion best appreciated in cine studies (Line et al. 1981), and because of the great diversity of liver anatomy among human beings.

The liver does not resemble the head or kidney with a regular shape, nor is it caught within a cage like the lungs. Not only is the tissue itself highly variable in shape and size, but the normal voids within it vary also. These are caused by separation of lobes, gallbladder and kidney impressions, ligamentum teres, ligamentum venosum, hepatic veins, and vena cava, so that a diagnostician must gain experience and confidence with SPECT liver images before attempting to use them in critical situations (Keyes et al. 1983). Pettigrew and colleagues (1984) studied five healthy individuals with both technetium-99m sulfur colloid and red blood cells at separate times. Their analysis of the images in three planes shows the defects caused by vascular structures in the liver in the colloid images. To overcome the problems the blood vessels may cause in the diagnosis of liver disease, they suggested (1) thorough knowledge of liver vasculature, (2) examination of each defect in multiple orthogonal planes, and (3) performance of labeled red cell studies in inconclusive cases. These authors suggested that dual-nuclide examinations would allow the simultaneous acquisition of both RE cell and vascular data. After processing, the two nuclide images could be overlaid in color to identify the structures. Three-dimensional display methods would be very helpful in distinguishing blood vessels and other structures from liver lesions. Familiarity with x-ray CT images of the liver is a practical first step. Since SPECT images have greater contrast and fewer landmarks, they are more difficult to read; it has been suggested that lesions and structure seen on SPECT images may be profitably checked using either ultrasound or x-ray CT. Buell and associates (1983b) said that ultrasound should be the first examination. followed by SPECT in equivocal instances, and that SPECT should be used for follow-up because it is reproducible. Strauss, Bostel, and Clorius (1983) pointed out in addition that in the presence of fatty infiltration of the liver, x-ray CT images may be difficult to intrepret, so SPECT should be used in these cases as the modality of choice. Retrospective studies of SPECT liver imaging (Croft and Teates 1983) led to a certain reluctance to overcall the images. On the other hand, an examination of the combined statistics of five laboratories comparing conventional planar liver scintigraphy and SPECT leads to the overwhelming conclusion that SPECT is the better modality. Each of the laboratories whose numbers contribute to Table 8–5 found it to be so. Table 8–6 shows the experience of one laboratory (Biersack et al. 1983) with large numbers of patients. These results were reported in an abstract; the difficulties they experienced with nonfocal liver disease and SPECT are not spelled out. Since the size of a liver lesion may affect its visibility, this has been addressed in Table 8–7.

In addition, liver-spleen SPECT has been useful in children after abdominal trauma; now that surgeons are more cautious about removing ruptured spleens, the procedure may be used to follow trauma victims to eventual recovery (D. L. Gilday, personal communication, 1983).

The technique for performing liver SPECT examinations varies from one laboratory to the next, but there are certain common themes. The first is that in imaging the liver, a large, thick organ moving with a regular plastic motion, in which small lesions must be distinguished from normal anatomy and artifacts, very careful technique and quality control are required. Everyone who writes on this topic reiterates these points (Keyes et al. 1983; Todd-Pokropek 1983; Croft, Teates, and Honeyman 1982) The examination is conducted after intravenous injection of 2 to 8 mCi (75 to 300 MBq) of a technetium-99m-labeled colloid. The patient is positioned on his back on the table with his arms over his head so they do not attenuate the radiation and widen the cross-section needlessly. If the system requires, the patient's cross-sectional ellipse is located for the computer. An elliptical or concentric circle orbit to match the patient's shape is much preferred to the smallest circular orbit that will encompass the patient because resolution is improved by having the radioactivity close to the collimator face. The examination is usually structured to last 20 to 40 minutes. One may use a 64 × 64 matrix or a 128 × 128 matrix and any number of angular increments from 60 to 120. Since the FWHM is about 1.5 cm in the trunk of a patient, the 64 × 64 matrix has adequate resolution. An all-purpose or high-

TABLE 8–5.—Diagnostic Accuracy of Liver Imaging

	SENSITIVITY	SPECIFICITY	ACCURACY	REFERENCE
Conventional imaging	147/196 (75%)	155/188 (82%)	302/384 (79%)	Yamamoto et al. 1983; Berche et al. 1983a; Israelsson et al. 1981; Strauss et al. 1982
SPECT alone or with conventional imaging	209/229 (91%)	248/270 (92%)	457/499 (92%)	Yamamoto et al. 1983; Berche et al. 1983a; Israelsson et al. 1981; Strauss et al. 1982; Croft and Teates 1983

TABLE 8–6.—Sensitivity and Specificity of SPECT*

	SENSITIVITY		SPECIFICITY
	Focal	Cirrhosis/fibrosis	
Conventional imaging	74/96 (77%)	.../169 .../34	418/498 (84%)
Conventional imaging plus SPECT	85/96 (88%)	SPECT was no additional help	438/498 (88%)

*From Biersack et al. 1983.

TABLE 8–7.—Size Sensitivity of SPECT

	<2 CM	2–4 CM	4–6 CM	TOTAL	REFERENCES
Conventional imaging	0/17	17/35	45/46	42/78	Yamamoto et al. 1983
SPECT	25/66 (38%)	82/104 (79%)	81/84 (96%)	168/234 (72%)	Yamamoto et al. 1983; Strauss et al. 1982

resolution collimator is used. The Anger camera window is typically centered, with a width of 15% to 20%. A narrower window rejects scattered radiation. A suitable uniformity correction matrix of 30 M counts should be stored for the correction of acquired data. Two to four sources are placed on the patient, safely out of the field of view of the liver, to be used for positional quality control. Ideally, one of more of these sources should be in view at all times. Before reconstruction, uniformity correction and image displacement should be attended to.

During reconstruction, the planar data should be corrected for attenuation and filtered according to laboratory practice. Some (Keyes et al. 1983) use smooth filters to remove any excess noise in the liver, while others (Larsson 1980; Croft, Teates, and Honeyman 1982, 1983) prefer a higher-bandpass filter to be sure of seeing fine-grained structure. Sinograms of the liver and the test sources should be formed to be sure the patient did not move during the examination. The cine presentation should be viewed for light that it may throw on patient movement and diagnosis. Test sources should be reconstructed, as well as the liver, for signs of difficulty with the center of rotation. Slice thickness of the transaxial images is also a matter of balancing large numbers of counts against thin slices with the least possibility for partial voluming, unless sagittal and coronal views are desired, in which case the transaxial slices should be one pixel thick. After reconstruction, slices should be added together and even averaged with a running average for better statistical precision. Some software (Larsson 1980) does not permit this unless extra hardware is available to the computer or unless the images have been manipulated prior to reconstruction to trick the computer, in which case the sagittal and coronal images, in their turn, must be manipulated to remove the effects of the "trick."

Photographic protocols must be developed to transfer the greatest amount of information to the hard copy. The films should encompass a long gray range. Detail overexposed or underexposed is detail lost. When either the spleen or the liver has much more activity per pixel than the other, some form of windowing must be used to make detail in both organs visible. This may necessitate two sets of film images; one for the liver and the other for the spleen. The formatter may be made to produce images of approximately the same size as those from the x-ray CT scanner so that the films may be overlaid. In some laboratories, hardware may be interfaced so that overlays from x-ray CT images can be put onto SPECT images (Yui and Akiyama 1983).

There has been an undercurrent of interest in liver volume as a measurement of therapeutic effect and drug toxicity (Strauss, Georgi, and Frank 1983; Kan and Hopkins 1979). It would seem from phantom calibration experiments (Tauxe et al. 1982) that liver volume could be measured using a 45% threshold to represent the edge of the organ, so that outlines need not be traced by hand except in special circumstances. On any particular system, the outline threshold would have to be established (Tauxe and Todd-Pokropek 1983).

Liver imaging can be used in ingenious ways, as in the identification of hemangiomata (Croft, Teates, and Honeyman 1982) (Fig 8–7) or of hepatic vessels (Pettigrew et al. 1983, 1984) using a combination of colloid and labeled red blood cells. Injection of labeled microspheres into the arterial circulation of the liver (Ziessman et al. 1983) allowed the visualization of 26 colorectal tumor nodules in 18 patients; the tumor:normal liver ratio was always greater than 1,

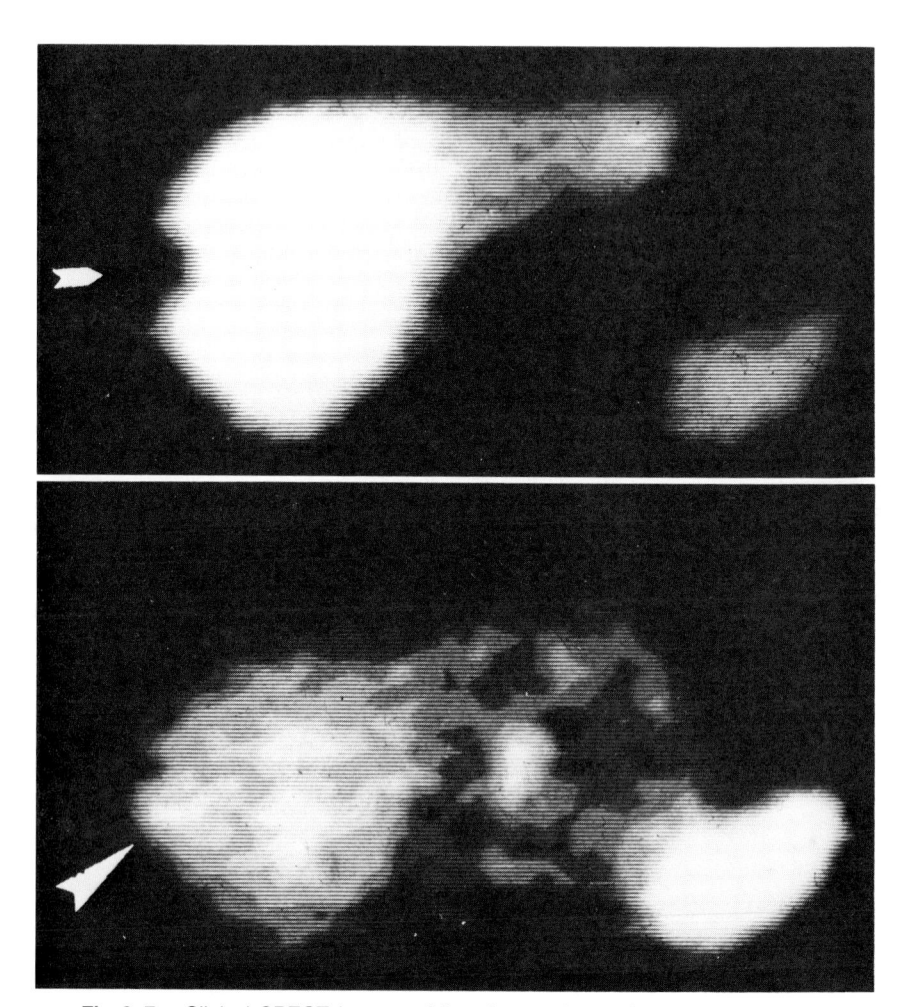

Fig 8–7.—Clinical SPECT images of liver hemangioma. On the **top** is a transaxial image of Tc-99m sulfur colloid, showing a defect. The patient was injected with 8 mCi of Tc-99m sulfur colloid; 64 20–second SPECT images were collected in a 64 × 64 matrix. The slice thickness is 1.2 cm. On the **bottom** is the corresponding transaxial image of the Tc-99m red blood cell distribution in the liver, showing activity in the area of the lesion. The patient was injected with 20 mCi of Tc-99m pertechnetate after a previous pyrophosphate injection, for red cell labeling.

with a median of 2.7. In addition, 14 carcinoid tumors were studied in five patients; again the tumor:normal liver ratio was greater than 1, with a median of 4.4. Large masses of both of these types seemed to have "cold" centers, while smaller masses appeared solid. In one hepatoma, the tumor:normal liver ratio was greater than 20 in three small nodules.

Because of its speed of rotation and sensitivity, Anger-camera-based SPECT is not normally used dynamically, but it can be. A dual-headed system (Nakamura et al. 1983) has been employed to follow the concentration and excretion of technetium-99m N-pyridoxylamine (PM). Two millicuries were injected and an imaging sequence of one minute on and one minute off over 51 minutes was followed, with 180 degrees of rotation being collected during the imaging minutes. The 26 reconstructed images were formed into time-to-maximum and half-time functional images to be displayed in color. The time-to-maximum estimates in healthy subjects ranged from 7.5 to 11.5 minutes, while half-times ranged from 15.5 to 21.5 minutes. The serial images afforded good views of sites of obstruction, while the functional images helped evaluate liver function on a regional basis. The same group (Nakamura et al. 1985) has also used SPECT images at two and four minutes after the injection of technetium-99m PM to estimate liver blood flow. The dynamic use of SPECT has only begun.

BONE

The excellent localization of the technetium-99m phosphate bone-imaging agents makes them good candidates for any kind of imaging. A three-dimensional picture is achieved with SPECT where planar images would not show the whole nature of the problem; for example, we are able to see deep inside the body to get details of uptake on the anterior spine.

Facial bones have been studied extensively with SPECT. By allowing the separation of deep from surface structures (Keyes 1980), SPECT truly does add another dimension to bone imaging in the head. Positioning is critical if the transaxial slices are to have the same meaning in and among patients. All patients must be positioned in the same way and care taken to understand the anatomy of the position used. The cine presentation is useful in showing the extent of a lesion. A three-dimensional image would also be helpful, since the substitution of transaxial slices for plane projection images may not solve all the problems of anatomic location.

In the section of this chapter that treats brain imaging, there is a discussion of the collimators and positioning required to image the head with good resolution. Use of a specially shaped Anger camera or the angulated collimator (Esser et al. 1983, 1984) allows the close approach of the camera to the head. Since the size of the human head does not exploit the whole of the large-field Anger camera, a fan-beam collimator would increase the sensitivity for head imaging.

The group at Columbia used the angulated collimator (Mitnick et al. 1983; Esser et al. 1983, 1984) to image heads in patients with sinusitis three hours after the injection of 20 mCi of technetium-99m diphosphonate. An acquisition time of 20 seconds per angle was used for 60 or 90 angles. Reconstructed slices were 1.24 cm thick. Their findings strongly suggest that SPECT is more sensitive than planar imaging.

Temporomandibular (TM) joints can be studied with SPECT (O'Mara et al. 1983). When technetium-99m phosphate perfusion, immediate and delayed images of the mouth open and closed, and SPECT were all compared, the delayed open-mouth images and the SPECT images were the most diagnostic. The bone scan images were compared with x-ray findings and surgical results: SPECT yielded more diagnostic results than multidirectional x-ray tomography for minimal and severe internal derangement of the TM joint. In addition, SPECT is the most sensitive indicator of degenerative change.

Bones throughout the body are good candidates for SPECT imaging. In the spine, for example, it may be possible to differentiate benign from malignant disease by observing the location of the lesion in the bone (Fig 8–8). Britton (1982) pointed out that since the strong point of SPECT is its ability to separate activity at one depth from that at another, it should be most used in parts of the body where there are layered structures, such as in the neck, thoracic inlet, and the pelvis at the level of the bladder.

The avascular necrosis of the femoral head has been diagnosed more accurately by SPECT (Collier et al. 1984); the criterion for positive diagnosis was the presence of a photopenic defect.

Jacobsson and co-workers (1984) used SPECT and a super high-resolution collimator in the diagnosis of ankylosing spondylitis. Especially well visualized was uptake in anterior spondylitis and intervertebral arthritis.

Fig 8–8.—Clinical image of spine after injection of 20.2 mCi of Tc-99m MDP (methylenediphosphonate). The patient was referred for a metastatic survey following diagnosis of cancer of the prostate. Tomography was performed to evaluate whether the lumbar uptake was within the vertebral bodies or the epiphyseal joints. The patient was imaged for 64 angular intervals of 20 seconds each with storage of information in a 64 × 64 matrix. The reconstructed slices were filtered with a lowpass filter in keeping with the poor statistical quality of the information. Each slice was 1.2 cm thick; no attenuation correction was used. On the **top** is a posterior planar view of the patient. On the **bottom** is a transaxial image through the spine and kidney at the L4 level. The uptake appears to be mainly posterior, more in keeping with degenerative changes in the epiphyseal facets.

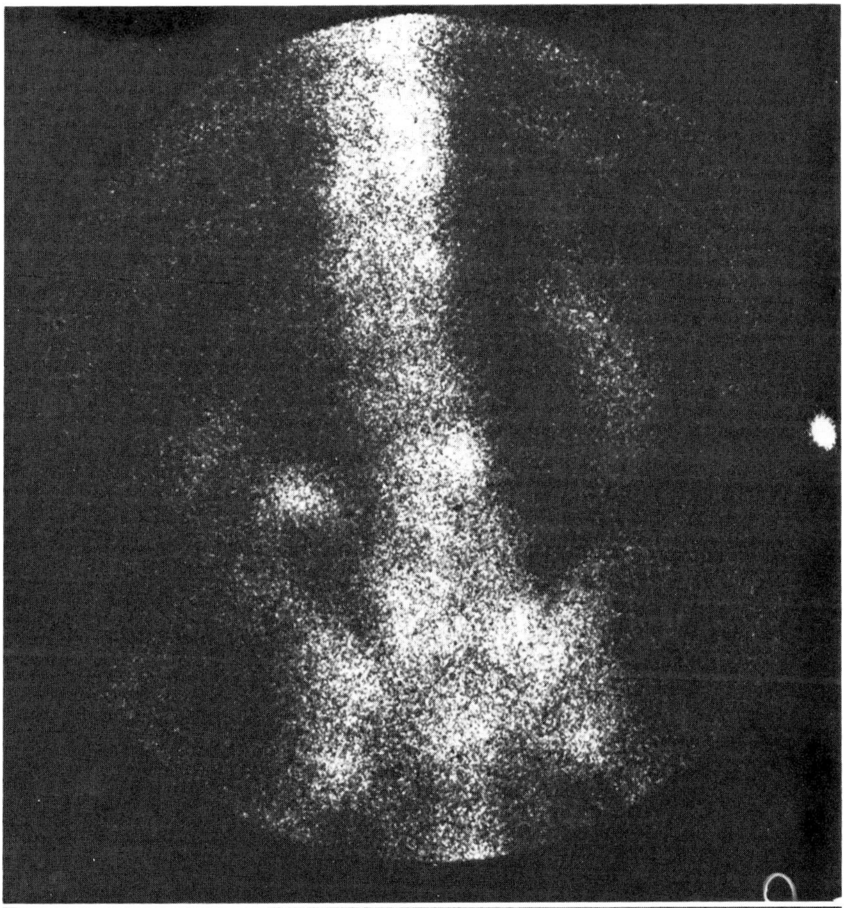

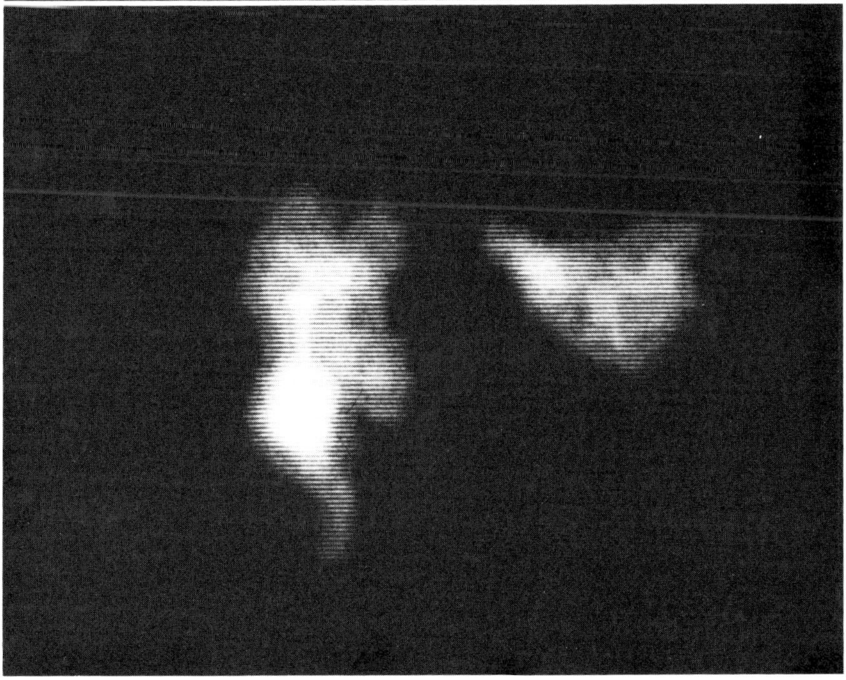

Quantification of bone uptake by comparison with some internal or external standard is important in metabolic bone disease (Britton 1982). Many internal standards are flawed because the disease may affect the relationship of the bone to soft tissues or may afflict the bone chosen as the standard. An external source or a realistic ring phantom (Ell, Deacon, and Jarritt 1980) permits the assessment of metabolic bone disease and its quantification over time (Ell et al. 1984).

The knee joint is a complex area that has been examined with SPECT (Collier et al. 1983). All joint derangements were correctly identified as to compartment when compared to arthroscopy. The SPECT technique is now being used to screen patients for arthroscopy and to point out areas requiring careful inspection during that procedure.

Bone marrow concentrates labeled colloids. Thus, SPECT may profitably be used to image marrow distribution in the major bones.

GALLIUM AND TUMOR IMAGING

Abscesses are currently being imaged either with the FDA-approved radiopharmaceutical gallium-67 citrate or with the investigative material indium-111 oxine that labels leukocytes. Neither of these nuclides exhibits gamma energies in the optimum range for the Anger camera, either for resolution or for collimation. Because of radiation dose considerations, the activities administered are not large enough to yield count rates that make them good candidates for SPECT; however, there is such a need for three-dimensional information in the diagnosis of abscesses that SPECT is used anyway. Dual windows and imaging times as long as possible are used to improve statistics. The collimators used for gallium-67 and indium-111 should be examined to be sure they are optimum; if its holes can be resolved by the camera, the collimator is not optimum. Septal penetration also makes a collimator less than optimum.

What SPECT has to offer is the possibility of separating abscess and tumor activity from that of overlying structures, such as a surgical incision, and of separating activity from background (DeLand and Shih 1984). It could even make possible the diagnosis from images created soon after injection.

Soft-tissue tumor imaging has been done with gallium-67 citrate, a well-studied radiopharmaceutical in this application. The technique and images are similar to those for the diagnosis of abscesses. Japanese clinicians (Yui and Akiyama 1983) examined 68 patients with malignant disease (mostly lung and uterine cancer and malignant lymphoma) and had positive SPECT findings in 60; SPECT had the same sensitivity as their planar imaging system but individual cases showed differences. Also, SPECT helped resolve questions of depth and extent of lesions. In one illustrated case, x-ray CT of the chest was used to make an outline of the heart and lung fields, which could be overlaid on a gallium SPECT image. A dual-headed SPECT instrument was employed so that imaging for a total of 40 minutes at 6–degree intervals allowed the acquisition of a relatively large number of counts; 1.62–cm-thick transaxial slices were created.

The sensitivity of SPECT imaging of gallium-67 citrate was greatly increased over that of planar imaging in a more recent series of 33 patients with lymphoma, infection, and lung cancer (Harwood et al. 1984).

Gallium imaging of esophageal cancer (Hattori et al. 1983) has been done with dual-camera SPECT. Total acquisition time was eight to 15 minutes, with imaging performed three days after a dose of 2 to 4 mCi of gallium-67 citrate. To identify the location of the esophagus, the patient was imaged twice, once in the ordinary way and once with a plastic tube filled with gallium-67 in the esophagus. The tube provided an anatomic landmark to relate the tumor to the esophagus; SPECT helped to separate the tumor from other structures, such as the hilum, sternum, vertebrae, and liver. Some tumors, invisible on planar imaging because of overlying structures, became visible on SPECT.

Lung metastases of osteosarcoma accumulate technetium-99m dimercaptosuccinic acid (Ohta et al. 1985); SPECT imaging separates the tumor activity from the background.

Imaging tumors with radiolabeled antibodies to the tumor is now being explored (Berche et al. 1983b; Chatal et al. 1983; Carasquillo et al. 1983; Granowska et al. 1983; Halpern et al. 1983). Typically, the antibodies are labeled with iodine-131, although technetium-99m, indium-111, gallium-67, and iodine-123 are possible. A quantity of 2.5 mCi of iodine-131–labeled antibody is injected and the distribution imaged at 24 hours after the injection (Vinocur 1984). The SPECT examination greatly aids the search for tumor sites and evaluation of tumor volume, and can help with estimates of absolute distribution of activity, but the statistical quality of the images may be poor. A great deal of experience is necessary to make proper use of antibody imaging (Delaloye et al. 1984).

When background is such a problem that it must be subtracted, the nuclides used as labels for the tumor antibody and normal IgG should be as similar as they can be in half-life and energy and still be imaged simultaneously (Perkins, Hardy, and Hardcastle 1983). Gallium-67 and indium-111 are suggested as complementary radionuclides. In addition, the use of indium-111 instead of iodine-131 avoids the problem of deiodination, which plagues iodine-131 antibody imaging (Halpern et al. 1983). In patients with melanoma, 5 mCi of indium-111 is used with about 5 mg of antibody. Part of the antibody is administered to saturate binding sites in normal tissue. Lesions of 1 cm at depth and 1.5 cm at the surface have been detected with SPECT (Halpern 1984). Subtraction is necessary in the liver. European researchers (Berche et al. 1983b) found that SPECT correctly imaged 16 of 17 tumor sites compared to the much poorer performance of the rectilinear scanner. Estimation of absolute distribution of activity is currently a bit beyond the capabilities of SPECT, but should become possible after sufficient modeling and phantom experimentation.

During treatment of hepatic tumors with intra-arterial chemotherapeutic agents, it is helpful to know whether the arterial circulation is also supplying nonhepatic structures. Technetium-99m-MAA injected intra-arterially and imaged with SPECT helps to delineate the organs that are perfused (Gyves et al. 1984). The stomach may be defined with gas bubbles, as in some radiologic gastrointestinal examinations.

In all nonorgan whole-body imaging, anatomic landmarks must be carefully sought and markers used for positioning. The superposition of the calculated or observed body outline around the image will help orientation. Similarly, a few sources placed strategically on the patient could help. Discrete markers on the tip of the sternum, umbilicus, iliac crests, and symphysis pubis could be useful. The sources must be of appropriate activity so that their presence does not interfere with the reconstructed images of the activity distribution in the patient.

KIDNEYS

Much of the practice of renal nuclear medicine is concentrated on the function of renal tubules or glomeruli through activity-vs.-time studies that are completed in 30 minutes. The current Anger-camera–based SPECT system, even in its most ambitious dynamic use (Nakamura et al. 1983), is not equal to dynamic imaging of the kidneys. Some of the multiple-probe scanner systems might be able to cope with the postpeak situation or to make running averages, which could be of some use, but all such efforts might be counted as using SPECT where it is really not necessary. In functional renal work, the patient is being compared with himself at two different times, and/or relative activities of kidney and bladder are being compared. The shape of the curves has been as important in assessing the patient's status as the numbers of counts associated with them.

The kidney is a complex layered organ that all too often is considered to be equivalent to its plane projection. Since this is really not the case, SPECT could give a three-dimensional picture of the functioning parts of the kidney if sufficient resolution could be mustered. Can sufficient resolution be achieved at this time, or what would be required? The typical normal kidney has a volume of 150 to 250 cc and therefore a length of 7 to 10 cm and a cross-section 5 to 6 cm in diameter, or about 60 to 80 square pixels in transaxial cross-section in a 64 × 64 matrix. This is about four to five resolution distances across. This relationship of the size of the organ to the resolution of the instrument does not allow a great deal of estimation of activity per unit volume in small regions to separate the kidney into layers. Better resolution is needed from the system to delineate the parts of the kidney in three dimensions. To the extent that smaller, slimmer bodies allow better resolution, renal work in children may be more promising.

There are other reasons for imaging kidneys: to show an anatomic variant (Veluvolu et al. 1984), an infarcted region, renal trauma, or tumor (Fig 8–9) (Teates et al. 1983), or to establish renal volume in order to compare it with itself over time as in renal transplantation; SPECT can do these tasks well. Technetium-99m compounds such as glucoheptonate allow high count rates from the kidneys. Also, SPECT may allow the appreciation of small amounts of activity in a kidney that might otherwise be considered to be nonfunctioning or absent. The technique is much like that for liver imaging. Kidney volume may be estimated from SPECT images after careful volume calibration of the clinical SPECT unit. A method has been described (Tauxe et al. 1982) that finds renal volume based on an edge determined by the 45% threshold; the system was calibrated for volumes from 53 to 5,000 cc. It has been pointed out that the correct threshold level must be determined for each system, since another system required the use of the 36% threshold level (Tauxe and Todd-Pokropek 1983). The measurements of volume should be made from any of the standard orthogonal images, not from an oblique image (Soderborg et al. 1983), because of interpolation.

282 Chapter 8

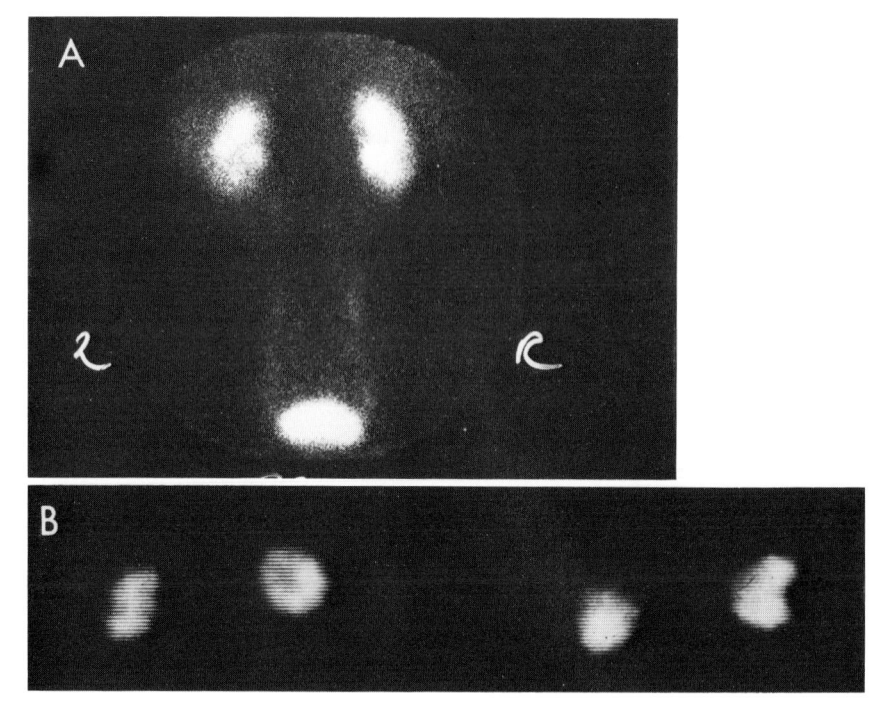

Fig 8–9.—Clinical SPECT images of Tc-99m glucoheptonate distribution in the kidneys. The patient, a 71-year-old male, was referred for a radioactive renal study after several episodes of pain which led to ultrasonography. The ultrasound images showed a solid mass on the anterior surface of the right kidney. Tomographic imaging was performed ater the intravenous injection of 15.3 mCi of Tc-99m glucoheptonate. Sixty-four 20–second images were collected in a 64 × 64 matrix format. Transaxial images were reconstructed using a modified Shepp-Logan filter (see Fig 2–5) and an attenuation coefficient of 0.12 reciprocal centimeters; slices were 1.2 cm thick. **A,** is a 20–minute posterior image; **B,** are two of the central slice images, showing lesions in both kidneys. The pathologic diagnosis of tissue samples taken at subsequent surgery and biopsy showed oncocytoma in both kidneys.

THYROID

The location of the thyroid in the neck makes its imaging with current SPECT instruments difficult because the camera cannot get close enough to the organ for good resolution. The problem is more acute for SPECT than for planar imaging because not only the head but the shoulders intervene. Since the thyroid is a small organ in which detail matters, it must be well resolved. A generation of Anger cameras tailored for the specific needs of head and neck SPECT should make three-dimensional imaging of the thyroid possible. The images can be used in all the ways planar images are, including formation of estimates of thyroid volume (Britton 1982). Of course when volume estimates are being made, the system should be calibrated with a phantom that attempts to mimic the human anatomy. Satisfactory calibration can be achieved using the ordinary thyroid neck phantom with a plastic bottle filled with a known volume of liquid containing realistic amounts of radioactivity, imaged at realistic distances for approximately the same number of counts and reconstructed in the same fashion as the thyroid would be. The planar projection may be used (Britton 1982) to determine the long axis of the thyroid, while the short axes are found from the SPECT transaxial images.

Not all of the uncertainty in thyroid treatment arises from that related to thyroid volume or mass; the patient's response to radioactivity and the future course of the disease are factors of which the physician has incomplete knowledge and incomplete control. Expending great efforts to find thyroid volume in order to titrate the dose of radioiodine may be futile in the face of greater unknowns.

GASTROINTESTINAL TRACT

Technetium-99m has been labeled to sucralfate, a drug used to treat ulcers (Vasques et al. 1983). The sucralfate becomes viscous in dilute acid and coats ulcer sites. The labeled drug makes it possible to visualize ulcer sites as small as 0.5 mm. In clinical work, planar imaging of the background of the unbound material makes image interpretation difficult. It is possible that SPECT could help to separate the activity of stomach contents from that of the peptic ulcer lesion. Radionuclidic peptic ulcer imaging may offer an alternative to endoscopy.

Because labeled food can be used for radionuclide imaging of the gastrointestinal tract rather than the nonphysiologic material used for x-ray contrast examinations, three-dimensional SPECT images may reveal phenomena not previously seen on images. The gastric bands described by Alazraki and co-authors (1984) represent such a case. The bands have been seen in humans at autopsy and in animals, but have not been previously imaged.

RADIOTHERAPEUTIC RADIOPHARMACEUTICALS AND FUTURE USES

Except for thyroid therapy with radioiodine, there are very few current uses of radiopharmaceuticals for radiotherapy. Monoclonal or polyclonal antibodies may be made practical for therapy by attaching cytotoxic drugs or radionuclides to them (Carrasquillo et al. 1983; Fawwaz et al. 1983). If drugs attached to antibodies are successful in treatment, they will be much easier to use than radioactive materials because of the shelf-life, contamination, shielding, and disposal problems of the latter.

There is every expectation that preparation for therapy and monitoring the distribution of the therapeutic dose would be undertaken with radionuclides, even if they are not actually used to kill the tumor cells, because of their ability to be imaged noninvasively. After the patient's initial diagnosis, particular antibodies to the tumor in question will be selected. They will be labeled with radioactivity (preferably technetium-99m or some nuclide of similar energy and a half-life consonant with the localization time of the antibodies) and injected. After SPECT imaging is performed, very possibly with some attendant background imaging using another radiopharmaceutical for background subtraction, a complete picture of the distribution of activity will be made. Tumor volume will be assessed, as well as distant metastases. The images will be compared to a complete set of x-ray CT images to learn how the tumor is positioned around other organs.

With respect to therapy, if a cytotoxic agent is to be radioactive, a set of isodose curves is made, preferably with a three-dimensional display technique (Batnitsky et al. 1982); these are inspected to be sure the radiation dose to nearby organs, seen on the x-ray CT images, is acceptable at the intended activity level. The need for accurate quantitative SPECT data in the case of radiotherapeutic antibodies is obvious; proper isodose curves can only be made from accurate information. Extensive work with phantoms will yield correction factors that will permit absolute quantification of SPECT.

Of all the nuclear medical techniques, only SPECT has even a chance of accurately determining such distributions (Schwinger et al. 1984). Whether the treatment is a drug or radioactivity, a tracer dose of gamma-emitting labeled antibodies might well be administered with the treatment to monitor the actual distribution. Of course such radioactive antibodies could be used to gauge therapeutic success and for later follow-up.

BIBLIOGRAPHY

Alazraki, N., et al. Visualization of gastric bands on radionuclide gastric emptying studies (abstract). *J. Nucl. Med.* 25:P95, 1984.

Alcidi, L., et al. Quantitative evaluation of left ventricular ejection fraction with single photon emission tomography. In *Nuclear Medicine and Biology Advances*, ed. C. Raynaud. Oxford: Pergamon, 1983, pp. 1289–1292.

Ashburn, W. L. Infarct-avid imaging. Presented at Selected Topics in Nuclear Medicine course, San Diego, February 1984.

Atkins, H. L., et al. Thallium-201 for medical use. Part 3. Human distribution and physical imaging properties. *J. Nucl. Med.* 18:133–140, 1977.

Barat, J. L., et al. Quantitative analysis of left-ventricular function using gated single photon emission tomography. *J. Nucl. Med.* 25:1167–1174, 1984.

Batnitsky, S., et al. Three-dimensional computer reconstructions of brain lesions from surface contours provided by computed tomography: a prospectus. *Neurosurgery* 11:73–84, 1982.

Berche, C., et al. Clinical interest of tomoscintigraphy in liver metastatic diseases and comparison with other diagnostic techniques. In *Nuclear Medicine and Biology Advances*, ed. C. Raynaud. Oxford: Pergamon, 1983a, pp. 2228–2231.

Berche, C., et al. Cancer detection by tomoscintigraphy with radiolabelled antibodies against carcinoembryonic antigen. In *Nuclear Medicine and Biology Advances*, ed. C. Raynaud. Oxford: Pergamon, 1983b, pp. 3674–3677.

Berger, H. J., et al. New vistas in cardiovascular nuclear medicine. *J. Nucl. Med.* 25:1254–1258, 1984.

Biersack, H. J., et al. Single photon emission computed tomography of the lung: preliminary results. *Eur. J. Nucl. Med.* 7:166–170, 1982.

Biersack, H. J., et al. Improvement of scintigraphic liver imaging by SPECT—a review of 797 cases (abstract). *J. Nucl. Med.* 24:P29, 1983.

Biersack, H. J. SPECT of myocardium and (gated) cardiac blood pool. In *Nuclear Medicine and Biology Advances*, ed. C. Raynaud. Oxford: Pergamon, 1983, pp. 1191–1194.

Bonte, F. J., et al. Single-photon tomography of regional brain blood flow in patients with arteriovenous malformations (abstract). *J. Nucl. Med.* 24:P105, 1983.

Bonte, F. J., and Stokely, E. M. Single-photon tomographic study of regional cerebral blood flow after stroke: concise communication. *J. Nucl. Med.* 22:1049–1053, 1981.

Borrello, J. A., et al. Oblique-angle tomography: a restructuring algorithm for transaxial tomographic data. *J. Nucl. Med.* 22:471–473, 1981.

Britton, K. E. Quantitation: clinical application. In *Computed Emission Tomography*, ed. P. J. Ell and B. L. Holman. London: Oxford University Press, 1982, pp. 521–536.

Britton, K. E., and Shapiro, R. Single photon emission tomography of the pituitary: preliminary communcation. *J. R. Soc. Med.* 74:667–669, 1981.

Budinger, T. F. Revival of clinical nuclear medicine brain imaging. *J. Nucl. Med.* 22:1094–1097, 1981.

Buell, U., et al. Evaluation of Xe-133 DSPECT in unilateral cerebrovascular disease. A comparative study to transmission CT and X-ray angiography (abstract). *J. Nucl. Med.* 24: P6, 1983a.

Buell, U., et al. Re: single-photon emission computed tomography (SPECT) for assessment of hepatic lesions: its role in the diagnostic workup (letter). *J. Nucl. Med.* 24: 746, 1983b.

Buell, U., et al. I-123 amphetamine vs Xe-133 SPECT. A comparative study in patients with unilateral disease (CVD) (abstract). *J. Nucl. Med.* 26:P25, 1985.

Burdine, J. A.; Murphy, P. H.; and DePuey, E. G. Radionuclide computed tomography of the body using routine radiopharmaceuticals. II. Clinical applications. *J. Nucl. Med.* 20:108–114, 1979.

Caldwell, J. H., et al. Regional distribution of myocardial blood flow measured by single-photon emission tomography: comparison with in vitro counting. *J. Nucl. Med.* 23:490–495, 1982.

Caldwell, J. H., et al. Quantification of thallium-201 myocardial perfusion defect size by single photon emission computed tomography (SPECT) (abstract). *J. Nucl. Med.* 23:P29, 1983.

Carrasquillo, J. A., et al. Localization and therapy of melanoma with I-131 (anti-p97) Fab (abstract). *J. Nucl. Med.* 24:P14, 1983.

Carril, J. M., et al. Cranial scintigraphy: value of adding emission computed tomographic sections to conventional pertechnetate images (512 cases). *J. Nucl. Med.* 20:1117–1123, 1979.

Chang, W., and Henkin, R. E. Photon attenuation in Tl-201 myocardial SPECT and quantitation through an empirical correction. In *Emission Computed Tomography: Current Trends*, ed. P. D. Esser. New York: Society of Nuclear Medicine, 1983, pp. 123–133.

Chatal, J. F., et al. Is immunoscintigraphy using radioiodinated monoclonal antibodies useful to cancer diagnosis? (abstract). *J. Nucl. Med.* 24:P14–15, 1983.

Coleman, R. E., et al. Collimation for I-123 imaging with SPECT. In *Emission Computed Tomography: Current Trends*, ed. P. D. Esser. New York: Society of Nuclear Medicine, 1983, pp. 135–145.

Coleman, R. E.; Drayer, B. P.; and Jaszczak, R. J. Studying regional brain function: a challenge for SPECT. *J. Nucl. Med.* 23:266–270, 1982.

Coleman, R. E., and Jaszczak, R. J. Tl-201 single-photon emission computed tomography (SPECT) (letter). *J. Nucl. Med.* 24:273–274, 1983.

Coleman, R. E.; Jaszczak, R. J.; and Cobb, F. R. Comparison of 180° and 360° data collection in thallium-201 imaging using single-photon emission computerized tomography (SPECT): concise communication. *J. Nucl. Med.* 23:655–660, 1982.

Collier, B. D., et al. Detection of avascular necrosis in adults by single photon emission computed tomography (abstract). *J. Nucl. Med.* 24:P25, 1983.
Collier, B. D., et al. Single photon emission computed tomography in suspected internal derangements of the knee (abstract). *J. Nucl. Med.* 24:P41, 1983.
Croft, B. Y., and Teates, C. D. Experience with single photon emission computed tomography of the liver. In *Emission Computed Tomography: Current Trends*, ed. P. D. Esser. New York: Society of Nuclear Medicine, 1983, pp. 155–162.
Croft, B. Y.; Teates, C. D.; and Honeyman, J. C. Single-photon emission computed tomography of the liver. In *Digital Imaging: Clinical Advances in Nuclear Medicine*, ed. P. D. Esser. New York: Society of Nuclear Medicine, 1982, pp. 271–282.
Croft, B. Y.; Teates, C. D.; and Honeyman, J. C. Single-photon emission computed tomography and albumin colloid imaging of the liver. In *Diagnostic Imaging in Medicine*, ed. R. C. Reba, D. J. Goodenough, and H. F. Davidson. The Hague: Martinus Nijhoff, 1983, pp. 590–600.
Delaloye, B., et al. SPECT with I-123 labeled F(ab')2 fragments from monoclonal anti-CEA antibodies in colon carcinoma (abstract). *J. Nucl. Med.* 25:P17, 1984.
DeLand, F. H., and Shih, W.-J. The status of SPECT in tumor diagnosis. *J. Nucl. Med.* 25:1375–1379, 1984.
Dendy, P. P., et al. An evaluation of transverse axial emission tomography of the brain in the clinical situation. *Br. J. Radiol.* 50:555–561, 1977.
Devous, M. D., et al. Single-photon tomographic determination of regional cerebral blood flow in psychiatric disorders (abstract). *J. Nucl. Med.* 25:P57–58, 1984.
Doherty, P. W.; King, M. A.; and Schwinger, R. B. Tomographic gated blood pool studies: the parameters for collection and reconstruction (abstract). *J. Nucl. Med.* 25:P85, 1984.
Donaldson, R. M., et al. Emission tomography in embolic lung disease: angiographic correlations. *Clin. Radiol.* 33:389–393, 1982.
Drayer, B., et al. Muscarinic cholinergic receptor binding: in vivo depiction using single photon emission computed tomography and radioiodinated quinuclidinyl benzilate. *J. Comput. Assist. Tomogr.* 6:536–543, 1982.
Eisner, R. L., et al. Effects of 180° acquisition on tomographic image quality (abstract). *J. Nucl. Med.* 25:P30–31, 1984.
Ell, P. J., et al. The MDP skull uptake test: a new diagnostic tool (abstract). *J. Nucl. Med.* 25:P24, 1984.
Ell, P. J.; Deacon, J. M.; and Jarritt, P. H. *Atlas of Computerized Emission Tomography*. London: Churchill Livingstone, 1980.
Epps, L. A., et al. Synthesis and characterization of a neutral oxotechnetium(V) diaminodithiol complex (abstract). *J. Nucl. Med.* 24:P10, 1983.
Esser, P. D., et al. Initial experiences with an intelligent gantry system for single photon emission computed tomography. In *Emission Computed*

Tomography: Current Trends, ed. P. D. Esser. New York: Society of Nuclear Medicine, 1983, pp. 105–119.

Esser, P. D., et al. Angled-collimator SPECT (A-SPECT): an improved approach to cranial single photon emission tomography. *J. Nucl. Med.* 25:805–809, 1984.

Fawwaz, R. A., et al. In vivo binding of In-111 labeled monoclonal antibody (MoAB) to a human high molecular weight melanoma-associated antigen (HMW-MAA) (abstract). *J. Nucl. Med.* 24:P78, 1983.

Fazio, F., et al. Tomographic assessment of cerebral perfusion using a single photon emitter (krypton-81m) and a rotating gamma camera. *J. Nucl. Med.* 21:1139–1145, 1980.

Fazio, F., et al. Single photon emission computerized tomography (SPECT) evaluation of the brain imaging agent (I-123) HIPDM in man with rotating gamma camera (abstract). *J. Nucl. Med.* 24:P5, 1983a.

Fazio, F., et al. Evaluation of cerebrovascular disorders using the brain imaging agent (I-123) HIPDM, and single photon emission computerized tomography (SPECT) (abstract). *J. Nucl. Med.* 24:P5–6, 1983b.

Fazio, F., et al. Tomographic assessment of regional cerebral perfusion using intravenous I-123 HIPDM and a rotating gamma camera. *J. Comput. Assist. Tomogr.* 8:911–921, 1984.

Friedman, J., et al. Motion detection and correction in Tl-201 SPECT imaging: a simple, practical method (abstract). *J. Nucl. Med.* 25:P70, 1984.

Garcia, E., et al. Quantification of rotational thallium-201 myocardial tomography. *J. Nucl. Med.* 26:17–26, 1985.

Garcia, E., et al. Accuracy of rotation tomography for predicting absolute Tl-201 concentrations (abstract). *J. Nucl. Med.* 25:P70, 1984.

Gatley, S. J., et al. On the rate-limiting step in myocardial clearance of label from 16–iodohexadecanoic acid (IHDA) (abstract). *J. Nucl. Med.* 24:P12, 1983.

Gelfand, M. J., et al. Quantitative I-123–HIPDM single-photon emission computed tomography (SPECT) (abstract). *J. Nucl. Med.* 25:P109, 1984.

Gibson, R. E., et al. The characteristics of I-125 4–IQNB and H-3 QNB in vivo and in vitro. *J. Nucl. Med.* 25:214–222, 1984.

Gilday, D. L., et al. Effective image filtration of pediatric single photon emission tomograms (abstract). *J. Nucl. Med.* 25:P58, 1984.

Go, R. T., et al. Comparative accuracy of stress and redistribution thallium-201 cardiac single photon emission transaxial tomography and planar imaging in the diagnosis of myocardial ischemia (abstract). *J. Nucl. Med.* 23:P25, 1982.

Go, R. T., et al. False-positive perfusion defects and image distortions of 180 degree acquired thallium-201 myocardial SPECT images with and without attenuation correction (abstract). *J. Nucl. Med.* 25:P61, 1984.

Go, R. T., et al. Transaxial SPECT myocardial imaging with thallium-201: instrumentation, technical, and clinical aspects. In *Nuclear Medicine Annual, 1985,*, ed. L. M. Freeman and H. S. Weissman. New York: Raven Press, 1985.

Gould, K. L., and Mullani, N. Dynamic cardiac imaging. *J. Nucl. Med.* 25:1380–1386, 1984.

Graham, L. S., and Zielinski, F. W. Scintillation camera imaging with I-123. *Radiology* 130:519–523, 1979.

Graham, M. M., and Caputo, G. R. Measurement of left ventricular volume using emission computed tomography. In *Emission Computed Tomography: Current Trends*, ed. P. D. Esser. New York: Society of Nuclear Medicine, 1983, pp. 147–153.

Granowska, M., et al. Ovarian cancer: diagnosis using I-123 monoclonal antibody in comparison with surgical findings (abstract). *J. Nucl. Med.* 24:P15, 1983.

Guthaner, D. F., et al. Quantitative evaluation of left ventricular function using computed tomography. *Med. Phys.* 12:333–338, 1985.

Gyves, J. W., et al. Definition of hepatic tumor microcirculation by single photon emission computerized tomography (SPECT). *J. Nucl. Med.* 25:972–977, 1984.

Halpern, S. E., et al. The clinical evaluation of 111–indium labeled monoclonal anti-melanoma antibodies (111-In-anti mel) for tumor scanning (abstract). *J. Nucl. Med.* 24:P15, 1983.

Halpern, S. E. The case for radioimmunoscintigraphy using 111–In-labeled monoclonal antibodies. Presented at the Selected Topics in Nuclear Medicine course, San Diego, February, 1984.

Han, K. S., and Song, H. B. Oblique angle display of ECT images. In *Emission Computed Tomography: Current Trends*, ed. P. D. Esser. New York: Society of Nuclear Medicine, 1983, pp. 177–191.

Harwood, S. J., et al. Efficacy of 67 gallium ECT imaging in lymphoma, infection, and lung carcinoma (abstract). *J. Nucl. Med.* 25:P44, 1984.

Hattori, T., et al. Gallium imaging of esophageal cancer using emission computed tomography. In *Nuclear Medicine and Biology Advances*, ed. C. Raynaud. London: Pergamon, 1983, pp. 158–161.

Higa, T., et al. Superimposition of krypton-81m single photon emission CT and x-ray CT images for cerebral blood flow evaluation. *J. Comput. Assist. Tomogr.* 7:37–41, 1983.

Hill, T. C. Teaching editorial: single-photon emission computed tomography to study cerebral function in man. *J. Nucl. Med.* 21:1197–1199, 1980.

Hill, T. C., et al. Early clinical experience with a radionuclide emission computed tomographic brain imaging system. *Radiology* 128:803–806, 1978.

Hill, T. C., et al. Initial experience with SPECT (single-photon computerized tomography) of the brain using N-isopropyl I-123 iodoamphetamine: concise communication. *J. Nucl. Med.* 23:191–195, 1982.

Hill, T. C.; Lovett, R. D.; and McNeil, B. J. Observations on the clinical value of emission computed tomography. *J. Nucl. Med.* 21:613–616, 1980.

Hoffman, E. J. 180° compared with 360° sampling in SPECT. *J. Nucl. Med.* 23:745–747, 1982.

Holman, B. L., ed. *Radionuclide Imaging of the Brain.* New York: Churchill Livingstone, 1985.

Holman, B. L., et al. Tc-99m pyrophosphate transaxial emission computed tomography in patient with acute myocardial infarction (abstract). *J. Nucl. Med.* 21:P69, 1980.

Holman, B. L., et al. Quantitation of perfused myocardial mass using Tl-201 and emission computed tomography (abstract). *J. Nucl. Med.* 23:P25, 1982.

Holman, B. L., et al. A comparison of two cerebral blood flow tracers, *N*-isopropyl I-123 *p*-iodoamphetamine and I-123 HIPDM (abstract). *J. Nucl. Med.* 24:P6, 1983.

Holman, B. L., et al. A new Tc-99m-labeled myocardial imaging agent, hexakis(*t*-butylisonitrile)-technetium(I) (Tc-99m TBI): initial experience in the human. *J. Nucl. Med.* 25:1350–1355, 1984.

Holman, B. L.; Hill, T. C.; and Magistretti, P. L. Brain imaging with emission computed tomography and radiolabeled amines. *Invest. Radiol.* 17:206–215, 1982.

Hosain, P., and Hosain, F. Revision of gonadal radiation dose to man from thallium-201. In *Third International Radiopharmaceutical Dosimetry Symposium*, ed. E. E. Watson et al. Washington, D.C.: U. S. Government Printing Office, HHS Publication FDA 81–8166, 1981, pp. 333–344.

Hutton, B. F., et al. Estimates of left ventricular volumes by equilibrium radionuclide angiography: importance of attenuation correction (letter). *J. Nucl. Med.* 26:317–319, 1985.

Israelsson, A., et al. Detection of space occupying lesions of the liver and spleen: a comparison of emission computed reconstructive tomography and conventional gamma camera scintigraphy. In *Emission Computed Tomography: The Single Photon Approach*, ed. P. Paras and E. A. Eikman. Washington, D.C.: U. S. Government Printing Office, HHS Pub. FDA 81–8177, 1981, pp. 171–176.

Jacobsson, H., et al. The application of single photon emission computed tomography to the diagnosis of ankylosing spondylitis of the spine. *Br. J. Radiol.* 57:133–140, 1984.

Jaszczak, R. J., et al. Radionuclide emission computed tomography of the head with Tc-99m and a scintillation camera. *J. Nucl. Med.* 18:373–380, 1977.

Jaszczak, R. J.; Chang, L.-T.; and Murphy, P. H. Single photon emission computed tomography using multi-slice fan beam collimators. *IEEE Trans. Nucl. Sci.* 26:610–618, 1979.

Jaszczak, R. J.; Greer, K.; and Coleman, R. E. SPECT system misalignment: comparison of phantom and patient images. In *Emission Computed Tomography: Current Trends*, ed. P. D. Esser. New York: Society of Nuclear Medicine, 1983, pp. 57–70.

Kan, M. K., and Hopkins, G. B. Measurement of liver volume by emission computed tomography. *J. Nucl. Med.* 20:514–520, 1979.

Kearfott, K. J.; Rottenberg, D. A.; and Knowles, R. J. R. A new headholder for PET, CT, and NMR imaging. *J. Comput. Assist. Tomogr.* 8:1217–1220, 1984.

Keyes, J. W., Jr. Tomographic applications: thyroid and facial bones. In

Emission Computed Tomography: The Single Photon Approach, ed. P. Paras and E. A. Eikman. Washington, D.C.: U. S. Government Printing Office, HHS Pub. FDA 81-8177, 1981, pp. 141-146.

Keyes, J. W., Jr., et al. The Humongotron—a scintillation-camera transaxial tomograph. *J. Nucl. Med.* 18:381-387, 1977.

Keyes, J. W., Jr., et al. Calculation of viable and infarcted myocardial mass from thallium-201 tomograms. *J. Nucl. Med.* 22:339-343, 1981.

Keyes, J. W., Jr., et al. SPECT studies of liver and spleen—technique and normal anatomy. In *Nuclear Medicine and Biology Advances,* ed. C. Raynaud. Oxford: Pergamon, 1983, pp. 2232-2235.

Keyes, W. I. A practical approach to transverse-section gamma-ray imaging. *Br. J. Radiol.* 49:62-70, 1976.

Khan, O., et al. Radionuclide section scanning of the lungs in pulmonary embolism. *Br. J. Radiol.* 54:586-591, 1981.

Kilbourn, M. R., and Zalutsky, M. R. Research and clinical potential of receptor based radiopharmaceuticals. *J. Nucl. Med.* 26:655-662, 1985.

Kipper, S. L. Ultra-short lived radionuclides for first pass angiocardiography. Presented at Selected Topics in Nuclear Medicine course, San Diego, February 1984.

Kirsch, C.-M., et al. In vivo assessment of infarct size in dogs using a transaxial single photon emission computed tomographic system (abstract). *J. Nucl. Med.* 22:P53, 1981.

Kirsch, C.-M., et al. Detection of severe coronary heart disease with Tl-201: comparison of resting single photon emission tomography with invasive arteriography. *J. Nucl. Med.* 24:761-767, 1983.

Kuhl, D. E., et al. The Mark IV system for radionuclide computed tomography of the brain. *Radiology* 121:405-413, 1976.

Kuhl, D. E., et al. Mapping local cerebral blood flow by means of emission computed tomography of N-isopropyl- p(I-123)-iodoamphetamine (IMP) (abstract). *J. Nucl. Med.* 22:P16, 1981.

Kuhl, D. E., et al. Quantifying local cerebral blood flow by N-isopropyl-p-(I-123)iodoamphetamine (IMP) tomography. *J. Nucl. Med.* 23:196-203, 1982.

Kuhl, D. E. Imaging local brain function with emission computed tomography. *Radiology* 150:625-631, 1984.

Kuhl, D. E., and Edwards, R. Q. Cylindrical and section radioisotope scanning of the liver and brain. *Radiology* 83:926-936, 1964.

Kuhl, D. E., and Sanders, T. P. Characterizing brain lesions with the use of transverse section scanning. *Radiology* 98:317-328, 1971.

Kung, H. F., et al. Synthesis and biodistribution of neutral lipid-soluble Tc-99m complexes which cross the blood-brain barrier (abstract). *J. Nucl. Med.* 24:P23-24, 1983.

Larsson, S. A. Gamma camera emission tomography. *Acta Radiol.* (Suppl.) 363:1-75, 1980.

Larsson, S. A., et al. A special cut-off gamma camera for high-resolution SPECT of the head. *J. Nucl. Med.* 25:1023-1030, 1984.

Lassen, N. A. Dynamic emission tomography of regional cerebral blood flow. In *Diagnostic Imaging in Medicine,* ed. R. C. Reba, D. J. Goodenough, and H. F. Davidson. The Hague: Martinus Nijhoff, 1983, pp. 436–444.

Lassen, N. A., et al. Cerebral blood-flow tomography: xenon-133 compared to isopropyl-amphetamine-iodine-123: concise communication. *J. Nucl. Med.* 24:17–21, 1983.

Lassen, N. A.; Henriksen, L.; and Paulson, O. Regional cerebral blood flow in stroke by Xe-133 inhalation and emission tomography. *Stroke* 12:284–288, 1981.

Lavender, J. P.; Al-Nahhas, A. M.; and Myers, M. J. Ventilation perfusion ratios of the normal supine lung using emission tomography. *Br. J. Radiol.* 57:141–146, 1984.

Lazewatsky, J. L., and Tow, D. E. Multiple gated single photon emission tomographic (SPECT) ventriculography (abstract). *J. Nucl. Med.* 24:P91–92, 1983.

Lee, R. G. L., et al. Comparison of N-isopropyl (I-123) p-iodoamphetamine brain scans using Anger camera scintigraphy and single-photon emission tomography. *Radiology* 145:789–793, 1982a.

Lee, R. G. L., et al. N-isopropyl (I-123) p-iodoamphetamine brain scans with single-photon emission tomography: discordance with transmission computed tomography. *Radiology* 145:793–799, 1982b.

Lee, R. G. L., et al. The predictive value of sizing of perfusion defects using N-isopropyl I-123 p-iodoamphetamine brain scans in acute stroke (abstract). *J. Nucl. Med.* 24:P6, 1983.

LeJeune, J. J., et al. Emission computed tomography vs perfusion scanning in lung disease. *Eur. J. Nucl. Med.* 7:171–173, 1982.

Lewis, M. H., et al. Work in progress: a comparison of data collection protocols for single photon emission tomography: 180° versus 360°. *Radiology* 145:501–504, 1982.

Lewis, M. H., et al. Planar versus tomographic imaging with Tc-99m PPi for detection of acute myocardial infarction in patients (abstract). *J. Nucl. Med.* 24:P38, 1983.

Line, B. R., et al. Radionuclide cinepneumography: flow-volume imaging of the respiratory cycle. *J. Nucl. Med.* 21:219–244, 1980.

Line, B. R., et al. Effect of respiration and patient position on liver-spleen scans determined by multigated image analysis. In *Functional Mapping of Organ Systems,* ed. P. D. Esser. New York: Society of Nuclear Medicine, 1981, pp. 65–81.

Liu, P., et al. Dual label single photon emission tomography: a new method to assess redistribution in regional coronary blood flow after nitroglycerin (abstract). *J. Nucl. Med.* 25:P28, 1984.

MacIntyre, W. J., et al. Evaluation of 180° and 360° reconstruction of the heart by single photon emission transaxial tomography with 201–thallium (abstract). *J. Nucl. Med.* 23:P53–54, 1982.

Maeda, H., et al. Determination of the pleural edge by gamma-ray transmission computed tomography. *J. Nucl. Med.* 22:815–817, 1981.

Maeda, T., et al. Three-dimensional regional cerebral blood perfusion images with single-photon emission computed tomography. *Radiology* 140:817–822, 1981.

Magistretti, P. L., et al. Computed tomographic cerebral blood flow studies, electroencephalography and transmission computed tomography in epileptics (abstract). *J. Nucl. Med.* 23:P57, 1982.

Maublant, J. C. Tl-201 single-photon emission computed tomography (SPECT) (letter). *J. Nucl. Med.* 24:273, 1983.

Maublant, J., et al. A comparison between conventional scintigraphy and emission tomography with thallium-201 in the detection of myocardial infarction: concise communication. *J. Nucl. Med.* 23:204–208, 1982.

Maublant, J., et al. Feasibility of gated single-photon emission transaxial tomography of the cardiac blood pool. *Radiology* 146:837–839, 1983.

Mena, I., et al. Ultra-short lived gold-195m: use in the simultaneous evaluation of left ventricular function and myocardial perfuson with thallium-201 (abstract). *J. Nucl. Med.* 24:P76, 1983.

Mitnick, R. J., et al. Comparison of planar bone scintigraphy and single photon emission computed tomography (SPECT) in evaluation of patients with paranasal sinus disease (abstract). *J. Nucl. Med.* 24:P58, 1983.

Moore, M. L.; Murphy, P. H.; and Burdine, J. A. ECG-gated emission computed tomography of the cardiac blood pool. *Radiology* 134:233–235, 1980.

Moretti, J. L., et al. I-123 *N*-isopropyl amphetamine (I-123 AMP) SPECT in epilepsy and cerebral ischemia (abstract). *J. Nucl. Med.* 24:P108, 1983.

Mukai, T., et al. ECG-gated emission computed tomograhy of the cardiac blood-pool using rotating gamma camera (abstract). *J. Nucl. Med.* 23:P53, 1982.

Nakajima, K., et al. Tomographic phase analysis to detect the site of accessory conduction pathway in Wolff-Parkinson-White syndrome (abstract). *J. Nucl. Med.* 25:P86, 1984.

Nakamura, K., et al. Evaluation of dynamic SPECT in the hepatobiliary scintigraphy (abstract). *J. Nucl. Med.* 24:P99, 1983.

Nakamura, K., et al. Estimation of total and regional hepatic blood flow (EHBF) by SPECT, using a hepatobiliary agent (abstract). *J. Nucl. Med.* 26:P94, 1985.

O'Donnell, J. K., et al. Improved diagnostic accuracy of lung perfusion imaging using Tc-99m MAA SPECT (abstract). *J. Nucl. Med.* 25:P67–68, 1984a.

O'Donnell, J. K., et al. Clinical evaluation of thallium-201 SPECT with cardiac short axis display (abstract). *J. Nucl. Med.* 25:P61, 1984b.

Ohta, H., et al. Is ECT imaging with Tc(V)-99m dimercaptosuccinic acid useful to detect lung metastases of osteosarcoma? *Clin. Nucl. Med.* 10:13–15, 1985.

Olson, D. O., et al. Calculation of transverse ventricular sections from transaxial ECT reconstruction of the myocardium. In *Functional Mapping of Organ Systems and Other Computer Topics*, ed. P. D. Esser. New York: Society of Nuclear Medicine, 1981, pp. 167–183.

O'Mara, R. E., et al. Skeletal imaging in temporomandibular joint (TMJ) disease (abstract). *J. Nucl. Med.* 24:P42, 1983.
Osborne, D., et al. Single photon emission computed tomography in the canine lung. *J. Comput. Assist. Tomogr.* 5:684–689, 1981.
Osborne, D., et al. In vivo regional quantitation of intrathoracic Tc-99m using SPECT: concise communication. *J. Nucl. Med.* 23:446–450, 1982.
Osborne, D. R., et al. Detection of pulmonary emboli in dogs: comparison of single photon emission computed tomography, gamma camera imaging, and angiography. *Radiology* 146:493–497, 1983.
Osborne, D., et al. SPECT quantification of technetium-99m microspheres within the canine lung. *J. Comput. Assist. Tomogr.* 9:73–77, 1985.
Osborne, D. R.; Jaszczak, R.; and Coleman, R. E. Single photon emission computed tomography and its application in the lung. *Radiol. Clin. North Am.* 21:789–800, 1983.
Parodi, O., et al. Cardiac emission computed tomography: underestimation of regional tracer concentrations due to wall motion abnormalities. *J. Comput. Assist. Tomogr.* 8:1083–1092, 1984.
Patton, D. D.; Cardell, G. C.; and Woolfenden, J. M. Experience with gamma camera (GC) measurement of regional cerebral blood flow (rCBF) (abstract). *J. Nucl. Med.* 24:P108, 1983.
Perkins, A. C.; Hardy, J. G.; and Hardcastle, J. D. The optimization of dual isotope imaging techniques in immunoscintigraphy (abstract). *J. Nucl. Med.* 24:P15, 1983.
Pettigrew, R., et al. Single photon emission computed tomography (SPECT) compared to planar Tc-99m pyrophosphate infarct-avid scintigraphy (abstract). *J. Nucl. Med.* 24:P18–19, 1983a.
Pettigrew, R., et al. Vascular intrahepatic defects in single photon emission computed tomography (SPECT) of the normal liver as defined by Tc-99m RBCs and sulfur colloid (abstract). *J. Nucl. Med.* 24:P30, 1983b.
Pettigrew, R. I., et al. Single photon emission computed tomograms of the liver: normal vascular intrahepatic structures. *Radiology* 150:219–223, 1984.
Phelps, M. E.; Kuhl, D. E.; and Mazziotta, J. C. Metabolic mapping of the brain's response to visual stimulation: studies in humans. *Science* 211:1445–1448, 1981.
Phillippe, L., et al. Tomographic measurement of left ventricular ejection fraction and comparison with conventional projections. In *Nuclear Medicine and Biology Advances*, ed. C. Raynaud. Oxford: Pergamon, 1983, pp. 1285–1288.
Phillippe, L., and Itti, R. Premiers resultats de gamma-tomographie dynamique des cavites cardiaques. *Compt. Rend. Acad. Sci. Paris* 292 (Ser. III):673–676, 1981.
Pistolesi, M., et al. Chest tomography by gamma camera and external gamma source: concise communication. *J. Nucl. Med.* 19:94–97, 1978.
Pistolesi, M., et al. Lung distribution and kinetics of I-123 HIPDM: a poten-

tial agent for early detection of lung cellular injury (abstract). *J. Nucl. Med.* 24:P71, 1983.

Prigent, F., et al. Comparison of rotational tomography with planar imaging for Tl-201 stress myocardial scintigraphy (abstract). *J. Nucl. Med.* 24:P18, 1983.

Prigent, F., et al. Quantification of the extent and severity of myocardial ischemia in single-vessel disease using stress-redistribution thallium-201 single-photon emission computerized tomography (abstract). *J. Nucl. Med.* 25:P60–61, 1984.

Raff, U.; Nelson, T. R.; and Ritenour, E. R. Improvement of SPECT imaging for myocardial perfusion studies using a median filter preprocessing technique (abstract). *J. Nucl. Med.* 25:P14, 1984.

Ravert, H. T., et al. Synthesis of neutral, lipid soluble technetium complexes of bis(2–mercaptoethyl)amines (abstract). *J. Nucl. Med.* 24:P10, 1983.

Rellas, J. S., et al. Quantitative tomographic imaging evaluation of myocardial clearance of I-123 phenyl pentadecanoic acid in acute myocardial infarction (abstract). *J. Nucl. Med.* 24:P12, 1983.

Reske, S. N., et al. Myocardial turnover of *p*-I-123–phenylpentadecanoic acid (I-PPA) in patients with valvular heart and coronary artery disease. In *Radioaktiv Isotope in Klinic und Forschung*, ed. R. Hofer and H. Bergmann. Vienna: Egermann, 1982, pp. 243–247.

Reske, S. N., et al. Flow-dependence of uptake of (I-123–phenyl)-pentadecanoic acid (IP) in the canine heart (abstract). *J. Nucl. Med.* 24:P12–13, 1983a.

Reske, S. N., et al. Clearance-patterns of 15(*p*-I-123 phenyl-) pentadecanoic acid (IP) in patients with CAD after bicycle exercise (abstract). *J. Nucl. Med.* 24:P13, 1983b.

Rezai, K., et al. Regional cerebral blood flow (rCBF) measurements by SPECT analysis of xenon-133 transit: validation of technique and clinical correlation (abstract). *J. Nucl. Med.* 25:P8, 1984.

Rothenberg, H. P., Devenney, J.; and Kuhl, D. E. Transverse-section radionuclide scanning in cisternography. *J. Nucl. Med.* 17:924–929, 1976.

Schwinger, R. B., et al. Validation of a rotating camera based SPECT system for dosimetry applications (abstract). *J. Nucl. Med.* 25:P94, 1984.

Smalling, R. W. The SPECTrum of Tl-201 imaging in coronary artery disease. *J. Nucl. Med.* 24:854–858, 1983.

Soderberg, B., et al. Re: determination of organ volume by single photon emission tomography (reply to letter to the editor). *J. Nucl. Med.* 24:1197, 1983.

Stokely, E. M. A contiguous-slice design for single photon emission tomography (SPECT). *J. Nucl. Med.* 23:355–356, 1982.

Stokely, E. M., et al. A single photon dynamic computer assisted tomograph (DCAT) for imaging brain function in multiple cross sections. *J. Comput. Assist. Tomogr.* 4:230–240, 1980.

Strauss, L., et al. Single-photon emission computed tomography (SPECT) for assessment of hepatic lesions. *J. Nucl. Med.* 23:1059–1065, 1982.

Strauss, L.; Bostel, F.; Clorius, J. H. Re: single-photon emission computed tomography (SPECT) for assessment of hepatic lesions: its role in the diagnostic workup (reply to letter to the editor). *J. Nucl. Med.* 24:746–747, 1983.

Strauss, L.; Georgi, P.; and Frank, T. Single-photon- emission-computed-tomography (SPECT) used for automatic calculation of liver and spleen volumes. In *Nuclear Medicine and Biology Advances*, ed. C. Raynaud. Oxford: Pergamon, 1983, pp. 2963–2965.

Summerville, D. A., et al. Noninvasive quantitative assessment of pacing induced ischemia in coronary artery disease patients using SPECT imaging with thallium-201 (abstract). *J. Nucl. Med.* 25:P61, 1984a.

Summerville, D. A., et al. SPECT quantification of myocardial mass with thallium-201: comparison of 180° vs 360° acquisitions (abstract). *J. Nucl. Med.* 25:P107, 1984b.

Tamaki, N. Tl-201 single-photon emission computed tomography (SPECT) (reply to letter to the editor). *J. Nucl. Med.* 24:274–275, 1983.

Tamaki, N., et al. Clinical evaluation of thallium-201 emission myocardial tomography using a rotating gamma camera: comparison with seven-pinhole tomography. *J. Nucl. Med.* 22:849–855, 1981.

Tamaki, N., et al. Comparative study of thallium emission myocardial tomography with 180° and 360° data collection. *J. Nucl. Med.* 23:661–666, 1982.

Tamaki, N., et al. Values and limitations of segmental analysis of stress and redistribution Tl ECT for locations of coronary artery disease (abstract). *J. Nucl. Med.* 24:P18, 1983.

Tamaki, N., et al. Value of quantitative stress thallium-201 emission CT for localization of coronary artery disease: comparison with qualitative analysis (abstract). *J. Nucl. Med.* 25:P61, 1984.

Tauxe, W. N., et al. Determination of organ volume by single-photon emission tomography. *J. Nucl. Med.* 23:984–987, 1982.

Tauxe, W. N., and Todd-Pokropek, A. E. Re: determination of organ volume by single photon emission tomography (reply to letter to the editor). *J. Nucl. Med.* 24:1197–1199, 1983.

Teates, C. D., et al. Emission tomography of the kidney. *South. Med. J.* 76:1499–1502, 1983.

Todd-Pokropek, A. E. The mathematics and physics of emission computerized tomography (ECT). In *Emission Computed Tomography: Current Trends*, ed. P. D. Esser. New York: Society of Nuclear Medicine, 1983, pp. 3–31.

Touya, J. J., et al. Pulmonary extraction of N-isopropyl-p-I-123–amphetamine (IMP) measured by multiple indicator dilution technique (abstract). *J. Nucl. Med.* 24:P71, 1983.

Troutner, D. E., et al. A tetradentate amine oxime complex of Tc-99m (abstract). *J. Nucl. Med.* 24:P10, 1983.

Underwood, S. R., et al. ECG-gated blood pool tomography in the determination of left ventricular volume, ejection fraction, and wall motion (abstract). *J. Nucl. Med.* 25:P87, 1984.

Van Herk, G., et al. Gated tomography of the heart with a rotating gamma camera: physical characteristics and clinical results. In *Nuclear Medicine and Biology Advances,* ed. C. Raynaud. Oxford: Pergamon, 1983, pp. 1278–1279.

Vasques, T. E., et al. Work in progress. Gastrointestinal ulcerations: detection using a technetium-99m labeled ulcer-avid agent. *Radiology* 148:227–231, 1983.

Veluvolu, P., et al. False-positive planar bone image due to horse shoe kidney. *Clin. Nucl. Med.* 10:292–293, 1984.

Vinocur, B. Final obstacles confront monoclonal imaging. *Diagnostic Imaging,* Feb. 1984, 56–61.

Visser, F. C., et al. Free fatty acid scintigraphy in patients with successful thrombolysis after acute myocardial infarction (abstract). *J. Nucl. Med.* 24:P5, 1983.

Von Schulthess, G. K., et al. Regional quantitative noninvasive assessment of cerebral perfusion and function with N-isopropyl-(I-123)*p*-iodoamphetamine. *J. Nucl. Med.* 26:9–16, 1985.

Wackers, F. J., et al. Rapidly alternating gated cardiac blood pool and myocardial perfusion imaging using gold-195m and thallium-201 (abstract). *J. Nucl. Med.* 24:P76, 1983.

Watson, D.D., et al. Defect perception in myocardial perfusion images (abstract). *J. Nucl. Med.* 21:P61–62, 1980.

Watson, N. E., et al. A comparison of brain imaging with gamma camera, single-photon emission computed tomography, and transmission computed tomography: concise communication. *J. Nucl. Med.* 21:507–511, 1980.

Winchell, H. S.; Baldwin, R. M.; and Lin, T. H. Development of I-123 labeled amines for brain studies: localization of I-123 iodophenylalkyl amines in rat brain. *J. Nucl. Med.* 21:940–946, 1980.

Wolfe, C. L., et al. Determination of left ventricular mass in man using single photon emission computed tomography (abstract). *J. Nucl. Med.* 25:P61–62, 1984.

Woolley, J. L.; Williams, B.; and Venkatesh, S. Cranial isotopic section scanning. *Clin. Radiol.* 28:517–528, 1977.

Yamamoto, K., et al. Clinical usefulness of emission computed tomography for liver scintigraphy. In *Nuclear Medicine and Biology Advances,* ed. C. Raynaud. Oxford: Pergamon, 1983, pp. 2866–2869.

Yasuda, T., et al. Quantitation of myocardial necrosis with Tc-99m-monoclonal antimyosin Fab and single photon emission tomography (abstract). *J. Nucl. Med.* 24:P37, 1983.

Yasuda, T., et al. Prediction of infarct volume in patients undergoing reperfusion therapy by Tc-99m antimyosin SPECT (abstract). *J. Nucl. Med.* 25:P20, 1984.

Yui, N., and Akiyama, Y. Emission computed tomography using gallium-67 citrate in the diagnosis of malignant tumor. In *Nuclear Medicine and Biology Advances,* ed. C. Raynaud. Oxford: Pergamon, 1983, pp. 170–173.

Ziessman, H. A., et al. Microcirculation of hepatic tumors studied by SPECT and intra-arterial Tc-99m MAA (abstract). [i]J. Nucl. Med.[r] 24:P51, 1983.

Index

A

Aberdeen Sectional Scanner (ASS), 84–85, 88
Abscess imaging, 278
Acceptance testing, 179, 218–228
Accuracy, 23, 27–32
Air conditioning and humidity control, 58, 104, 171, 180, 184
Aliasing, 36
Analog-to-digital converter (ADC), 102, 111, 197–202, 205, 229
Anger camera, 54–67
   analog, 110
   cable (see Gantry, cabling)
   collimator, 64–67, 125–127, 190, 196
      angulated, 65–67, 95, 127, 140, 238, 240, 275
      coded-aperture, 96
      fan-beam, 65, 66, 127, 241, 275
      for gold-198—thallium-201, 268
      for I-123, 67, 125, 250
      line-spread function, 126, 213
      long-bore, 66
      low-energy all-purpose, 65, 250
      point-spread function, 126
      septal penetration, 125–127
      seven-pinhole, 95
   count rate limitations, 129, 132, 170, 191, 238
   dead time, 62, 191, 212
   depth response, 12
   digital, 111
   dual heads, 76, 81, 135, 163, 170, 267
   energy setting, 10, 62, 128, 182, 184–186, 189, 228, 237
   energy spectral response, 59–63, 129, 184–186, 222–223
   energy window, 10, 60, 63, 67, 128, 130, 170, 184–186, 228, 237
      offset window, 130, 131, 170, 182, 185, 190, 213
   gantry (see Gantry)
   gravitational effect, 63, 210, 221–222
   level head, 80, 140, 141, 208, 230
   light guide, 59, 61, 183
   linearity, 11, 61, 123, 171, 182, 183, 193–195, 206, 213, 229–231
      correction, 61, 183, 193, 194
   magnetic field effects and shielding, 63, 64, 210, 221–223
   magnification or zoom acquisition, 141
   microprocessor-based corrections, 60, 61, 62, 124, 130, 183
   photomultiplier (PM) tube, 56, 59, 60, 62, 185, 222
      coupling, 56, 63, 193, 198, 216, 222

299

Anger camera *(cont.)*
  voltage, 59
  position switches, 67, 124, 202, 216
  quality control, 181–196, 220
  resolution, 55, 66, 125, 132, 182, 183
    testing, 195–196, 206, 213, 229–231
  sensitivity, 58, 59, 66, 125, 182, 183, 186–193, 201, 206, 210, 212, 228, 230, 231
  shaped camera head, 64, 238, 240, 241, 275
  shielding, 63, 222–223
  stability, 58, 62, 179, 190, 198
  three heads, 81, 170
  uniformity, 11, 58–64, 171, 182, 186–193
    correction, 58–59, 107, 108, 123–124, 186, 189, 204, 206, 210, 216, 237, 272
      skimming, 59, 61
    testing, 62, 187, 201, 228–232
      intrinsic, 187, 189, 194, 195
      extrinsic, 187, 189, 194, 195
Angular increment, 111, 132, 133, 203, 227, 237
Antibody SPECT, 172, 284
  heart imaging, 268–269
  tumor imaging, 279–280, 284
Archival storage, 112, 119, 164–165, 237
Artifact, 133, 136, 142, 164, 182, 192, 214, 215–218, 226
Attenuation, 15–19, 27, 38, 169, 170, 172, 254
  coefficient, 39, 149, 152, 218, 225, 241, 254, 256, 261
    for head, 241
    for heart, 261
    for lungs, 254
  correction, 15–19, 27, 39, 40, 43, 48, 108, 116, 125, 138, 149, 151, 160, 170, 204, 209, 212, 215, 226, 231, 237, 239, 241, 259, 261, 272
    Chang, 17–19, 41, 150, 151
    iterative, 116, 149, 150, 254
  modeling, 19, 151, 241, 261

Averaging, 11, 133, 145, 146
  arithmetic, 37, 146, 226
  geometric, 12, 37, 38, 48, 146, 226
Axis of rotation, 136, 140, 143, 219, 238, 262

B

Back projection, 3, 11, 19–20, 32, 35, 152–155, 225, 227, 237
  analytic solutions, 34
  attenuation-corrected filtered back projection, 33, 38–43
  comparison of results, 49–51
  filtered back projection, 32, 33, 35, 43
  filtration of back-projected images, 43
  interpolation, 21, 22, 38, 152, 153, 217, 225, 226
  iterative solution (see also Iterative solution), 34, 45–47
  Novak algorithm, 38, 154–155, 226
  simple back projection, 19, 20, 34, 35
Bone SPECT, 217, 275–278
  marrow, 278
  quantification, 278
Buying a SPECT system, 110, 118–122, 173–176

C

Camera-computer interface, 110–111, 196–204
  analog-to-digital converter (ADC) (see also Analog-to-digital converter), 111, 201–202, 229
  alignment of PM tubes in computer matrix, 197–200
  distance calibration, 124, 200, 204, 230
  gantry control, 110, 232
  quality control, 196, 220, 229
  timing, 196, 200–201, 232
Center of rotation, 124, 197–200, 216, 217, 219, 230, 241, 273

Index   **301**

Chang (see Attenuation correction)
Cine presentation, 113, 119, 140, 143, 144, 158, 159, 208, 215, 238, 239, 255, 256, 267
Circular-elliptical orbit, 77–79, 143
Cleon 710, 84–85, 89, 118, 247
Cleon 711, 84–85, 90, 118, 256
Collimator (see Anger camera, collimator)
Compton imaging, 82–83, 255
Computer, 101–122
   acquisition units, 117, 119
   arithmetic logic unit, 102, 103
   array processor, 102, 103, 107, 115, 116
   assembly language, 106
   bit, 103
   bit-slice processor, 103, 117
   buffers, 111, 201
   byte, 103
   central processing unit (CPU), 102–107, 114
    cycle time, 104
    Data General Nova 4, 104, 116
    Intel 8086, 104, 117
    LSI 11/23, 104, 116
    memory, 102–104, 115–117
    Micro Vax II, 118
    Motorola 68000, 104
    PDP 11/34, 104, 115
    T-11, 117
   compiler, 103, 106
   device driver, 103, 105, 114
   documentation, 113, 204, 224
   dynamic acquisition (see also Dynamic SPECT), 111, 113
   floating-point processor, 103
   gated acquisition (see Gated SPECT)
   hardware, 102
   higher language, 106
    Ada, 106
    APL, 106
    BASIC, 106, 115–117
    FORTRAN, 106, 115–117
    Pascal, 106
    structured or modular programs, 106, 114
   imaging station, 118, 119, 121, 122, 157, 158, 164
   interface to Anger camera (see Camera-computer interface)
   interpreter, 103, 106
   joystick, 105, 113
   list mode acquisition, 111, 113, 132, 267
   machine language, 105
   matrix size, 132, 133, 227, 237
   memory
    nonvolatile, 103, 108
    random-access (RAM), 102, 103, 107
    read-only (ROM), 103
    volatile, 103
   microprocessor (see also Anger camera, microprocessor), 103
   modular programming, 106, 114
   networking, 112, 122
   operating system, 105–106, 110, 115–117
   operations, 118–122, 223–225
   processing time, 103, 107
   programmable, 105, 107
   software, 102, 105, 112
    ADAC, 116
    CD&A, 117
    Donner Laboratory, 118
    Elscint, 117
    General Electric, 116
    Medical Data Systems, 115–116
    for quality control, 180, 205–206
    quality control of, 223–227
    Siemens, 117
   SPECT acquisition, 113–114, 123–141
   SPECT processing, 114, 138, 142–164
   SPETS, 115, 116
   x-axis offset correction, 125, 198
   word, 103, 104
Concentric-circles orbit, 76–81, 144
Continuous data, 15, 21
Continuous rotation, 20–21, 73, 110, 111, 113, 115–117, 132, 202, 227
Contrast enhancement, 111, 122, 156–157

302 *Index*

Convolution, 13, 35
  kernel, 13, 36, 37, 43
Coordinate system, 4–7, 22
Cormack, A. M., 3

D

Data acquisition, 123–141
Discontinuous or digital data, 15, 21
Display and photographic presentation, 111–112, 157–160, 229, 230
Dual nuclides, 110, 128, 186, 268, 270
Dwell time, 111, 132, 133–134, 203, 227
Dynamic SPECT, 91, 109, 111, 172, 275, 280

E

Economics of SPECT, 168
Edge detection, 149, 162
Electrical power, 57, 104, 171, 180, 184
EM algorithm, 48
Esophageal source, 254, 279

F

Film, 112, 157, 158, 160, 164, 165, 214–215, 237
Filtering, filtration, 3, 12–16, 23, 28, 35–37, 43, 108, 146–149, 152, 172, 213, 225–227, 237, 261
Filter, 13–16, 27, 28, 36, 114, 162, 216, 239, 240, 256, 262
  bandpass, 256, 262, 272
  Butterworth, 35
  continuous, 15
  discontinuous or discrete, 15
  Hamming, 35, 37
  Hann or von Hann, 37
  "hanning," 37
  nonlinear, 147, 149
  ramp, 14–16, 27, 35, 36, 44
  rectangular, 152
  Shepp-Logan, 14, 16, 35, 40, 282
  triangular, 13, 152

Formatter, 111, 158, 214–215, 240, 263
Four-dimensional display, 160, 258
Fourier space or frequency space, 13, 35, 96, 155
  methods for back projection, 43–45, 118, 155
  rho-filtered layergram, 44

G

Gallium SPECT, 128, 155, 190, 195, 278–280
  efficacy, 279
Gammatom-1, 86–87
Gantry, 68–75
  cabling, 73–74, 201
  design, 69–72
  installation, 218
  orbit
    circular-elliptical, 77–79, 143
    concentric-circles, 76–81, 144
    elliptical, 79
    rotation (see also Continuous rotation, Step-and-shoot rotation), 21, 73, 110–111, 113, 207
  shielding, 68
Gastrointestinal tract SPECT, 283
Gated SPECT, 109–111, 113, 134–135, 160, 196–197, 203–204, 232, 254–255, 258, 264, 266–268
  data storage requirements, 109–110, 267

H

Harvard Body Scanner, 84–85, 90
Harvard Head Scanner, 84–85, 89, 118, 243, 247
Head SPECT, 65–67, 84–87, 89, 127, 137, 151, 161, 172, 240–253
  blood-brain barrier, 242–245
  efficacy of SPECT, 243
  Caldwell position, 242
  cerebral blood flow, 90, 245–250
    quantification, 248–250
  cisternography, 251
  Compton scatter device, 82–83

HIPDM (2-hydroxy-3-methyl-5-(I-123) (iodobenzyl)-1,3-propanediamine), 249–250
IMP (N-isopropyl (I-123) p-iodoamphetamine), 247–250
pituitary gland, 251, 253
radioactive gases, 90, 246–247, 249
receptor binding, 250–251
Townes position, 155, 242
HEADTOME II, 86–87, 92–94
Heart SPECT, 132, 155, 171, 257–269
  antimyosin antibodies, 268
  gated blood pool (see also Gated SPECT), 134, 171, 266–268
    dual nuclide, 268
    Fourier analysis, 268
  infarct-avid imaging, 268
  metabolic imaging, 269
  perfusion imaging, 172, 257–266
    hexakis (t-butylisonitrile) Tc(I) (TBI), 266
    human albumin microspheres (HAM), 266
    thallium-201 (see also Thallium-201)
      180- vs. 360-degree imaging, 133, 137, 259–261
      attenuation correction, 259–261
      dosimetry, 259
      efficacy, 265–266
      filtering, 261, 262
      model, 261
      quantification, 259–261, 264, 266
      short-axis projection, 155, 262–263
      technique, 258
Hounsfield, G. N., 3
Hybrid tomographic instruments, 92–94

I

Image enhancement (see Filtering)
Interpolation (see Back projection, interpolation)

Iodine-123, 93
  collimator questions, 66–67, 125, 250
  heptadecanoic acid, 269
  HIPDM (2-hydroxy-3-methyl-5-(I-123) (iodobenzyl)-1,3-propanediamine), 249–250, 255
  IMP (N-isopropyl (I-123) p-iodoamphetamine), 247–250, 255
  phenylpentadecanoic acid, 269
  purity, 247–248, 269
  quinuclidinyl-(3-iodo-4-hydroxybenzilate) (QNB), 250–251
Iterative solution, 45–47
  algebraic reconstruction techniques, 47
  least-square iterative technique, 48
  simultaneous iterative reconstruction techniques (SIRT), 48

K

Kidney SPECT, 280–282
  dynamic, 280–281
  volume, 162, 171, 281
Krypton-81m, 247, 255
Kuhl, D. E., 2, 4, 34, 83–88, 240, 242, 245

L

Limited-angle tomography, 4, 94–96
Line voltage (see Electrical power)
Liver SPECT, 25, 132, 139, 150, 269–275
  anatomy, 270, 271
  dynamic, 275
  efficacy, 271–274
  filters, 272
  reconstruction protocol, 272–273
  technique, 271–272
  volume, 273
Lung SPECT, 132, 135, 151, 171, 253–257
  Compton imaging, 82, 255
  metabolic imaging, 255

304 Index

Lung SPECT *(cont.)*
  perfusion imaging
    attenuation correction, 256
    efficacy, 256
    quantification, 171, 254
    technique, 255
  respiratory motion, 254
  transmission imaging, 254
  ventilation imaging, 255
  volume, 257

M

Magnetic flux, 184
Magnetic media and storage, 105, 107–110, 112, 115–118, 164
  capacity, 109–110, 267
  environmental requirements, 109
  floppy disk, 108, 122, 164
  hard disk, 108, 164
  tape, 108, 112, 122, 267
Mark IV scanner (Kuhl), 83–88, 94, 245
Maximum likelihood method, 48–49
Moire effect, 194, 214
Multiple nuclides, gamma energies (see also Dual nuclides), 128, 186, 190, 195
Multiprobe SPECT, 2, 4, 83–94, 96, 118, 172, 240, 242, 243, 245–249, 251, 253
MUMPI, 86–87

N

NEMA standards, 181, 182, 192–195, 206, 220
Networking, 164
Nuclear magnetic resonance (NMR), 173, 222, 242

P

Paper tape, 3, 83, 108
Partial voluming, 23, 164, 210, 250, 259, 264, 268, 273
Patient
  body contouring of, for data acquisition, 65, 75–81, 90, 114, 135–136, 171, 207
  data acquisition protocol, 123–141, 227–228, 236–239, 271–272
  marker sources, 124, 136, 138, 139, 140, 143, 145, 215, 237, 238, 255, 272
  motion, 10, 132, 133, 136, 144, 170, 215, 217, 238
  outline of, for attenuation correction, 15, 17, 42, 108, 138, 149, 150, 215, 217, 231
  positioning, 124, 136–140, 228, 236–238
  safety, 79, 136, 171, 207, 227, 229
  selection, 171, 236
  typical examination, 134, 238
Pediatric SPECT
  kidney, 281
  liver-spleen, 271
PETT III, 94
Phantom, 141, 214, 284
  Alderson liver, 32, 214
  bar, 180, 194, 229, 230
  cobalt-57, 187, 188
  cardiac, 204, 261
  cylinder, 30, 39–40, 210, 211, 218, 225–227, 230
  Hine-Duley bar, 194
  line-source, 125, 194, 195, 198, 229
  NEMA, 194
  orthogonal-hole, 194, 229
  parallel-line equal-spacing (PLES), 194
  point-source, 125, 127, 133, 141, 163, 187, 188, 190, 228, 230
  quality control, 180
  ring, for bone quantification, 278
  uniformity, 185–187, 189, 190, 194, 204, 228–230
Photomultiplier tube (see Anger camera, photomultiplier tube)
Picture archiving and communications systems (PACS), 112, 122
Pituitary gland SPECT, 251, 253
Pixel size, 124, 200, 204
Poisson statistics, effects of, 10, 23, 47, 96, 132, 169–170

Positron emission tomography (PET), 4, 86, 88, 93–94, 245, 250, 269
Precision, uncertainty, 24–29
 Budinger equation, 26, 27
  effect of attenuation correction, 27
 effect of SPECT on, 26
 Jaszczak treatment, 27, 163
  effect of filtration on precision, 27
Projections, sagittal, coronal, oblique, short-axis, 20, 108, 110, 155–156, 162, 237, 239, 256, 262–263, 273
Purchasing a SPECT system (see Buying a SPECT system)

Q

Quality assurance, 177–234, 239
Quality control (see also Acceptance testing), 123, 124, 171, 177, 181–232, 237
 human factors, 178
 protocols, 181, 184, 190, 228–232
 record keeping, 180, 228
 software, 180, 205–206
Quantification, 28–32, 42, 160, 162–164, 171–172
 contrast, 30–31
 edge detection, 138, 149, 162
 radiometric, 29, 30, 162, 213, 249, 254, 260–261, 264, 266
 volumetric, 29–31, 160, 162, 213, 230, 231, 257, 264, 266, 268, 269, 281

R

Radiopharmaceutical
 dose, 132, 134, 227
 dosimetry, 134, 236, 247–248, 259, 284
 selection, 236
 therapeutic, 284
Radon, J., 3, 44, 45, 50
 projections, 3, 44
Reconstruction (see Back projection)

Rectilinear scanner, 2, 83, 86, 95, 156–157, 263, 280
Resolution, 10, 24, 28, 153, 160, 170, 261
 resolution cell, 26
Rho-filtered layergram, 44
Ringing, 14, 147, 164
ROC analysis, 50, 168–169

S

Scatter, 10, 15, 39, 41, 126, 128–132, 169–171, 264
 correction, 38, 41–42, 149, 152, 160
Sensitivity, 80, 153, 160, 170
Seven-pinhole collimator, 95–96
Signal-noise ratio, 23
Sinogram, 140, 144–145, 208, 215, 238, 239, 256, 273
Slice thickness, 21, 155, 164, 193, 225, 226, 237, 239, 256, 259, 273
Smoothing, 11, 29, 156, 225, 226, 256
Software (see Computer, software)
SPECT, early instruments, 2, 84–86
Speed, 80
Spleen SPECT, 269–275
SPRINT (single photon ring tomograph), 4, 84–85, 91
Step-and-shoot rotation, 73, 110, 113, 115–117, 132, 202, 227
Summing (see Averaging)

T

Table, imaging (see also Gantry), 74–80, 110, 135, 171, 238, 241
 head holder, 74, 238, 241
 installation, 219–220
Technetium-99m compounds, 250, 281
 colloid, 270–273
 DMSA, 279
 DTPA, 109, 251
 glucoheptonate, 245, 282
 HSA, 267
 MAA, 254, 255, 280

Technetium-99m compounds *(cont.)*
  MDP, 217, 276–277
  microspheres (HAM), 254, 255, 266, 273–274
  pertechnetate, 251–252
  phosphate, 275
  N-pyridoxylamine (PM), 275
  red blood cells, 245, 267, 270, 273, 274
  sucralfate, 283
  sulfur colloid, 270, 274
  TBI (hexakis(t-butylisonitrile)-Tc(I)), 266
Three-dimensional display, 112, 144, 158–160, 258, 284
Thyroid SPECT, 172, 282–283
Tomographic process, 11
Tomomatic 64 (Medimatic), 86–87, 90, 118, 246
Tomoscanner, Tomogscanner, 84–85
Transmission SPECT, 19, 139, 151, 237, 254, 255
Troubleshooting from clinical examinations, 215–218, 239–240
Tumor imaging with SPECT, 278, 284
  intra-arterial particles, 273–274, 280

U

Ultrasound, 164, 173, 178, 270

V

Videotape, 119, 122, 158
Voxel size (see Pixel size, Slice thickness)

X

X-axis offset (see Axis of rotation, Center of rotation, Software, x-axis offset), 124, 142, 197–200, 204, 205, 230
X-ray transmission CT, 3, 4, 18, 38, 54, 68, 81, 107, 139, 151, 155, 157, 160, 164, 172, 173, 178, 188, 208, 242, 243, 247, 249, 252, 253, 270, 279, 284
Xenon-127, 247
Xenon-133, 246, 249

Y

Ytterbium-169 DTPA, 251, 252